ACP | MKSAP® 18
Medical Knowledge Self-Assessment Program®

Neurology

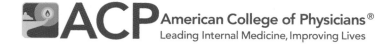

ACP American College of Physicians®
Leading Internal Medicine, Improving Lives

Welcome to the Neurology Section of MKSAP 18!

In these pages, you will find updated information on headache and facial pain, head injury, epilepsy, stroke, cognitive disorders, movement disorders, multiple sclerosis, disorders of the spinal cord, neuromuscular disorders, and neuro-oncology. All of these topics are uniquely focused on the needs of generalists and subspecialists *outside* of neurology.

The core content of MKSAP 18 has been developed as in previous editions—all essential information that is newly researched and written in 11 topic areas of internal medicine—created by dozens of leading generalists and subspecialists and guided by certification and recertification requirements, emerging knowledge in the field, and user feedback. MKSAP 18 also contains 1200 all-new peer-reviewed, psychometrically validated, multiple-choice questions (MCQs) for self-assessment and study, including 96 in Neurology. MKSAP 18 continues to include *High Value Care* (HVC) recommendations, based on the concept of balancing clinical benefit with costs and harms, with associated MCQs illustrating these principles and HVC Key Points called out in the text. Internists practicing in the hospital setting can easily find comprehensive *Hospitalist*-focused content and MCQs, specially designated in blue and with the 🄷 symbol.

If you purchased MKSAP 18 Complete, you also have access to MKSAP 18 Digital, with additional tools allowing you to customize your learning experience. MKSAP Digital includes regular text updates with new, practice-changing information, 200 new self-assessment questions, and enhanced custom-quiz options. MKSAP Complete also includes more than 1200 electronic, adaptive learning–enhanced flashcards for quick review of important concepts, as well as an updated and enhanced version of Virtual Dx, MKSAP's image-based self-assessment tool. As before, MKSAP 18 Digital is optimized for use on your mobile devices, with iOS- and Android-based apps allowing you to sync between your apps and online account and submit for CME credits and MOC points online.

Please visit us at the MKSAP Resource Site (mksap.acponline.org) to find out how we can help you study, earn CME credit and MOC points, and stay up to date.

On behalf of the many internists who have offered their time and expertise to create the content for MKSAP 18 and the editorial staff who work to bring this material to you in the best possible way, we are honored that you have chosen to use MKSAP 18 and appreciate any feedback about the program you may have. Please feel free to send any comments to mksap_editors@acponline.org.

Sincerely,

Patrick Alguire

Patrick C. Alguire, MD, FACP
Editor-in-Chief
Senior Vice President Emeritus
Medical Education Division
American College of Physicians

Neurology

Committee

Robert G. Kaniecki, MD, Section Editor[2]
Director, The Headache Center
Chief, Headache Division
Assistant Director, Neurology Residency Training Program
Director, Headache Fellowship Program
Assistant Professor of Neurology
University of Pittsburgh School of Medicine
Pittsburgh, Pennsylvania

Amar Bharat Bhatt, MD[1]
Program Director, Neurology Residency
Assistant Professor, Epilepsy Section
Rush University Medical Center
Chicago, Illinois

Daniel Harrison, MD[2]
Assistant Professor
University of Maryland Center for Multiple Sclerosis
    Treatment and Research
University of Maryland School of Medicine
Baltimore, Maryland

Houman Homayoun, MD[1]
Assistant Professor
University of Pittsburgh Medical Center
Pittsburgh, Pennsylvania

Eric McDade, DO[2]
Assistant Professor
Washington University School of Medicine
St. Louis, Missouri

Joshua Z. Willey, MD[2]
Assistant Professor of Neurology
Columbia University
New York, New York

Editor-in-Chief

Patrick C. Alguire, MD, FACP[2]
Senior Vice President Emeritus, Medical Education
American College of Physicians
Philadelphia, Pennsylvania

Deputy Editor

Robert L. Trowbridge, Jr, MD, FACP[2]
Associate Professor of Medicine
Tufts University School of Medicine
Maine Medical Center
Portland, Maine

Neurology Reviewers

Thomas P. Bleck, MD, FACP[2]
Jorge H. Bordenave, MD, FACP[1]
Amar R. Chadaga, MD, FACP[1]
Marilou I. Ching, MD, FACP[1]
S. Claudia Didia, MD, FACP[1]
Richard E. Ferguson, MD, FACP[1]
Stella J. Fitzgibbons, MD, FACP[1]
Erich W. Garland, MD, FACP[1]
Peter Glusker, MD, FACP[1]
Philip B. Gorelick, MD, FACP[2]

Hospital Medicine Neurology Reviewers

Alan J. Hunter, MD, FACP[1]
Suresh Kumar, MBBS FACP[2]

Neurology ACP Editorial Staff

Ellen McDonald, PhD[1], Senior Staff Editor, Self-Assessment
    and Educational Programs
Margaret Wells[1], Director, Self-Assessment and Educational
    Programs
Becky Krumm[1], Managing Editor, Self-Assessment and
    Educational Programs

ACP Principal Staff

Davoren Chick, MD, FACP[2]
Senior Vice President, Medical Education

Patrick C. Alguire, MD, FACP[2]
Senior Vice President Emeritus, Medical Education

Sean McKinney[1]
Vice President, Medical Education

Margaret Wells[1]
Director, Self-Assessment and Educational Programs

Becky Krumm[1]
Managing Editor

Valerie Dangovetsky[1]
Administrator

Ellen McDonald, PhD[1]
Senior Staff Editor

Acknowledgments

The American College of Physicians (ACP) gratefully acknowledges the special contributions to the development and production of the 18th edition of the Medical Knowledge Self-Assessment Program® (MKSAP® 18) made by the following people:

Graphic Design: Barry Moshinski (Director, Graphic Services), Michael Ripca (Graphics Technical Administrator), and Jennifer Gropper (Graphic Designer).

Production/Systems: Dan Hoffmann (Director, Information Technology), Scott Hurd (Manager, Content Systems), Neil Kohl (Senior Architect), and Chris Patterson (Senior Architect).

MKSAP 18 Digital: Under the direction of Steven Spadt (Senior Vice President, Technology), the digital version of MKSAP 18 was developed within the ACP's Digital Products and Services Department, led by Brian Sweigard (Director, Digital Products and Services). Other members of the team included Dan Barron (Senior Web Application Developer/Architect), Chris Forrest (Senior Software Developer/Design Lead), Kathleen Hoover (Senior Web Developer), Kara Regis (Manager, User Interface Design and Development), Brad Lord (Senior Web Application Developer), and John McKnight (Senior Web Developer).

The College also wishes to acknowledge that many other persons, too numerous to mention, have contributed to the production of this program. Without their dedicated efforts, this program would not have been possible.

MKSAP Resource Site (mksap.acponline.org)

The MKSAP Resource Site (mksap.acponline.org) is a continually updated site that provides links to MKSAP 18 online answer sheets for print subscribers; access to MKSAP 18 Digital; Board Basics® e-book access instructions; information on Continuing Medical Education (CME), Maintenance of Certification (MOC), and international Continuing Professional Development (CPD) and MOC; errata; and other new information.

International MOC/CPD

For information and instructions on submission of international MOC/CPD, please go to the MKSAP Resource Site (mksap.acponline.org).

Continuing Medical Education

The American College of Physicians is accredited by the Accreditation Council for Continuing Medical Education (ACCME) to provide continuing medical education for physicians.

The American College of Physicians designates this enduring material, MKSAP 18, for a maximum of 275 *AMA PRA Category 1 Credits*™. Physicians should claim only the credit commensurate with the extent of their participation in the activity.

Up to 22 *AMA PRA Category 1 Credits*™ are available from July 31, 2018, to July 31, 2021, for the MKSAP 18 Neurology section.

Learning Objectives

The learning objectives of MKSAP 18 are to:

- Close gaps between actual care in your practice and preferred standards of care, based on best evidence
- Diagnose disease states that are less common and sometimes overlooked and confusing
- Improve management of comorbid conditions that can complicate patient care
- Determine when to refer patients for surgery or care by subspecialists
- Pass the ABIM Certification Examination
- Pass the ABIM Maintenance of Certification Examination

Target Audience

- General internists and primary care physicians
- Subspecialists who need to remain up to date in internal medicine
- Residents preparing for the certifying examination in internal medicine
- Physicians preparing for maintenance of certification in internal medicine (recertification)

ABIM Maintenance of Certification

Check the MKSAP Resource Site (mksap.acponline.org) for the latest information on how MKSAP tests can be used to apply to the American Board of Internal Medicine (ABIM) for Maintenance of Certification (MOC) points following completion of the CME activity.

Successful completion of the CME activity, which includes participation in the evaluation component, enables the participant to earn up to 275 medical knowledge MOC points in the ABIM's MOC program. It is the CME activity provider's responsibility to submit participant completion information to ACCME for the purpose of granting MOC credit.

Earn Instantaneous CME Credits or MOC Points Online

Print subscribers can enter their answers online to earn instantaneous CME credits or MOC points. You can submit your answers using online answer sheets that are provided at mksap.acponline.org, where a record of your MKSAP 18 credits will be available. To earn CME credits or to apply for MOC points, you need to answer all of the questions in a test and earn a score of at least 50% correct (number of correct answers divided by the total number of questions). Please note that if you are applying for MOC points, you must also enter your birth date and ABIM candidate number.

Take either of the following approaches:

1. Use the printed answer sheet at the back of this book to record your answers. Go to mksap.acponline.org, access the appropriate online answer sheet, transcribe your answers, and submit your test for instantaneous CME credits or MOC points. There is no additional fee for this service.
2. Go to mksap.acponline.org, access the appropriate online answer sheet, directly enter your answers, and submit your test for instantaneous CME credits or MOC points. There is no additional fee for this service.

Earn CME Credits or MOC Points by Mail or Fax

Pay a $20 processing fee per answer sheet and submit the printed answer sheet at the back of this book by mail or fax, as instructed on the answer sheet. Make sure you calculate your score and enter your birth date and ABIM candidate number, and fax the answer sheet to 215-351-2799 or mail the answer sheet to Member and Customer Service, American College of Physicians, 190 N. Independence Mall West, Philadelphia, PA 19106-1572, using the courtesy envelope provided in your MKSAP 18 slipcase. You will need your 10-digit order number and 8-digit ACP ID number, which are printed on your packing slip. Please allow 4 to 6 weeks for your score report to be emailed back to you. Be sure to include your email address for a response.

If you do not have a 10-digit order number and 8-digit ACP ID number, or if you need help creating a username and password to access the MKSAP 18 online answer sheets, go to mksap.acponline.org or email custserv@acponline.org.

Disclosure Policy

It is the policy of the American College of Physicians (ACP) to ensure balance, independence, objectivity, and scientific rigor in all of its educational activities. To this end, and consistent with the policies of the ACP and the Accreditation Council for Continuing Medical Education (ACCME), contributors to all ACP continuing medical education activities are required to disclose all relevant financial relationships with any entity producing, marketing, re-selling, or distributing health care goods or services consumed by, or used on, patients. Contributors

are required to use generic names in the discussion of therapeutic options and are required to identify any unapproved, off-label, or investigative use of commercial products or devices. Where a trade name is used, all available trade names for the same product type are also included. If trade-name products manufactured by companies with whom contributors have relationships are discussed, contributors are asked to provide evidence-based citations in support of the discussion. The information is reviewed by the committee responsible for producing this text. If necessary, adjustments to topics or contributors' roles in content development are made to balance the discussion. Further, all readers of this text are asked to evaluate the content for evidence of commercial bias and send any relevant comments to mksap_editors@acponline.org so that future decisions about content and contributors can be made in light of this information.

Resolution of Conflicts

To resolve all conflicts of interest and influences of vested interests, ACP's content planners used best evidence and updated clinical care guidelines in developing content, when such evidence and guidelines were available. All content underwent review by peer reviewers not on the committee to ensure that the material was balanced and unbiased. Contributors' disclosure information can be found with the list of contributors' names and those of ACP principal staff listed in the beginning of this book.

Hospital-Based Medicine

For the convenience of subscribers who provide care in hospital settings, content that is specific to the hospital setting has been highlighted in blue. Hospital icons (H) highlight where the hospital-only content begins, continues over more than one page, and ends.

High Value Care Key Points

Key Points in the text that relate to High Value Care concepts (that is, concepts that discuss balancing clinical benefit with costs and harms) are designated by the HVC icon [HVC].

Educational Disclaimer

The editors and publisher of MKSAP 18 recognize that the development of new material offers many opportunities for error. Despite our best efforts, some errors may persist in print. Drug dosage schedules are, we believe, accurate and in accordance with current standards. Readers are advised, however, to ensure that the recommended dosages in MKSAP 18 concur with the information provided in the product information material. This is especially important in cases of new, infrequently used, or highly toxic drugs. Application of the information in MKSAP 18 remains the professional responsibility of the practitioner.

The primary purpose of MKSAP 18 is educational. Information presented, as well as publications, technologies, products, and/or services discussed, is intended to inform subscribers about the knowledge, techniques, and experiences of the contributors. A diversity of professional opinion exists, and the views of the contributors are their own and not those of the ACP. Inclusion of any material in the program does not constitute endorsement or recommendation by the ACP. The ACP does not warrant the safety, reliability, accuracy, completeness, or usefulness of and disclaims any and all liability for damages and claims that may result from the use of information, publications, technologies, products, and/or services discussed in this program.

Publisher's Information

Disclaimer Regarding Direct Purchases from Online Retailers

CME and/or MOC for MKSAP 18 is available only if you purchase the program directly from ACP. CME credits and MOC points cannot be awarded to those purchasers who have purchased the program from non-authorized sellers such as Amazon, eBay, or any other such online retailer.

Unauthorized Use of This Book Is Against the Law

MKSAP 18 ISBN: 978-1-938245-47-3
(Neurology) ISBN: 978-1-938245-52-7

Printed in the United States of America.

For order information in the U.S. or Canada call 800-ACP-1915. All other countries call 215-351-2600, (Monday to Friday, 9 AM – 5 PM ET). Fax inquiries to 215-351-2799 or email to custserv@acponline.org.

Errata

Errata for MKSAP 18 will be available through the MKSAP Resource Site at mksap.acponline.org as new information becomes known to the editors.

Table of Contents

Neurology High Value Care Recommendations

The American College of Physicians, in collaboration with multiple other organizations, is engaged in a worldwide initiative to promote the practice of High Value Care (HVC). The goals of the HVC initiative are to improve health care outcomes by providing care of proven benefit and reducing costs by avoiding unnecessary and even harmful interventions. The initiative comprises several programs that integrate the important concept of health care value (balancing clinical benefit with costs and harms) for a given intervention into a broad range of educational materials to address the needs of trainees, practicing physicians, and patients.

HVC content has been integrated into MKSAP 18 in several important ways. MKSAP 18 includes HVC-identified key points in the text, HVC-focused multiple choice questions, and, for subscribers to MKSAP Digital, an HVC custom quiz. From the text and questions, we have generated the following list of HVC recommendations that meet the definition below of high value care and bring us closer to our goal of improving patient outcomes while conserving finite resources.

High Value Care Recommendation: A recommendation to choose diagnostic and management strategies for patients in specific clinical situations that balance clinical benefit with cost and harms with the goal of improving patient outcomes.

Below are the High Value Care Recommendations for the Neurology section of MKSAP 18.

- Imaging is not indicated for patients with stable migraine and a normal neurologic examination.
- Imaging is not indicated for tension-type headache.
- Head CT is the most appropriate initial study for an unprovoked, first-time seizure (see Item 7).
- Lumbar puncture after a first seizure is recommended only if an infectious cause is suspected.
- Transesophageal echocardiography is not routinely indicated for the evaluation of acute stroke.
- Do not administer platelet transfusion for intracerebral hemorrhage in patients treated with antiplatelet agents.
- Internal carotid artery revascularization for primary prevention of stroke is not indicated unless stenosis is greater than 80% or rapid progression of stenosis is documented.
- Aspirin monotherapy is a first-line antiplatelet regimen for secondary stroke prevention.
- Do not stent symptomatic high-grade intracranial arterial stenosis.
- Do not obtain specialized genetic or cerebrospinal fluids tests for dementia unless diagnosis is uncertain.
- No treatments or primary prevention interventions are currently approved for mild cognitive impairment.
- A positive pull test is the most reliable predictor of backward falls in Parkinson disease.
- Proper application of diagnostic criteria for multiple sclerosis can prevent unnecessary neurologic testing, referrals, and misdiagnoses.
- Exclude transient symptoms associated with increased body temperature before treating an apparent multiple sclerosis exacerbation.
- Using agents other than ocrelizumab and mitoxantrone for progressive forms of multiple sclerosis increases cost and unnecessary risk.
- Routine electromyography is not necessary for patients with slowly progressive distal symmetric sensory neuropathy and a negative family history.
- Clinical diagnosis and supportive care is appropriate for carpal tunnel syndrome with mild symptoms.
- Brain imaging and laboratory testing is not required for the diagnosis of classic Bell palsy.
- Prophylactic antiepileptic drugs are not recommended for central nervous system tumors in the absence of seizures.
- Reassurance is the best management for periodic limb movements of sleep if no associated sleep disorder is present (see Item 46).
- Most patients with chronic cervical and lumbar stenosis do not require surgery (see Item 79).

Neurology

Headache and Facial Pain

🅗 Approach to the Patient with Headache

Formal classification of headache disorders identifies three headache subtypes: primary headaches, secondary headaches, and painful cranial neuralgias. Primary headaches, or those in which the symptoms are due to a specific headache disorder, are more commonly seen in practice, and are defined by clinical criteria. Primary headache disorders include migraine, tension-type headache, cluster headache, and the other trigeminal autonomic cephalalgias. Secondary headaches result from another underlying process and are defined by that causative disease process (**Table 1**); these headaches may be associated with significant morbidity and mortality and require early identification. Patients with serious secondary headaches typically have acute or subacute symptoms and a headache pattern that is progressive or unstable; suspicion of a secondary headache is heightened in the presence of the following clinical "red flags":

- First or worst headache
- Abrupt-onset or thunderclap attack
- Progression or fundamental change in headache pattern
- Abnormal physical examination findings
- Neurologic symptoms lasting longer than 1 hour
- New headache in persons younger than 5 years or older than 50 years
- New headache in patients with malignancy, coagulopathy, immunosuppression, or pregnancy
- Association with alteration in or loss of consciousness
- Headache triggered by exertion, sexual activity, or Valsalva maneuver

A detailed headache history (**Table 2**) is the most valuable clinical assessment tool in the evaluation of headaches. Neurologic examination with funduscopic testing is essential, and brain imaging is the most important diagnostic study. Imaging is indicated for suspected secondary headaches and for some of the uncommon primary syndromes (such as trigeminal autonomic cephalalgias). Stable headaches meeting criteria for most primary headaches usually do not require imaging. Head CT is indicated in the assessment of acute, severe headaches, and brain MRI is used when indicated for subacute or chronic headaches, given its greater sensitivity and safety. Additional testing is determined by differential diagnostic considerations and may include erythrocyte sedimentation rate determination, C-reactive protein measurement, lumbar puncture, serum chemistries, or toxicology screens. There is no indication for electroencephalography in the assessment of headache disorders. 🅗

TABLE 1. Secondary Headache and Associated Syndromes
Posttraumatic headache
Head injury
Whiplash injury
Headache attributed to cranial or cervical vascular disorder
Ischemic stroke or transient ischemic attack
Parenchymal or subarachnoid hemorrhage
Unruptured vascular malformation or aneurysm
Intracranial or extracranial arteritis
Arterial dissection
Venous or sinus thrombosis
Headache attributed to nonvascular intracranial disorders
Intracranial hypotension or hypertension
Brain neoplasia
Noninfectious inflammatory disorders (sarcoidosis)
Chiari malformation
Headache attributed to substance use or withdrawal
Medication adverse event (nitrates)
Alcohol
Caffeine withdrawal
Medication overuse headache
Headache attributed to infection
Intracranial infection (meningitis, encephalitis, brain abscess)
Extracranial infection (systemic bacterial infection, viral syndrome)
Headache attributed to disorder of homeostasis
Hypertensive crisis, dialysis, hypoxia, hypercapnia, hypothyroidism
Headache attributed to disorder of the neck, eyes, ears, nose, sinuses, teeth, or mouth
Headache attributed to a psychiatric disorder

Adapted with permission of Sage Publications LTD., London, Los Angeles, New Delhi, Singapore and Washington DC, from Headache Classification Committee of the International Headache Society (IHS). The International Classification of Headache Disorders, 3rd edition (beta version). Cephalalgia. 2013 Jul;33(9):683. [PMID: 23771276] doi:10.1177/0333102413485658. Copyright SAGE Publications LTD., 2013.

TABLE 2. Headache History
Headache Temporal Profile
Onset of the condition
When did these headaches first develop?
How long have the headaches been occurring at the frequency reported presently?
Monthly headache frequency over past 3 months
Total headache days?
Severe headache days?
Headache days requiring medication?
Duration of headache episodes
Untreated?
Treated?
Headache Symptom Profile
Pain
Location of pain
Quality of pain
Severity of pain
Effect of routine physical activity on pain
Associated features
Precursor symptoms
Sensitivities to light, sound, smell
Nausea, vomiting
Neurologic or visual complaints
Cranial autonomic features (tearing, nasal congestion or rhinorrhea, ptosis, conjunctival injection)
Contributing Clinical Factors
Family history
Provocative or palliative features
Detailed medication history

KEY POINTS

- Early identification of secondary headaches is essential because of their potentially significant morbidity and mortality; patients with serious secondary headaches typically have acute or subacute symptoms and a headache pattern that is progressive or unstable.
- Stable headaches meeting criteria for most primary headaches usually do not require imaging.

HVC

Secondary Headache

Thunderclap Headache

Thunderclap headache is defined as a severe attack of headache pain developing abruptly and reaching maximum intensity within 1 minute. Although occasionally of primary origin, thunderclap headache is a medical emergency that warrants immediate diagnostic evaluation. Noncontrast head CT should be performed without delay. Lumbar puncture with measurement of opening pressure, cell counts, and xanthochromia should be performed if the head CT is nondiagnostic. Contrast-enhanced brain MRI and noninvasive vascular imaging (magnetic resonance angiography [MRA] or CT angiography [CTA]) of cranial and cervical vessels should be performed in patients with a normal CT scan and normal results of cerebrospinal fluid (CSF) analysis. **Table 3** lists essential considerations in the differential diagnosis.

Subarachnoid hemorrhage (SAH), the most common cause of thunderclap headache, is discovered in nearly 25% of affected patients. The headache associated with SAH may be described as the worst the patient has ever experienced, although the specificity of this finding is limited. Mortality is 50%, with an additional 25% of affected patients experiencing significant morbidity. In the presence of a normal neurologic examination, the following features increase the likelihood of a diagnosis of SAH: age 40 years or older, onset during exertion, witnessed loss of consciousness, or concomitant neck pain. Estimates vary widely, but many patients describe a past headache consistent with a sentinel leak within the previous 1 to 2 weeks; these leaks typically involve abrupt, severe, transient headaches that may be focal or global. Sensitivity of head CT is approximately 95% at 12 hours but decreases to 50% at 1 week. Lumbar puncture in SAH typically reveals a CSF erythrocyte count greater than 10,000/µL (10,000 × 10⁶/L) and an elevation in protein level. CSF xanthochromia may take 4 hours or more to develop but is nearly 100% sensitive

TABLE 3. Possible Causes of Thunderclap Headache
Secondary Headache Disorders
Subarachnoid or parenchymal hemorrhage
Intracranial venous or sinus thrombosis
Cervical artery dissection
Reversible cerebral vasoconstriction syndrome
Posterior reversible encephalopathy syndrome
Ischemic stroke or transient ischemic attack
Spontaneous intracranial hypotension
Subdural hematoma
Pituitary apoplexy
Pheochromocytoma
Colloid cyst of third ventricle
Acute hydrocephalus
Subdural hematoma
Acute angle-closure glaucoma
Primary Headache Disorders
Primary thunderclap headache
Primary stabbing headache

between 12 hours and 7 days. Urgent neurosurgical consultation is required.

Headache is the most common symptom and may be the only presenting manifestation with thrombosis of the intracranial veins and sinuses. The pain is typically of sudden onset and is unremitting. Clinical symptoms may be related to the resulting increase in intracranial pressure and include pain exacerbation with the Valsalva maneuver, pulsatile tinnitus, and diplopia. Nonspecific findings of increased intracranial pressure include papilledema, decreased mentation, and seizures. Abducens nerve (cranial nerve VI) palsy secondary to increased intracranial pressure may falsely indicate a focal lesion (falsely localizing abducens nerve palsy). Specific findings may help localize the thrombosis. Cavernous sinus thrombosis usually involves extension of dental or sinus bacterial infection and manifests as acute-onset headache, proptosis, periorbital edema, and ophthalmoplegia; this disorder requires immediate administration of antibiotics, often with surgical drainage. Other forms of cerebral venous thrombosis are not related to infection and often occur in the presence of hypercoagulable states, thrombophilia, pregnancy (and the puerperium), oral contraceptive use, or dehydration. Anticoagulation is recommended even in those patients with hemorrhagic parenchymal lesions. Treatment with low-molecular-weight heparin results in lower hospital mortality than treatment with unfractionated heparin. Anticoagulation with warfarin is generally continued for a minimum of 3 to 6 months. Extended anticoagulation should be considered in those with severe hypercoagulable states, myeloproliferative disorders, or recurrence and perhaps in those with idiopathic thrombosis.

Dissections of the cervical vessels (**Figure 1**) often present with acute pain in the head and neck, typically occur in younger patients, and may develop spontaneously or as a result of trauma, which may be minor. Risk factors include hypertension, migraine, polycystic kidney disease, and connective tissue disorders. Extracranial dissections are a common cause of stroke in persons younger than 50 years. Dissections of the carotid artery often present with orbital pain, partial Horner syndrome (ptosis and miosis only), and ipsilateral signs of cerebral or retinal ischemia. Those with dissections of the vertebral arteries may describe occipital and neck pain and posterior fossa symptoms, such as dysarthria, dysphagia, ataxia, and hemifield visual loss. Brain MRI may show a tapered arterial lumen or increased arterial diameter with an intramural hematoma. Noninvasive vessel imaging with MRA or CTA is typically sufficient. Comparative trials have not documented the superiority of anticoagulation in patients with dissections, and many are treated with aspirin.

Reversible cerebral vasoconstriction syndrome is characterized by recurrent thunderclap headache and multifocal constriction of intracranial vessels normalizing within 3 months of onset. Predisposing factors are listed in **Table 4**. It is the second most frequent source of thunderclap headache. The headaches may be triggered by exertion, Valsalva maneuvers, emotion, or bathing. Focal deficits, encephalopathy, and

seizures are seen in a minority of patients. Diagnostic evaluation should include noninvasive imaging of the brain and neck vessels with MRA or CTA and CSF analysis. Digital subtraction angiography has been associated with transient neurologic deficits and is typically avoided. Results of head CT and lumbar puncture are both typically normal. Brain MRI is more sensitive and may show areas of white matter edema primarily in the occipital and parietal lobes compatible with posterior reversible encephalopathy syndrome. Areas of ischemia or hemorrhage may be seen in the parenchyma, and a subdural or subarachnoid hemorrhage also may be found in some patients. Management begins with resolution of predisposing factors, avoidance of physical exertion, and management of blood pressure. Verapamil and nimodipine are the drugs of choice. Glucocorticoids may worsen the clinical course and should be avoided. Repeat MRA or CTA is necessary at 12 weeks to document resolution of vasospasm, at which time medication is tapered.

KEY POINTS

- Thunderclap headache is a medical emergency that warrants immediate diagnostic evaluation; noncontrast head CT should be performed without delay.

- Subarachnoid hemorrhage is the most common cause of thunderclap headache.

- Cavernous sinus thrombosis manifests as acute-onset headache, proptosis, periorbital edema, and ophthalmoplegia; usually involves extension of dental or sinus bacterial infections; and requires immediate administration of antibiotics and frequently surgical drainage.

- Dissections of the cervical vessels often present with acute pain in the head and neck and are a common cause of stroke in patients younger than 50 years.

- Reversible cerebral vasoconstriction syndrome is characterized by recurrent thunderclap headache and is the second most frequent source of thunderclap headache.

Idiopathic Intracranial Hypertension

Increased intracranial pressure in the absence of any vascular or space-occupying lesion is the hallmark of idiopathic intracranial hypertension (IIH) (also known as pseudotumor cerebri). Approximately 90% of affected persons are women of childbearing age with an elevated BMI. IIH is associated with the following conditions:

- Hypervitaminosis A

- Use of the tetracycline class of antibiotics

- Retinoic acid use

- Kidney failure

- Endocrine disorders (hypoparathyroidism, Addison disease)

- Use of estrogen and progesterone supplements and pregnancy

- Glucocorticoid use or withdrawal

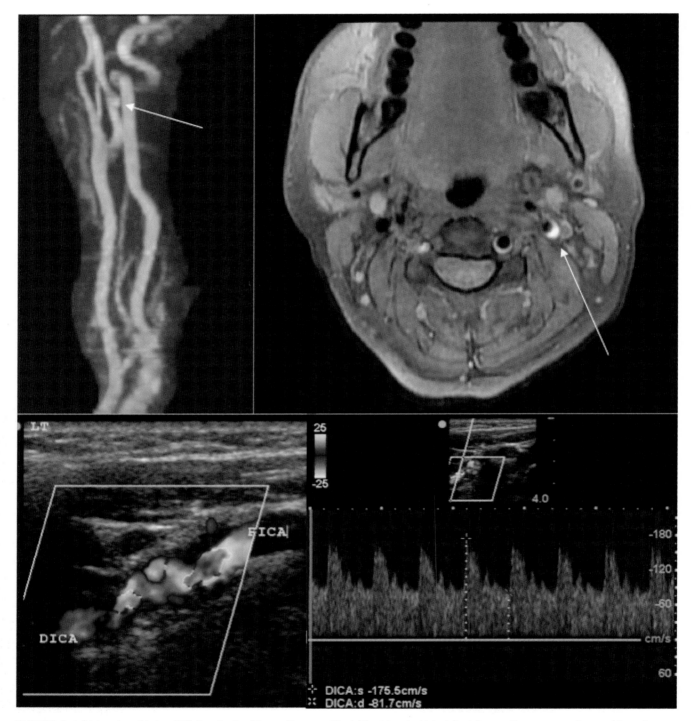

FIGURE 1. Left internal carotid artery (ICA) dissection in a 32-year-old woman with a left frontal cerebral infarct. *Top left*, magnetic resonance angiogram of the neck showing mild irregularity in the distal extracranial ICA with a possible pseudoaneurysm (*arrow*). *Top right*, T1-weighted MRI of the soft tissues in the neck showing a crescent-shaped hematoma (*arrow*) within the ICA wall. *Bottom*, carotid Duplex ultrasounds from the same patient showing turbulent flow in the mid to distal ICA with associated accelerated systolic and diastolic velocities. DICA = distal ICA; LT = left; PICA = proximal ICA.

CONT.

Headaches, visual symptoms, and intracranial noises (pulsatile tinnitus) are the most common presenting symptoms of IIH. Head pain is nonspecific and may be similar to that of tension-type headache or migraine. Vision may be blurred, doubled, or periodically dim in brief episodes known as visual obscurations. Visual field testing is essential in the initial and follow-up evaluations of IIH. Although only 25% of patients may report visual

TABLE 4. Predisposing Factors of Reversible Cerebral Vasoconstriction Syndrome
Vasoactive Drug Exposure
Sympathomimetic agents (amphetamines, pseudoephedrine, phenylpropanolamine)
Antidepressants (SSRIs, SNRIs, monoamine oxidase inhibitors)
Triptans or ergot alkaloid derivatives
Nicotine
Illicit drugs (cocaine, cannabis, ecstasy, methamphetamines)
Pregnancy and Puerperium
Preeclampsia, eclampsia
HELLP syndrome
Head and Neck Trauma and Surgery
Acute Cerebrovascular Disorders
Cervical artery dissection
Cerebral endovascular procedures or angiography
Cerebral vein or sinus thrombosis
Miscellaneous Conditions
Exposure to immunosuppressants or blood products
Meningitis
Catecholamine-secreting tumors

HELLP = Hemolysis, Elevated Liver enzymes, and Low Platelet count; SNRI = serotonin-norepinephrine reuptake inhibitor; SSRI = selective serotonin reuptake inhibitor.

CONT.

symptoms, 90% have some abnormality on visual perimetry. Typical findings include blind spot enlargement and peripheral field reduction. Patients with atypical presentations (men older than 50 years, patients with normal BMIs) are less likely to report headaches and have a more benign visual prognosis.

Findings on neurologic examination include papilledema and, occasionally, ophthalmoplegia. Enhanced brain MRI with magnetic resonance venography may reveal widening of the optic nerve sheaths or flattening of the posterior optic globes but is otherwise unremarkable. An elevation in CSF opening pressure of greater than 250 mm H_2O with normal CSF composition confirms the diagnosis.

Treatment of IIH is aimed primarily at preservation of vision. Patients with BMI elevation require introduction of a weight-loss program. Bariatric procedures have been shown to be helpful, when necessary. Acetazolamide is the drug of choice. Topiramate may be less effective but carries the potential added benefit of weight loss. Paresthesias, kidney stones, and taste perversion are possible adverse effects of both drugs. More immediate reduction in intracranial pressure may be accomplished through repeated lumbar punctures. Decompressive procedures, such as lumboperitoneal shunting or optic nerve fenestration, should be considered in patients with medically refractory IIH. **H**

Headaches from Intracranial Hypotension

The most common source of intracranial hypotension is leakage of CSF after a lumbar puncture. The cardinal feature is a postural headache, typically worsening within 20 seconds of sitting or standing. Tinnitus, diplopia, neck pain, nausea, photophobia, and phonophobia are additional symptoms. Risk of developing symptoms may be reduced by using a small-caliber atraumatic needle but is unaffected by bed rest postprocedure. More than 50% of these headaches resolve spontaneously by day 4 postprocedure, and more than 75% by day 7. Persistent symptoms are treated with an autologous epidural blood patch (EBP), which causes resolution of symptoms in 80% to 90% of patients. **H**

Spontaneous intracranial hypotension also classically presents with an orthostatic headache, but the interval between postural change and headache development is highly variable. When present for a period of weeks to months, the orthostatic component may fade completely. Associated symptoms are similar to those of post–dural-puncture headaches. Headache presentation may be thunderclap or subacute in nature. Diagnosis of intracranial hypotension can be confirmed by a CSF opening pressure of less than 60 mm H_2O, but lumbar puncture may introduce another site of potential CSF leakage. Most clinicians rely on the contrast-enhanced brain-MRI finding of diffuse nonnodular pachymeningeal enhancement seen in nearly 80% of patients. Cerebellar tonsillar descent similar to that of a Chiari malformation, subdural fluid collections, decreased ventricular size, and engorgement of the pituitary gland are other common findings on MRI. Identification of the source of CSF leakage may be challenging. Most cases are empirically treated with lumbar EBP procedures. The success rate with "blind" patches is approximately 30%, and repeat procedures are commonly required. If two to three patches do not relieve the condition, attempts are made to further localize the site of CSF leakage using spinal CT myelography. Noncontrast spine MRI is a noninvasive alternative that also may show an extradural fluid collection at the site of the leak. Once identified, the site may be treated with targeted EBP or surgical repair. If no leak is identified, the studies can be repeated in 4 to 6 months.

- The headache associated with intracranial hypotension caused by leakage of cerebrospinal fluid after a lumbar puncture is treated with an autologous epidural blood patch.
- The diagnosis of spontaneous intracranial hypotension is associated with the contrast-enhanced brain-MRI finding of diffuse nonnodular pachymeningeal enhancement in nearly 80% of patients.

Trigeminal Neuralgia

Trigeminal neuralgia is the most common and most intense cranial neuralgia. Incidence increases with advanced age. Multiple sclerosis should be considered in those with onset before age 50 years. Pain is typically unilateral and localized to the maxillary and mandibular branches of the trigeminal nerve (cranial nerve V). The pains are brief, "shock-like," or electric, lasting seconds to minutes. Paroxysms may be spontaneous or triggered by innocuous stimulation of the face. Refractory periods are common after a series of paroxysms. Ipsilateral autonomic features are rare. Neurologic examination is typically normal. Contrast-enhanced brain MRI detects nonvascular structural pathology (such as compressing and demyelinating causes) in 15% of patients. In the other 85%, brain MRA often identifies neurovascular contact between a loop of the superior cerebellar artery and the trigeminal nerve. Contact causing displacement or atrophy of the nerve has been associated with a greater likelihood of symptom development.

Management of trigeminal neuralgia begins with carbamazepine administration. Pain may resolve within a few days, although mild dizziness and drowsiness are common. Other adverse effects of the medication, including hyponatremia and agranulocytosis, are less common but necessitate intermittent monitoring. Alternative drugs are oxcarbazepine, baclofen, gabapentin, and lamotrigine. Approximately 30% of patients do not respond to trials of monotherapy or combined therapy. For those refractory to two-drug trials, surgical intervention should be considered. Nonsurgical options are effective in 50% of patients and include percutaneous radiofrequency coagulation, glycerol injection, or focused stereotactic (Gamma Knife) radiation. Posterior fossa microvascular decompression of the neurovascular contact zone is a more invasive and more effective option. It should be prioritized in those with low surgical risk.

- Contrast-enhanced brain MRI detects nonvascular structural pathology in 15% of patients with trigeminal neuralgia, and brain magnetic resonance angiography often identifies neurovascular contact between a loop of the superior cerebellar artery and the trigeminal nerve in the other 85%.

(Continued)

- Initial management of trigeminal neuralgia is with carbamazepine; if medical therapy fails, focused stereotactic (Gamma Knife) radiation, glycerol injection, or posterior fossa microvascular decompression may be effective.

Medication-Induced Headache

Headache is a potential effect of medication exposure or withdrawal. Oral contraceptives, phosphodiesterase inhibitors, β-adrenergic agonists, and nitrates are among the most commonly implicated drugs; they may cause headache de novo or aggravate an existing primary headache disorder. Withdrawal from caffeine or antidepressants also frequently provokes headache. Medication overuse headache (MOH), previously called "rebound" headache, is a highly prevalent condition affecting 1% of adults. This clinical syndrome may result from overtreatment with acute medication in patients with underlying migraine or tension-type headache. Use of triptans, ergot alkaloids, opioids, or combination analgesics for 10 or more days per month or simple analgesics for 15 or more days per month constitutes medication overuse. Affected patients often report daily or near-daily headache that is refractory to numerous treatment options. MOH is more common in midlife, in women, and in those with high baseline headache frequency. In those with migraine, opioids are associated with a 44% increase and butalbital compounds with a 70% increase in the risk of headache progression. These medications should be avoided in patients with recurrent primary headache disorders. Management of MOH involves discontinuation of the overused medication and the introduction of appropriate preventive medication directed at the primary headache disorder.

- Medication overuse headache can result from use of triptans, ergot alkaloids, opioids, or combination analgesic agents for 10 or more days per month or simple analgesic agents for 15 or more days per month; treatment includes discontinuation of the overused medication and use of appropriate preventive medication directed at the primary headache disorder.

Primary Headache
Migraine
Diagnosis

The International Classification of Headache Disorders (ICHD), third edition (beta version), recognizes several subtypes of migraine, including migraine without aura, migraine with aura, and chronic migraine. Each is characterized by episodes of disabling headache lasting hours to days. Accuracy of diagnosis and management is enhanced by the use of formal ICHD criteria, although the POUND mnemonic (Pulsatile quality of headache, One-day duration, Unilateral location, Nausea or vomiting, Disabling intensity) is a helpful means of recalling

CONT.

the symptoms typically associated with migraines. Because of the extensive phenotypic variation, nearly half of migraine presentations are misdiagnosed. Neck pain (75%) and "sinus" symptoms, such as tearing or nasal drainage (50%), are both more common than features felt to be characteristic of migraine, such as vomiting or aura. In the presence of a stable clinical pattern of migraine and a normal neurologic examination, brain imaging is not indicated.

Migraine without aura is the most prevalent migraine subtype (**Table 5**). Although clinicians often emphasize unilateral location or pulsatile characteristics, moderate to severe pain is the most sensitive feature, and worsening by routine physical activity is the most specific element among the pain criteria. Photophobia, phonophobia, and nausea are each reported by approximately 75% of patients with migraine without aura.

The diagnosis of migraine with aura is made after two discrete aura episodes have occurred (**Table 6**). Aura may occur in 20% to 30% of patients with migraine. It frequently precedes pain but may occur during or without head discomfort. Aura symptoms involve positive and negative neurologic phenomena developing gradually and evolving over a period of 5 to 60 minutes. Resolution is gradual and complete. ICHD criteria recognize a number of aura subtypes. Typical aura involves any combination of homonymous visual, hemisensory, or language symptoms. Brainstem aura is defined by the presence of two of the following brainstem symptoms: dysarthria, vertigo, tinnitus, hypacusis, diplopia, ataxia, or decreased level of

TABLE 6.	International Headache Society Criteria for Migraine With Aura

A. At least two attacks fulfilling criteria B and C

B. One or more of the following fully reversible aura symptoms:
  1. Visual
  2. Sensory
  3. Speech and/or language
  4. Motor
  5. Brainstem
  6. Retinal

C. At least two of the following four characteristics:
  1. At least one aura symptom spreads gradually over >5 minutes, and/or two or more symptoms occur in succession
  2. Each individual aura symptom lasts 5-60 minutes
  3. At least one aura symptom is unilateral
  4. The aura is accompanied, or followed within 60 minutes, by headache

D. Headache not better accounted for by another ICHD-3 diagnosis, and transient ischemic attack has been excluded

ICHD-3 = International Classification of Headache Disorders, 3rd edition (beta version).

Adapted with permission of SAGE Publications LTD., London, Los Angeles, New Delhi, Singapore and Washington DC, from Headache Classification Committee of the International Headache Society (IHS). The International Classification of Headache Disorders, 3rd edition (beta version). Cephalalgia. 2013 Jul;33(9):646. [PMID: 23771276] doi:10.1177/0333102413485658. Copyright SAGE Publications LTD., 2013.

TABLE 5.	International Headache Society Criteria for Migraine Without Aura

A. At least five attacks fulfilling criteria B-D

B. Headache attacks lasting 4-72 hours (untreated or unsuccessfully treated)

C. Headache with at least two of the following four characteristics:
  1. Unilateral location
  2. Pulsating quality
  3. Moderate or severe pain intensity that inhibits or prohibits daily activities
  4. Aggravation by walking up or down stairs or similar routine physical activity

D. During headache, occurrence of at least one of following symptoms:
  1. Nausea/vomiting
  2. Photophobia/phonophobia

E. Headache not better accounted for by another ICHD-3 diagnosis

ICHD-3 = International Classification of Headache Disorders, 3rd edition (beta version).

Adapted with permission of SAGE Publications LTD., London, Los Angeles, New Delhi, Singapore and Washington DC, from Headache Classification Committee of the International Headache Society (IHS). The International Classification of Headache Disorders, 3rd edition (beta version). Cephalalgia. 2013 Jul;33(9):645. [PMID: 23771276] doi:10.1177/0333102413485658. Copyright SAGE Publications LTD., 2013.

consciousness. Hemiplegic aura comprises any aura involving motor weakness. Both hemiplegic and brainstem auras are listed as contraindications for triptan use. Retinal aura involves monocular visual compromise. These auras need to be distinguished from ocular pathologies, such as retinal ischemia or detachment. Given an associated increased risk of stroke, estrogen-containing oral contraceptives should be avoided in women with migraine aura of all subtypes.

Chronic migraine is defined as headache for 15 or more days per month (**Table 7**). Transformation from acute to chronic migraine occurs in the general population at an annual rate of 3%. Older age, female sex, head trauma, major life changes or stressors, obesity, chronic pain, mood and anxiety disorders, and inadequate acute migraine management are risk factors. Acute migraine medication or caffeine overuse and exposure to nicotine may also raise the risk of or exacerbate chronic migraine; some patients with chronic migraine may have a secondary diagnosis of MOH. Patients with chronic migraine are more disabled and more likely to report migraine-related comorbidities (mood or anxiety disorders, sleep dysfunction, irritable bowel syndrome, fibromyalgia) than are those with episodic migraine.

Acute Migraine Management

The acute treatment of migraine aims to eliminate pain and restore function. Goals of care involve freedom from pain,

TABLE 7. International Headache Society Criteria for Chronic Migraine

A. Headache (tension-type-like and/or migraine-like) on at least 15 days per month for greater than 3 months and fulfilling criteria B and C

B. Occurring in a patient who has had at least five attacks fulfilling criteria B-D for migraine without aura and/or criteria B and C for migraine with aura

C. On at least 8 days per month for greater than 3 months, fulfilling any of the following:

    1. Criteria C and D for migraine without aura

    2. Criteria B and C for migraine with aura

    3. Believed by the patient to be a migraine at onset and relieved by a triptan or ergot alkaloid derivative

    4. The aura is accompanied, or followed within 60 minutes, by headache

D. Headache not better accounted for by another ICHD-3 diagnosis

ICHD-3 = International Classification of Headache Disorders, 3rd edition (beta version).

Adapted with permission of SAGE Publications LTD., London, Los Angeles, New Delhi, Singapore and Washington DC, from Headache Classification Committee of the International Headache Society (IHS). The International Classification of Headache Disorders, 3rd edition (beta version). Cephalalgia. 2013 Jul;33(9):650. [PMID: 23771276] doi:10.1177/0333102413485658. Copyright SAGE Publications LTD., 2013.

Triptans are selective agonists at 5-hydroxytryptamine 1B and 1D receptors. They are migraine-specific agents with direct impact on trigeminovascular activation associated with migraine attacks. Triptans reverse intracranial vasodilation (1B) and provide neuronal inhibition at peripheral and central trigeminal nerve circuitry (1D). Guidelines recommend the use of triptans in patients with moderate to severe migraine who have not responded to NSAID therapy over a series of at least three migraine attacks. Current evidence suggests that all oral triptans possess nearly similar clinical efficacy. Orally dissolvable tablets are intestinally absorbed; their only advantage is use without the need to drink liquids. Nasal spray options may have more rapid onset, bypassing the gastrointestinal tract. Outcomes are similar to those of oral agents, but unpleasant taste, nasal congestion, or burning may be limiting factors. Subcutaneous sumatriptan provides the most rapid onset and achieves the highest response rates among all triptan agents and formulations. Local site reactions and more prominent "triptan" sensations characteristic of the class (flushing, chest or throat tightness, paresthesias) may be noted. All triptans are

CONT. nausea, and sensory sensitivities within 1 to 2 hours and maintenance of such control through at least 24 hours. Because attack characteristics show significant inter-individual and intra-individual variability, different treatment options and strategies are required (**Table 8**). Guidelines recommend tailoring the treatments to the severity and symptomatology of the attack. Migraines awakening a patient from sleep or those associated with nausea and vomiting may require medication offered in parenteral or nasal formulations. Because consistency of response to any treatment rarely approaches 100%, most patients benefit from availability of two or more acute migraine therapies. Administration of medication at the time of mild pain has been shown to improve therapeutic outcomes when compared to treating moderate to severe headache; therefore, treatment should be started as early as possible in the disease course. Treatment should be limited to 10 days per month to avoid MOH.

Evidence-based guidelines recommend several simple and combination analgesic agents as first-line therapies for acute migraine. Acetaminophen has established efficacy only in migraine of mild to moderate intensity; data suggest the response may be enhanced by coadministration with metoclopramide. Aspirin administered alone or in combination with acetaminophen and caffeine also has established efficacy in acute migraine. The effectiveness of the NSAIDs ibuprofen, naproxen sodium, and diclofenac potassium is supported by strong evidence. Special formulations of these products have been shown to be more rapidly absorbed and effective than their standard tablet counterparts. These formulations include effervescent aspirin, solubilized ibuprofen, and diclofenac powder for oral solution.

TABLE 8. Acute Migraine Therapies

Drug	Recommended Dose
NSAIDs[a]	
Aspirin	325-900 mg
Ibuprofen	400-800 mg
Naproxen sodium	250-1000 mg
Combination of acetaminophen-aspirin-caffeine	2 tablets
Diclofenac potassium (oral solution)	50 mg
Migraine-Specific Oral Agents[a]	
Almotriptan	6.25-12.5 mg
Eletriptan	20-40 mg
Frovatriptan	2.5 mg
Naratriptan	1-2.5 mg
Rizatriptan	5-10 mg
Sumatriptan	25-100 mg
Sumatriptan-naproxen	85-500 mg
Zolmitriptan	2.5-5 mg
Nonoral Agents[a]	
Dihydroergotamine	1 mg nasally
Dihydroergotamine	1 mg subcutaneously
Prochlorperazine	10 mg intravenously
Sumatriptan	5-20 mg nasally
Sumatriptan	4-6 mg subcutaneously
Zolmitriptan	5 mg nasally

[a]Doses listed may be administered once or twice daily.

CONT.

contraindicated in the presence of coronary, cerebral, or peripheral vascular disease; uncontrolled hypertension; or migraine with brainstem or hemiplegic auras. Different formulations of one triptan may be used safely within the same day, but using a different triptan or an ergot alkaloid should be delayed by 24 hours. Despite labeling precautions, the concurrent use of triptans and selective serotonin reuptake inhibitors or serotonin-norepinephrine reuptake inhibitor antidepressants is safe in most cases.

Other agents also are effective in the management of acute migraine. Ergot alkaloids have been used for years but have been largely replaced by triptans, which have preferable safety and tolerability profiles; parenteral and nasal formulations of dihydroergotamine are the most available and effective options among the ergot alkaloids. Dopamine D_2 receptor antagonists (metoclopramide, prochlorperazine) are often used as adjuncts to analgesics or triptans. In addition to antiemetic properties, these agents can reduce migraine pain when delivered parenterally. Guidelines recommend avoiding the use of opioids and butalbital-containing compounds for acute migraine. In addition to the potential for dependence or addiction, use of these agents has been linked to an increased risk of transformation from episodic to chronic migraine. They should be used sparingly and only when more appropriate acute therapies are contraindicated.

Migraine with a duration lasting longer than 72 hours is known as status migrainosus. Many patients with this condition can be treated with several days of glucocorticoids. Severe cases of acute migraine or status migrainosus may require emergency department or inpatient management. The cornerstone of care in these settings is intravenous delivery of a dopamine antagonist. These are typically combined with intravenous diphenhydramine (to limit dystonic reactions), intravenous ketorolac, and hydration. Opioids may be associated with prolonged length of hospital stay and should be avoided. A more extended course of treatment involving repetitive intravenous dihydroergotamine with antiemetics over 2 to 3 days is very effective in the management of refractory status migrainosus.

Migraine Prevention

The goals of migraine prevention are the reduction of migraine frequency, intensity, and duration. None of the medications used for migraine prevention were designed for this specific purpose. The best agents may reduce migraine frequency by half in approximately half of the patients treated. Nonpharmacologic preventive measures are not only optimal but required. Trigger identification and avoidance are often helpful. Stress management techniques, such as relaxation therapy or biofeedback, have established efficacy. Regulation of sleep patterns, intake of small frequent meals, adequate hydration, and daily aerobic exercise are all extremely helpful. Regular work and school schedules should be encouraged. Stimulants (such as caffeine and nicotine) must be eliminated or limited. Diet should be modified to avoid additives or preservatives, such as monosodium glutamate and artificial sweeteners. There is good evidence to support the use of certain supplements, such as petasites (butterbur), magnesium, riboflavin, and feverfew.

Pharmacologic prophylaxis should be considered when the headache frequency reaches 5 days per month and almost always is initiated when the frequency exceeds 10 days per month. Data suggest preventive medication can reduce attack frequency and intensity, patient disability, and medical cost. Several weeks or months are often required before maximum benefit is achieved. Once a response occurs, the medications should be continued for a period of 6 to 12 months, at which point dose reduction or drug elimination may be considered. Evidence-based guidelines for pharmacologic prevention of episodic migraine have established Level A evidence supporting the use of five medications: three β-adrenergic blockers (propranolol, timolol, metoprolol) and two antiepileptic drugs (divalproex sodium and topiramate). Level B evidence is available for atenolol, two antidepressants (amitriptyline and venlafaxine), and several NSAIDs. No evidence supports the use of calcium channel blockers or selective serotonin reuptake inhibitor antidepressants in migraine prevention. Studies involving patients with chronic migraine are more limited, but efficacy in prevention has been shown with topiramate and onabotulinum toxin A. Treatment selection is informed by previous therapeutic trials, the presence of coexisting medical conditions, and patient preference.

KEY POINTS

- Because of the extensive phenotypic variation, nearly half of migraine presentations are misdiagnosed; the POUND mnemonic (Pulsatile quality of headache, One-day duration, Unilateral location, Nausea or vomiting, Disabling intensity) is a helpful means of recalling the symptoms typically associated with migraines. **HVC**

- In the presence of a stable clinical pattern of migraine and a normal neurologic examination, brain imaging is not indicated. **HVC**

- Given an associated increased risk of stroke, estrogen-containing oral contraceptives should be avoided in women with migraine aura of all subtypes.

- Triptans are migraine-specific agents that are useful in moderate to severe migraine that has not responded to NSAID therapy; they are contraindicated in the presence of coronary, cerebral, or peripheral vascular disease; uncontrolled hypertension; or migraine with brainstem or hemiplegic auras.

- Pharmacologic prophylaxis for migraine should be considered when headache frequency reaches 5 days per month and almost always is initiated when the frequency exceeds 10 days per month; propranolol, timolol, metoprolol, divalproex sodium, and topiramate are most effective for migraine prophylaxis.

Tension-Type Headache

The most prevalent primary headache condition, tension-type headache is defined by clinical criteria as a headache disorder that, unlike migraine, is mild to moderate in intensity and is not associated with nausea, severe sensory sensitivities, or neurologic symptoms (**Table 9**). Imaging is not indicated. Subclassification is based on monthly headache frequency: infrequent episodic (<1 day), frequent episodic (1-14 days), and chronic (15 or more days). Acetaminophen, aspirin, NSAIDs, and caffeine-containing compounds are effective acute treatments for tension-type headache. Amitriptyline and stress management techniques have modest benefit in prevention of tension-type headache, and some data support the use of acupuncture. Muscle relaxants, benzodiazepines, opioids, and onabotulinum toxin A have no role in the management of tension-type headache.

KEY POINTS

HVC

- Imaging is not indicated for tension-type headache.

- Acetaminophen, aspirin, NSAIDs, and caffeine-containing compounds are effective acute treatments for tension-type headache, but muscle relaxants, benzodiazepines, opioids, and onabotulinum toxin A have no role in the management of tension-type headache.

Trigeminal Autonomic Cephalalgias

Trigeminal autonomic cephalalgias (TACs) are the most severe and stereotypic primary headache disorders. Pain is severe, localized to the periorbital or temporal areas, and associated with pronounced ipsilateral cranial autonomic features, such as nasal congestion or rhinorrhea and ptosis or miosis. The TACs, which include cluster headache, chronic paroxysmal hemicrania (CPH), and short-lasting unilateral neuralgiform headache attacks with conjunctival injection and tearing (SUNCT), are differentiated by episode duration, frequency, and periodicity.

Cluster headache may last 15 to 180 minutes and recur one to eight times daily over a span of weeks to months; the shorter duration distinguishes cluster headache from migraine (**Table 10**). This headache is characterized by a cyclical nature in which periods of recurrent headache activity are interrupted by months to years of headache remission. Many of the attacks are nocturnal, and some may be provoked by alcohol ingestion. Episodes of CPH last 2 to 30 minutes and recur up to 40 times per day, whereas those of SUNCT last 1 to 600 seconds and may recur more than 100 times daily. SUNCT may be confused with trigeminal neuralgia, which is more likely mandibular or maxillary and lacks autonomic features. Unlike cluster headache, both CPH and SUNCT typically continue without periods of remission. Brain MRI should be performed initially to exclude structural lesions mimicking TACs.

Cluster headache has several acute and preventive options. Oxygen inhalation and subcutaneous sumatriptan are both effective in the treatment of attacks. A 2-week course of glucocorticoids may help reduce attack frequency at the onset

---

TABLE 9. International Headache Society Criteria for Tension-Type Headache

A. At least 10 attacks fulfilling criteria B-E

B. Headache attacks (untreated or unsuccessfully treated) lasting from 30 minutes to 7 days

C. Headache with at least two of the following four characteristics:

   1. Bilateral location

   2. Pressing/tightening (nonpulsating) quality

   3. Mild or moderate intensity

   4. Not aggravated by walking stairs or similar routine physical activity

D. Headache characterized by both of the following:

   1. No nausea/vomiting

   2. No more than one episode of photophobia or phonophobia

E. Not better accounted for by another ICHD-3 diagnosis

ICHD-3 = International Classification of Headache Disorders, 3rd edition (beta version).

Adapted with permission of SAGE Publications LTD., London, Los Angeles, New Delhi, Singapore and Washington DC, from Headache Classification Committee of the International Headache Society (IHS). The International Classification of Headache Disorders, 3rd edition (beta version). Cephalalgia. 2013 Jul;33(9):660-1. [PMID: 23771276] doi:10.1177/0333102413485658. Copyright SAGE Publications LTD., 2013.

TABLE 10. International Headache Society Criteria for Cluster Headache

A. At least five attacks fulfilling criteria B-D

B. Severe or very severe unilateral orbital, supraorbital, and/or temporal pain lasting 15-180 minutes (when untreated)

C. Either or both of the following:

   1. At least one of the following symptoms or signs, ipsilateral to the headache:

      a) conjunctival injection and/or lacrimation

      b) nasal congestion and/or rhinorrhea

      c) eyelid edema

      d) forehead and facial sweating

      e) forehead and facial flushing

      f) sensation of fullness in the ear

      g) miosis and/or ptosis

   2. A sense of restlessness or agitation

D. Attack frequency from one every other day to eight per day when the disorder is active

E. Headache not better accounted for by another ICHD-3 diagnosis

ICHD-3 = International Classification of Headache Disorders, 3rd edition (beta version).

Adapted with permission of SAGE Publications LTD., London, Los Angeles, New Delhi, Singapore and Washington DC, from Headache Classification Committee of the International Headache Society (IHS). The International Classification of Headache Disorders, 3rd edition (beta version). Cephalalgia. 2013 Jul;33(9):665-6. [PMID: 23771276] doi:10.1177/0333102413485658. Copyright SAGE Publications LTD., 2013.

of the cycle. Verapamil is the drug of choice for longer-term prevention of cluster headache. CPH is uniquely and universally responsive to indomethacin. Reports have suggested a small benefit from lamotrigine, but SUNCT is largely refractory to medical management.

KEY POINTS

- Trigeminal autonomic cephalalgias are the most severe and stereotypic primary headache disorders and include cluster headaches, chronic paroxysmal hemicrania, and short-lasting unilateral neuralgiform headache attacks with conjunctival injection and tearing.

- Cluster headache is treated with oxygen inhalation and subcutaneous sumatriptan.

- Chronic paroxysmal hemicrania is universally responsive to indomethacin; short-lasting unilateral neuralgiform headache attacks with conjunctival injection and tearing is largely refractory to medical management.

Other Primary Headache Syndromes

Primary stabbing headaches ("ice-pick headaches") are episodes of stabbing head pain lasting seconds and occurring in isolation or in series. There are no associated autonomic features. The location of pain is fixed in one third of patients and extratrigeminal in most patients. Those with migraine may be more likely to describe these attacks. Indomethacin can be helpful during cycles of more frequent attacks.

Cough headache develops abruptly with cough or Valsalva maneuvers and typically lasts seconds to minutes. Mild headache may continue for 1 to 2 hours. The severity of pain correlates with cough frequency. Advancing age and male sex may be risk factors. Brain MRI is indicated because secondary pathologies, most commonly a Chiari malformation, may be found in half of those affected. Indomethacin may reduce headache frequency during cycles of increased activity.

KEY POINT

- Brain MRI is indicated in patients with cough headache to identify possible secondary pathologies (such as a Chiari malformation), which may be found in 50% of affected patients.

Head Injury
Traumatic Brain Injury

Traumatic brain injury (TBI) results from biomechanical forces applied to the structures of the head and neck. Damage may be temporary or permanent and may arise from functional or structural alterations in the central nervous system. Severity is determined by clinical findings and imaging results. When indicated, noncontrast CT is the imaging modality of choice because it is more sensitive for bony injuries, less expensive, and more widely available than MRI. Mild TBI is associated with Glasgow

Coma Scale (GCS) scores of 13 to 15 with no or only a brief initial loss of consciousness; results of head CT are typically normal. Moderate TBI is associated with GCS scores of 9 to 12 and/or an initial loss of consciousness of 30 minutes to 24 hours. Severe TBI is associated with GCS scores of 3 to 8 and/or an initial loss of consciousness of more than 24 hours (**Table 11**). In moderate and severe TBI, head CT may reveal a skull fracture, cerebral contusions and edema, and intracranial hemorrhage.

Mild Traumatic Brain Injury

The terms mild TBI and concussion are often used interchangeably. Mild TBI is the most common presentation of TBI and frequently results from accidents, athletic activity, or military service activities. Guidelines for the use of head CT in mild TBI have been published by the Centers for Disease Activity and Prevention (**Table 12**). Although yet to be incorporated into management guidelines, serum measurements of brain-specific biomarkers released after mild TBI can help predict which patients may have intracranial lesions visible on CT scan. Elevated levels of ubiquitin carboxy-terminal hydrolase L1 and glial fibrillary acidic protein can be detected as early as 20 minutes after head injury. A recent study of patients within 12 hours of mild TBI (GCS scores of 9 to 15) showed that these elevated serum levels combined with certain clinical information had a sensitivity of 97.5% for predicting lesions visible on head CT scan; negative predictive value was 99.6%. Patients

TABLE 11.	Glasgow Coma Scale
Eye Opening	**Score**
Spontaneous	4
Response to verbal command	3
Response to pain	2
No eye opening	1
Best Verbal Response	
Oriented	5
Confused	4
Inappropriate words	3
Incomprehensible sounds	2
No verbal response	1
Best Motor Response	
Obeys commands	6
Localizing response to pain	5
Withdrawal response to pain	4
Flexion to pain	3
Extension to pain	2
No motor response	1
Total	

Data from: Teasdale G, Jennett B. Assessment of coma and impaired consciousness. A practical scale. Lancet 1974 Jul 13;2(7872); 81-4. [PMID: 4136544]

TABLE 12.	Indications for Head CT in Mild Traumatic Brain Injury[a]
Age >60 years	
Vomiting	
Headache	
Posttraumatic seizure	
Drug or alcohol intoxication	
Persistent drowsiness or short-term memory deficit	
"Dangerous" mechanisms of injury (fall from height greater than 3 feet or 5 steps, ejection from a vehicle, being struck by a vehicle as a pedestrian)	
Glasgow Coma Scale score <15	
Focal neurologic deficit	
Physical evidence of significant trauma to the head and neck	
Coagulopathy	

[a]CT scan should be obtained if any of the following findings are present.

TABLE 13.	Symptoms of Mild Traumatic Brain Injury
Physical	
Headache	
Nausea/vomiting	
Dizziness/vertigo	
Gait disturbance	
Photophobia or phonophobia	
Visual blurring	
Dysarthria	
Seizures	
Cognitive	
Poor concentration	
Mental "fogginess" or confusion	
Poor memory	
Learning impairment	
Slowed reaction times	
Psychological	
Irritability	
Depression	
Anxiety	
Sleep Associated	
Fatigue	
Insomnia	
Hypersomnia	
Drowsiness	
Vivid dreams	

with mild TBI, a normal neurologic examination, and (when necessary) a normal head CT scan may be safely discharged from the emergency department.

Symptoms following a mild TBI may be divided into four domains: physical, cognitive, psychological, and sleep-associated (**Table 13**). Most symptoms resolve spontaneously within 7 to 10 days. Headache is consistently the most common symptom and is among the most disabling sequelae. Head trauma may cause new headache or worsen a preexisting headache condition. A previous history of migraine has been linked with increased incidence and severity of postconcussion symptoms. Posttraumatic headaches most commonly have the characteristics of migraine and tension-type headaches.

Treatment is matched to the headache phenotype. Acetaminophen, aspirin, NSAIDs, and triptans are effective acute therapies; opioids and butalbital products should be avoided. β-Blockers, antidepressants, and antiepileptic drugs may be useful for headache prevention in patients with persistent posttraumatic headache. Treatment of other postconcussion symptoms is largely symptomatic and based on little evidence. Visual, vestibular, and cognitive therapies may be helpful in certain settings. Stimulants, such as amantadine, are sometimes given to patients with cognitive symptoms. Regulated sleep, graded return to exercise, and temporary modification of school or work schedules are often recommended.

KEY POINTS

- The symptoms of mild traumatic brain injury, which usually involves brief or no loss of consciousness, typically resolve spontaneously within 7 to 10 days.
- NSAIDs and triptans are effective acute therapies for mild traumatic brain injury–related headache, but opioids and butalbital products should be avoided.

Severe Traumatic Brain Injury

Severe TBI may present with an alteration in consciousness, seizures, repeated vomiting, or focal neurologic deficits. Bilateral periorbital or mastoid bruising and hemotympanum may be signs of basilar skull fracture.

The primary goal of initial management is prevention of hypotension and hypoxia. Normalization of blood oxygenation (arterial P_{O_2} > 60 mm Hg [8.0 kPa]) and blood pressure (systolic > 90 mm Hg) has been shown to improve outcomes. Early management of elevated intracranial pressure with head elevation and mannitol may be required; continuous measurement of intracranial pressure also may be necessary. Head CT is the preferred imaging study, and serial scans may be necessary. Penetrating injuries, depressed skull fracture, and intracranial hemorrhage all may require urgent surgery.

Medical management includes mechanical thromboprophylaxis (with intermittent pneumatic compression) for deep venous thrombosis prevention, glycemic control, and treatment of infectious or gastrointestinal complications. Nutritional support with full caloric replacement by day 7

CONT.

postinjury is recommended. Fever should be controlled aggressively, with some medical centers advocating induced hypothermia; acetaminophen is an appropriate initial treatment. Glucocorticoids worsen the prognosis of severe TBI and should be avoided.

KEY POINT

- Medical management in the treatment of severe traumatic brain injury includes normalization of blood oxygenation and blood pressure, correction of elevated intracranial pressure, mechanical thromboprophylaxis for deep venous thrombosis, glycemic control, and aggressive control of fever; glucocorticoids should be avoided.

Epidural and Subdural Hematoma

An epidural hematoma arises when an arterial structure is breached and blood collects between the dura mater and skull in a "lentiform" fashion (**Figure 2**). Most epidural hematomas involve a laceration of the middle meningeal artery from a temporal bone fracture. Lateral extension is limited by dural attachments at the skull sutures, and expansion occurs inward toward the brain parenchyma. Many patients with an epidural hematoma have a "lucid interval" followed by rapid neurologic compromise. Headache, vomiting, and declining mental status may occur early. Stupor or coma with ipsilateral occulomotor nerve (cranial nerve III) palsy and contralateral hemiparesis may signal transtentorial (uncal) herniation. Urgent surgical evacuation is recommended for those with a GCS score less than 9, anisocoria, or a hematoma greater than 30 mL in volume.

A subdural hematoma (**Figure 3**) is a collection of blood between the brain and dura mater. Rupture of bridging veins

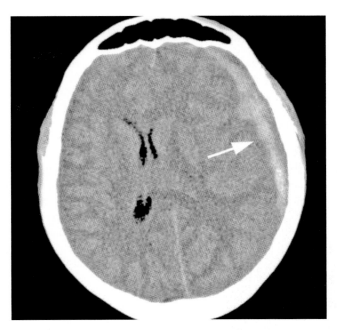

FIGURE 3. CT scan of a subdural hematoma. Note the crescent shape as blood under venous pressure separates the dura from the arachnoid membrane (*arrow*).

within this space is typically responsible. This may occur spontaneously, as a complication of anticoagulation, or after trauma. Because of cerebral atrophy and subsequent tension on the subdural bridging veins, older persons and those with alcoholism are particularly susceptible. Presentations may be acute, subacute, or chronic. Whereas acute subdural hematoma typically presents with coma or neurologic compromise, chronic hematoma may be associated with nonspecific symptoms, including altered mental status or somnolence, in addition to focal neurologic findings. In patients with acute subdural hematomas, a hematoma thickness greater than 10 mm, a score less than 9 on the GCS, and the presence of pupillary asymmetry or fixation are all indications for immediate surgical treatment. In patients with chronic hematomas, a hematoma thickness greater than 10 mm, a midline shift greater than 5 mm, and significant neurologic compromise are all indications for drainage.

KEY POINTS

- In patients with epidural hematoma, stupor or coma with ipsilateral occulomotor nerve palsy and contralateral hemiparesis may signal transtentorial herniation.

- Chronic subdural hematoma may be associated with nonspecific symptoms, including altered mental status or somnolence, in addition to focal neurologic findings.

- In patients with acute subdural hematomas, a hematoma thickness greater than 10 mm, a score less than 9 on the Glasgow Coma Scale, and the presence of pupillary asymmetry or fixation are indications for immediate surgical treatment.

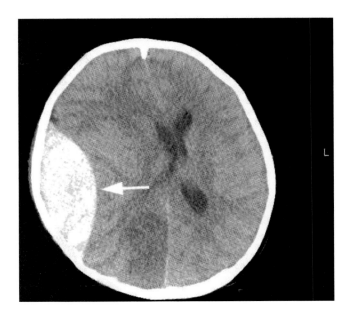

FIGURE 2. CT scan of an epidural hematoma. Note the biconvex lens appearance as blood under arterial pressure collects between the skull and outer margin of the dura (*arrow*).

Head Injury in Special Populations

Athletes

Any athlete suspected of sustaining a mild TBI should be immediately removed from play and assessed by a licensed health care provider trained in the evaluation and management of concussion. Guidelines recommend initial screening with a symptom checklist and neurologic examination involving specific cognitive evaluation and balance testing. Neuropsychological testing provides an objective and more sensitive measure of cognitive function; it should be employed as part of a comprehensive TBI management program for patients with persistent symptoms. Rest, both cognitive and physical, is required for the first days to weeks. Return to play requires the resolution of symptoms and normalization of cognition. The patient should progress through gradual stepwise increases in physical activity without the return of postconcussive symptoms before returning to play. There are no available guidelines for permanent disqualification from contact sports for athletes with mild TBI.

Chronic traumatic encephalopathy is being recognized with increasing frequency in athletes who play contact sports. The result of multiple concussions and head trauma, chronic traumatic encephalopathy may manifest as progressive neuropsychiatric symptoms, including depression and dementia, years after the inciting events. See Cognitive Impairment for more information.

KEY POINT

- Any athlete suspected of sustaining a mild TBI should be immediately removed from play and assessed by a licensed healthcare provider trained in the evaluation and management of concussion.

Military Personnel

TBI is a common consequence of service in the armed forces, particularly among those deployed to a combat theater. Mild TBI, which often lacks abnormalities on neurologic examination or imaging, is highly prevalent and accounts for 80% of TBI diagnoses. Guidelines recommend that military personnel undergo screening for TBI when exposed to trauma involving a direct blow to the head, a vehicular accident, or an explosive blast and when they are instructed to by a superior officer. The Military Acute Concussion Evaluation and a requisite 24-hour rest period are mandated, with return to duty requiring complete recovery. Headache is the most common symptom after TBI and the best prognostic indicator in returning service members. A posttraumatic headache still present at 1 year postinjury is likely to be permanent. Other sequelae of mild TBI in this population include posttraumatic stress disorder (PTSD), depression, anxiety, insomnia, and disorders of cognition and balance. The prevalence of PTSD is higher in military personnel with mild TBI than in civilians with mild TBI, and thus screening for PTSD in the former group is mandatory. Returning service members with any TBI are best managed through a multidisciplinary approach. Treatments are largely symptomatic and supportive.

KEY POINT

- The prevalence of posttraumatic stress disorder is higher in military personnel with mild traumatic brain injury (TBI) than in civilians with mild TBI.

Older Patients

Adults older than 75 years are at particular risk for hospitalization and death from TBI. Falls, motor vehicle accidents, and accidental blows to the head are the leading mechanisms of injury in this population. Prevention of these events is an essential aspect of geriatric medicine. See MKSAP 18 General Internal Medicine for more information.

Patients Receiving Anticoagulation

Anticoagulation is associated with an increased risk of intracranial hemorrhage after trauma. Intracranial hemorrhage in patients treated with warfarin has significant morbidity and a mortality as high as 50%; immediate correction of the INR limits hematoma expansion. Reversal of direct-acting anticoagulant agents with specific reversal agents, if available, also should be performed. The reinitiation of anticoagulation after intracranial hemorrhage is clinically challenging and is supported by scant empirical evidence. Hemorrhagic complications in this population appear to be greatest within the first 24 hours of injury, and the risk of thromboembolism is highest between days 3 through 5 after injury. For patients with lower risk of hematoma expansion (such as younger patients or those whose hemorrhage is small in size) and higher risk of thromboembolism (such as those with a mechanical heart valve), the optimal time to resume anticoagulation may be 72 hours after trauma. **H**

Seizures and Epilepsy

Clinical Presentation of Seizures

Epilepsy is defined as at least two unprovoked seizures more than 24 hours apart, or one unprovoked seizure with a risk of further seizures that is similar to the risk after two unprovoked seizures (at least 60%). The term "epileptic seizure" does not imply that the seizure is related to epilepsy; rather, it means that the seizure is "real"–that is, secondary to abnormal electrical activity in the brain and not to some other cause (such as syncope or psychiatric disease). The diagnosis of an epileptic seizure relies on a detailed patient history. The stereotyped nature of clinical events is characteristic of seizures; symptom variability from event to event suggests an alternative diagnosis. Epilepsy usually requires antiepileptic drug (AED) therapy, but isolated seizures may not, especially if provoked by reversible or preventable causes. The terminology of seizures is evolving, with more descriptive terms suggested as replacements for "simple partial seizures" and "complex partial seizures" (**Figure 4**).

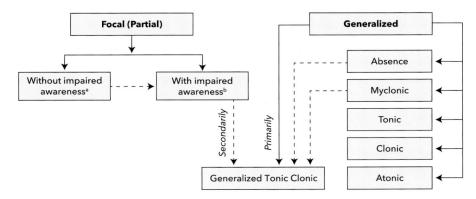

FIGURE 4. Common seizure types based on International League Against Epilepsy classification. The dashed arrows represent the possibility of one seizure type transitioning directly into another when a patient is seizing. Note that generalized tonic clonic seizures may start out focal or generalized.

[a]Formerly known as simple partial seizures.

[b]Formerly known as complex partial or focal dyscognitive seizures.

Focal Seizures

Focal seizures may occur without alteration of awareness (formerly, simple partial seizures) or with alteration of awareness (formerly, complex partial seizures). The first type includes auras, which are not just warning symptoms but actually very localized focal seizures (**Table 14**). Seizures involving impaired awareness may affect memory, responsiveness, language, or cognition. Both focal seizures and generalized absence seizures can present as "staring episodes" and must be carefully differentiated (**Table 15**).

Patients may not remember or volunteer a history of focal seizures because they may be unaware of the events. Therefore, it is important to ask about discrete episodes of memory loss or time lapses. A typical temporal lobe seizure, for example, may start with an aura of a rising feeling in the stomach, déjà vu, or fear, followed by altered awareness with staring, arrest of speech or behavior, and semipurposeful repetitive movements, called automatisms. Focal seizures also may present with autonomic symptoms, such as palpitations, sweating, and hot flashes. Whereas these symptoms also can be seen with psychiatric and cardiac disorders, focal seizures will typically have sudden onset, stereotyped symptoms, and a short duration.

Generalized Seizures

Generalized tonic-clonic seizures (GTCS) have a characteristic pattern of tonic activity followed by clonic activity. During the tonic phase, eyes are wide open while the entire body stiffens, and typically there is a single loud groan or "ictal cry" (not actual crying or sobbing) During the clonic phase, rhythmic jerking occurs synchronously in all limbs, initially at high frequency, with eventual slowing and cessation. This movement often is followed by stertor (deep, slow snoring). A postictal state with confusion, hypersomnolence, and fatigue is common and can persist for hours or even a day.

GTCS may be generalized at onset and are considered to be primarily generalized seizures. These may be preceded by

TABLE 14.	Examples of Focal Seizures Without Altered Awareness[a]
Lobe	**Clinical Presentation**
Frontal	Focal contralateral motor activity (clonic jerking)
Temporal	Epigastric rising sensation (nausea, butterflies); aphasia; déjà vu; fear; elation; auditory, olfactory[b], and gustatory[b] sensations
Parietal	Focal contralateral pain, numbness, or paresthesias
Occipital	Contralateral homonymous visual loss or nonformed hallucinations (dots, lines, flashes of light)

[a]Formerly known as simple partial seizures, which includes auras.

[b]Altered smell and taste also can be seen in psychogenic nonepileptic events.

TABLE 15.	Clinical Differentiation of Seizure Types Presenting As Staring Episodes	
Seizure Feature	**Absence Seizure**	**Focal Seizure With Altered Awareness[a]**
Aura	No	Possible
Onset	Abrupt	Gradual or abrupt
Duration	<15 s	>30 s
Termination	Abrupt	Usually gradual
Postictal state	Normal	Lethargy, confusion
Frequency	Multiple daily	Once weekly or monthly
Precipitated by hyperventilation	Usually	Unlikely
Associated seizure types	Generalized onset seizures (myoclonic, primarily generalized tonic-clonic, tonic, atonic)	Focal onset seizures (simple partial or secondarily generalized tonic-clonic)

[a]Formerly known as complex partial seizure, or focal dyscognitive seizure.

CONT.

other generalized events, such as absence or myoclonic seizures. Alternatively, GTCS may start as focal seizures with subsequent spread to both hemispheres (secondarily generalized). Aura or automatisms before GTCS and postictal unilateral weakness (Todd paralysis) suggest a focal onset.

Absence seizures are characterized by brief episodes of staring (see Table 15). Many patients are unaware of these seizures. They may occur as the only seizure type in school-age children and are often confused with attention deficit disorder. In adulthood, absence seizures most often occur in combination with other generalized seizure types, such as GTCS or myoclonic seizures.

Myoclonus is a single quick jerk of a limb or the entire body lasting less than a second and is not always associated with a seizure (see Movement Disorders). A diagnosis of myoclonic seizures can be confirmed by electroencephalography (EEG), with each jerk associated with a generalized spike-and-wave discharge (**Figure 5**). Myoclonic seizures also can occur repetitively and result in falls. Awareness is maintained and duration is very short (<1 second), which differentiates myoclonic seizures from GTCS.

Tonic seizures present as episodes of increased muscle tone, ranging from mild extension of the arms and head to a more severe stiffening of the entire body. Atonic seizures present with sudden loss of muscle tone. Both tonic and atonic

seizures occur with no warning, last a few seconds, and cause altered awareness, which often leads to falls and physical injuries; they lack postevent confusion. Prolonged episodes of increased or decreased tone with long duration of loss of consciousness are unlikely to represent seizures.

KEY POINTS

- Epilepsy is defined as at least two unprovoked seizures more than 24 hours apart, or one unprovoked seizure with a risk of further seizures that is similar to the risk after two unprovoked seizures (at least 60%).

- Focal seizures may present with autonomic symptoms, such as palpitations, sweating, and hot flashes, but will have sudden onset, stereotyped symptoms, and a short duration, which differentiate them from psychiatric and cardiac disorders.

- Generalized seizures consist of tonic-clonic, absence, myoclonic, tonic, and atonic seizures.

Epilepsy Syndromes
Focal Epilepsies

Identifiable causes of focal epilepsies include structural lesions, such as mesial temporal sclerosis, cavernous

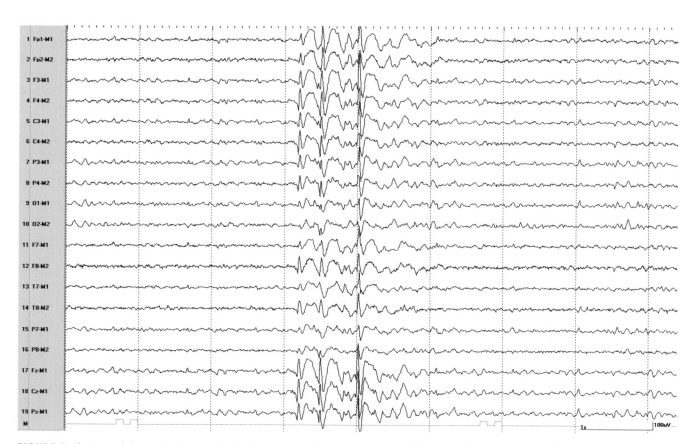

FIGURE 5. Electroencephalogram showing generalized spike-and-wave discharges. In an appropriate clinical setting, this strongly supports a diagnosis of generalized epilepsy.

malformations, cortical dysplasia, traumatic brain injury, stroke, and tumors, all of which may be seen on MRI (**Figure 6** and **Figure 7**). EEG may show focal spikes or sharp waves in the appropriate brain region (**Figure 8**). In most adults with focal epilepsy, however, brain MRI is normal and the cause is unknown.

Temporal lobe epilepsy is the most common adult-onset focal epilepsy. Typical symptoms include aura, loss of awareness, staring, behavior arrest, and amnesia. Automatisms, repetitive semipurposeful movements (such as lip smacking, chewing, and swallowing), and picking or grabbing movements with the ipsilateral arm are common. Speech arrest may be seen with involvement of the dominant hemisphere. Mesial temporal sclerosis with hippocampal atrophy is the most common cause of medication-resistant adult-onset focal epilepsy.

KEY POINTS

- Temporal lobe epilepsy is the most common adult-onset focal epilepsy; typical symptoms include aura, loss of awareness, staring, behavior arrest, and amnesia.
- Mesial temporal sclerosis with hippocampal atrophy is the most common cause of medication-resistant adult-onset focal epilepsy.

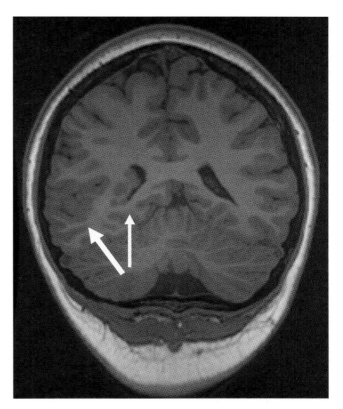

FIGURE 7. Focal cortical dysplasia with periventricular nodular heterotopia. Coronal MRI showing a focal area of thickened cortex in the right temporal region (*thick arrow*) and nodules of abnormal neuronal tissue along the ventricular surface (*thin arrow*).

Idiopathic (Genetic) Generalized Epilepsies

Idiopathic epilepsy is "pure" epilepsy without an underlying neurologic disorder. Newer classification schemes call this type of epilepsy "genetic," even in the absence of a positive family history, inheritability, or a single identifiable gene. In adults, juvenile myoclonic epilepsy (JME) is the most common form of idiopathic generalized epilepsy. JME seizures often are called "college seizures" because of the age of onset (teens or twenties) and associated triggers (sleep deprivation, alcohol use, and stress). Epilepsy may not be diagnosed until the first GTCS occurs because myoclonic seizures often remain unrecognized by patients, family, or friends until a physician takes a careful and complete history.

The presence of myoclonic seizures is required for the diagnosis of JME; patients may report dropping items from their hands, commonly a coffee cup or hairbrush, because myoclonic seizures in JME generally occur in the morning. Most affected patients have GTCS, and approximately 30% of patients have absence seizures. Patients are usually otherwise neurologically healthy and can live relatively normal lives because seizures are often controlled with one or two AEDs. Brain MRI is typically normal, and EEG may show generalized spike-and-wave discharges (see Figure 5). Lifelong AED therapy is typically required.

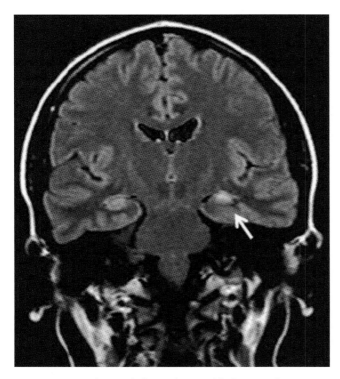

FIGURE 6. Mesial temporal sclerosis. The coronal fluid-attenuated inversion recovery MRI shows increased signal intensity and atrophy of the left mesial temporal lobe (*arrow*).

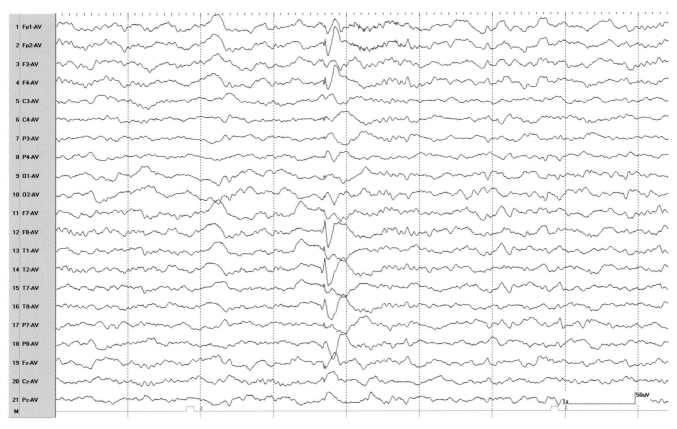

FIGURE 8. Electroencephalogram showing focal (left temporal) sharp waves. In an appropriate clinical setting, this strongly supports a diagnosis of temporal lobe epilepsy.

KEY POINTS

- The presence of myoclonic seizures is required for the diagnosis of juvenile myoclonic epilepsy (JME); JME often is not diagnosed, however, until the first generalized tonic-clonic seizure occurs because myoclonic seizures often remain unrecognized by patients, family, or friends until a physician takes a careful and complete history.

- Lifelong antiepileptic drug therapy is typically required for patients with juvenile myoclonic epilepsy.

Diagnostic Evaluation of Seizures and Epilepsy

Initial Approach to the Patient With a First Seizure

For any patient with a first seizure, obtaining a detailed history is crucial to distinguish seizures from other causes of symptoms. The distinction between seizure and nonseizure events and clarification of first-time versus recurrent episodes are key. A history of previous staring events or myoclonus may help identify patients with epilepsy and should be specifically sought out through careful questioning.

KEY POINT

- Obtaining a detailed history is critical in differentiating seizures from other causes of symptoms; a history of previous staring events or myoclonus may help identify patients with epilepsy.

Differential Diagnosis of Seizures

Many episodic disorders mimic seizures but are nonepileptic events. These include syncope, migraine, movement disorders (tremor, tics), sleep disorders, stroke, and psychogenic events. Seizures usually have positive symptoms, such as jerking, tingling, and visual flashes, whereas strokes have negative symptoms, such as weakness, numbness, and loss of vision. Normal mentation with a headache after the episode suggests migraine. Occurrence only in public suggests panic disorder with agoraphobia.

Associated lightheadedness or chest pain may suggest syncope or cardiac disease. Syncope often presents with shaking ("convulsive syncope") and must be differentiated from GTCS (**Table 16**). In one study, more than 90% of healthy volunteers had nonepileptic myoclonus (generalized or multifocal) when syncope was induced; only a minority had classic, motionless syncope. For distinguishing seizures from syncope

TABLE 16. Clinical Differentiation of Generalized Tonic-Clonic Seizures and Syncope

Seizure Feature	Generalized Tonic-Clonic Seizures	Syncope
Warning symptoms	Typical epileptic aura immediately before onset	Prodrome of lightheadedness, nausea, warmth, diaphoresis, blurred or tunnel vision, generalized weakness, palpitations, and a "faint" feeling
Self-protection	Aura may or may not be long enough to ensure patient safety, but seizure is not preventable	Lying or sitting down may prevent progression to LOC
Muscle tone	Generalized stiffening	Generalized loss of tone
Motor activity	Generalized clonic shaking (rhythmic, synchronous whole-body jerks)	Generalized myoclonic shaking (whole-body shaking or isolated subtle twitching of limbs)
Color	May have cyanosis	May have pallor
Duration of LOC	Usually >1 minute	Usually <1 minute
Postictal state	Confusion, lethargy, combativeness, somnolence	Normal, an other than situationally appropriate memory loss of event

LOC = loss of consciousness.

and psychogenic loss of consciousness, video EEG can be very useful, in combination with tilt-table testing, because it can specifically differentiate these events.

Psychogenic Nonepileptic Spells/Events

Psychogenic nonepileptic spells/events (PNES) were formerly called pseudoseizures or psychogenic nonepileptic seizures. These latter terms should be avoided because seizure is a misnomer in this context, and "pseudo" implies falseness of the symptoms. PNES are most often related to posttraumatic stress disorder or conversion disorder. Factitious disorder and malingering are rare. Patients often have a history of military combat, sexual or physical abuse, chronic medical illness, or prominent life stressors. PNES often mimic GTCS, but certain features help distinguish the diagnoses (**Table 17**). Event capture during video EEG monitoring usually is required to confirm the diagnosis.

> **KEY POINT**
> - Psychogenic nonepileptic spells/events are most often related to posttraumatic stress disorder or conversion disorder; factitious disorder and malingering are rare.

Diagnostic Evaluation

Neuroimaging is recommended for all patients with a first seizure. CT of the head is adequate initially to rapidly exclude emergent pathology, including hemorrhage, but MRI is required in most patients. Contrast-enhanced CT or MRI may be deferred unless infection, tumor, or vascular lesions are suspected. Because temporal lobe epilepsy is common, MRI sequences focusing on the hippocampus and temporal lobes are useful (coronal T2-weighted, fluid-attenuated inversion recovery, and

TABLE 17. Clinical Differentiation of GTCS and PNES

Seizure Feature	GTCS	PNES
Stereotyped	Yes	No (varies from event to event)
Eyelids	Open	Closed (may resist opening)
Color	May have cyanosis	May turn red
Vocalization	Ictal cry (sharp, loud, deep single inspiration against contracted epiglottis)	Intermittent breath holding alternating with gasping/rapid breaths, or crying/sobbing
Muscle tone	Starts with stiffening of all limbs (tonic)	Patients usually limp or limber; may resist movement or make atypical postures (fists, claws)
Motor activity	Synchronous shaking of all limbs (clonic)	Asynchronous flailing of variable limbs, side-to-side head shaking, pelvic thrusting[a]
Motor pattern	Shaking starts at high frequency and gradually slows down	Shaking may speed up or vary in frequency
Duration	Usually ends within <5 min	Prolonged, or waxes and wanes over >5 min or even hours
Consciousness/memory	Impaired/lost	May be retained (may hear or remember but not respond)
Postictal state	Confused, lethargic	May have relatively normal mental status despite high frequency of "seizures"
Postictal breathing	Slow, deep, loud, snoring-like stertor	Normal or rapid panting

GTCS = generalized tonic-clonic seizure; PNES = psychogenic nonepileptic spell/event.

[a]These typically psychogenic symptoms may be seen in true epileptic frontal lobe seizures.

CONT.

thin-slice T1-weighted imaging). Functional imaging (PET and single-photon emission CT) is considered when planning for epilepsy surgery but is not routinely indicated. H

Outpatient EEG also is recommended in patients with a first seizure. Because capture of an actual seizure is unlikely, the physician must rely on "epileptiform" abnormalities, such as focal sharp waves (see Figure 8) or generalized spike-and-wave discharges (see Figure 5). These findings are considered relatively specific for epilepsy; although not diagnostic, they may help support the diagnosis in an appropriate clinical context. A single routine EEG is only 40% to 50% sensitive for such findings, but the yield can increase to 80% to 90% with repeated studies, prolonged studies, and studies that capture sleep.

MRI and EEG can be performed at a follow-up evaluation, but the yield of EEG is higher within 24 hours of GTCS. Emergent lumbar puncture is recommended in adults only if an infectious cause, such as meningitis or encephalitis, is suspected.

Epilepsy Monitoring Units

A normal EEG does not rule out epilepsy. Capturing events during continuous 24-hour video EEG monitoring is the gold standard in diagnosis. Continuous video EEG monitoring is performed in an epilepsy-monitoring unit during a multiple-day elective hospitalization during which AEDs are decreased or withdrawn under close supervision. Patients who have not responded to two adequately dosed AEDs are considered to have refractory disease (see Intractable Epilepsy and Epilepsy Surgery) and also should be referred to an epilepsy center, where evaluation in an epilepsy-monitoring unit can both confirm the diagnosis of epilepsy and determine candidacy for epilepsy surgery.

Other Continuous Electroencephalographic Monitoring

Continuous video EEG monitoring also is useful in the ICU (**Table 18**). It can determine if episodic events are truly seizures, particularly in sedated or confused patients who cannot provide a history. This type of EEG additionally is the only method of diagnosing nonconvulsive status epilepticus. H

Provoked, Unprovoked, and Triggered Seizures

Provoking factors, risk factors, and triggers all can all lead to seizures (**Table 19**), and differentiating among them is essential. Provoking factors can cause seizures in patients with or

TABLE 18. Indications for Immediate Continuous Video Electroencephalographic Monitoring in the Critical Care Setting
AMS following CSE or clinical seizures
AMS with acute brain injury (such as hemorrhage, trauma, infection, stroke, hypoxia, cardiac arrest)
Unexplained AMS with subacute or chronic brain injury (tumor, history of epilepsy)
Unexplained AMS (or mental fluctuation) without acute brain injury (as in sepsis)
Unexplained AMS following a CNS procedure or CNS instrumentation
Pharmacologic coma and paralysis that limit the ability to perform a neurologic examination (as is used with therapeutic hypothermia, ECMO)
Clinical episodes concerning for seizures (such as unexplained muscle or eye movements)a

AMS = altered mental status; CNS = central nervous system; CSE = convulsive status epilepticus; ECMO = extracorporeal membrane oxygenation; EEG = electroencephalography.

aIf CSE is suspected, treatment should begin before EEG is performed or results are available; if nonconvulsive status epilepticus is suspected, treatment most often should await EEG results.

without epilepsy; avoidance of these provocations should prevent further seizures. Particular attention should be paid to the patient's medications, and drugs that can cause a seizure or lower seizure threshold (such as tramadol, meperidine, bupropion, fluoroquinolones, carbapenems, and cefepime) should be avoided. Risk factors increase the chance of developing epilepsy later in life; however, an acute symptomatic seizure (such as a seizure occurring in the first week after traumatic brain injury, stroke, or meningitis) may not necessarily lead to the development of epilepsy. Although triggers lead to seizures in patients with epilepsy, they are not the cause of epilepsy (and are not considered provoking factors).

Determining the risk of recurrence guides the decision to treat. The 2-year recurrence risk after a single unprovoked seizure is approximately 40%. Risk is lower (20%-30%) if there are no epilepsy risk factors and the MRI and EEG are normal. A first unprovoked seizure is often not treated; although treatment may reduce the risk of seizure over the next 2 years, it does not change a patient's long-term prognosis for developing epilepsy. In the setting of two unprovoked seizures or one unprovoked seizure with significant EEG or MRI abnormalities, recurrence risk is at least 60%, and treatment is recommended. H

TABLE 19. Potential Causes of Seizures or Epilepsy		
Seizure-Provoking Factors	**Epilepsy Risk Factors**	**Seizure Triggers**
Hypo- or hypernatremia	Febrile seizures	Sleep deprivation[b]
Hypo- or hypercalcemia	Family history (especially first-degree relatives)	Fever
Hypomagnesemia		Emotional stress
Hypoglycemia	Past meningitis/encephalitis	Acute infection (nonneurologic)
Hyperammonemia or hepatic failure	History of structural brain lesion (such as stroke, tumor)	Hyperventilation
Uremia or kidney failure	Past significant head trauma (loss of consciousness or amnesia >30 min, penetrating skull injury)	Photic stimulation
Acute head trauma, meningitis, encephalitis, stroke, or hypoxia/ischemia		Music, reading, eating (only in specific reflex epilepsies)
Alcohol intoxication or withdrawal	Preterm birth	
Recreational drug use	Birth injury, asphyxia, or stroke	
Benzodiazepine withdrawal	Neurologic developmental delay	
Baclofen withdrawal	Intellectual disability	
Fluoroquinolones	History of brain surgery	
Carbapenems		
Cefepime		
Metronidazole		
Tramadol		
Meperidine		
Morphine		
Bupropion		
Clozapine[a]		
Lithium[a]		
Tricyclic antidepressants[a]		
Typical antipsychotic agents[a]		

[a]Can be used in patients with epilepsy, if needed.

[b]Typically does not trigger seizures in patients without epilepsy and is not considered a provoking factor.

Treatment of Epilepsy

Antiepileptic Drug Therapy

Empiric pharmacologic treatment generally is not recommended unless the patient's history is strongly suggestive of seizures or epilepsy. The exception is convulsive status epilepticus, which must be treated emergently if clinically suspected. Similarly, prophylactic treatment is avoided except in specific situations, such as during the week after severe head trauma or brain tumor resection. Alcohol- or benzodiazepine-withdrawal seizures typically are not treated with AEDs.

Selection and Adverse Effects of Antiepileptic Drugs

Many AEDs are available for patients with epilepsy (**Table 20**). Newer AEDs, although not more effective in controlling seizures than older AEDs, are often preferred because they have fewer adverse effects, fewer drug interactions, and a reduced need for laboratory monitoring. The higher cost and shorter length of experience with the newer AEDs are disadvantages. Most often, treatment is guided by the seizure type rather than AED mechanism or epilepsy cause. When a patient has GTCS and focal onset is not certain, a broad-spectrum AED should be used. Focal seizure medications are also used for secondarily generalized seizures.

Most dangerous AED toxicities (rash, pancytopenia, hepatotoxicity) are idiosyncratic and not necessarily dose related. **Table 21** lists common adverse effects and laboratory monitoring recommendations. Key dose-dependent adverse effects include oxcarbazepine-related hyponatremia and valproic acid–related thrombocytopenia. Hyponatremia is a particular concern with oxcarbazepine and carbamazepine in older patients, especially with concomitant diuretic use. Enzyme-inducing AEDs (**Table 22**) increase statin clearance and necessitate higher doses or alternative options; they also can increase bone catabolism. Therefore, bone density testing and

TABLE 20. Spectrum of Use of Antiepileptic Drugs

Population	First-Line Agent	Second-Line Agent	Considerations
Patients with focal seizures	Lamotrigine Levetiracetam Oxcarbazepine	Carbamazepine Gabapentin Pregabalin Topiramate Zonisamide	Includes treatment of secondarily generalized tonic-clonic seizures
Patients with generalized seizures	Ethosuximide (absence only) Lamotrigine (may worsen myoclonic seizures) Levetiracetam Valproate	Topiramate Zonisamide	May be worsened by gabapentin, pregabalin, carbamazepine, and oxcarbazepine
Woman of childbearing age	Lamotrigine Levetiracetam	Oxcarbazepine	Avoid carbamazepine, phenobarbital, phenytoin, topiramate, and valproate
Older patients	Gabapentin Lamotrigine Levetiracetam		Higher risk for hyponatremia with carbamazepine and oxcarbazepine, especially with concomitant diuretics

TABLE 21. Adverse Effects of Selected Antiepileptic Drugs and Recommended Laboratory Monitoring

Drug	Common Adverse Effects	Serious Adverse Effects	Recommended Laboratory Monitoring
Phenobarbital	Sedation (but paradoxical hyperactivity in children)	Rash, pancytopenia, osteoporosis, hepatotoxicity	CBC, liver chemistry studies, bone density, serum drug level
Phenytoin	Sedation, nausea, ataxia, tremor, diplopia, imbalance, headache, and dose-dependent dizziness; if given IV, tissue necrosis (with extravasation), bradycardia, hypotension, and asystole	Rash, gingival hyperplasia, cerebellar atrophy, peripheral neuropathy, pancytopenia, osteoporosis, hepatotoxicity	CBC, liver chemistry studies, bone density, serum drug level
Valproic acid	Sedation, nausea, ataxia, tremor, diplopia, imbalance, headache, and dose-dependent dizziness; weight gain, hair loss, PCOS, and reversible parkinsonism with dementia	Pancytopenia, osteoporosis, hepatotoxicity, pancreatitis, hyperammonemia	CBC, liver chemistry studies, bone density, serum drug level, serum ammonia level in select cases
Carbamazepine and oxcarbazepine	Sedation, nausea, ataxia, tremor, diplopia, imbalance, headache, and dose-dependent dizziness	Hyponatremia, rash, pancytopenia, osteoporosis, hepatotoxicity	CBC, liver chemistry studies, bone density, serum drug level
Felbamate	Insomnia, weight loss, nausea, vomiting, and diarrhea	Aplastic anemia and hepatotoxicity[a]	CBC, liver chemistry studies
Lamotrigine	Sedation, nausea, ataxia, tremor, diplopia, imbalance, headache, insomnia, and dose-dependent dizziness	Rash	Serum drug level
Gabapentin and pregabalin	Sedation, weight gain, edema, and dose-dependent dizziness	—	—
Topiramate and zonisamide	Sedation, nausea, ataxia, tremor, diplopia, imbalance, headache, word finding difficulty, poor concentration, paresthesias, weight loss, anhidrosis, and dose-dependent dizziness	Nephrolithiasis, acute angle glaucoma, psychosis	BMP in select cases
Levetiracetam	Sedation, irritability, psychosis, and depression	Suicidal ideation[b] and thrombocytopenia (rare)	—
Tiagabine	Sedation, nausea, ataxia, tremor, diplopia, imbalance, headache, and dose-dependent dizziness	Acute confusion and encephalopathy	—
Lacosamide	Sedation, nausea, ataxia, tremor, diplopia, imbalance, headache, dose-dependent dizziness, and PR-interval prolongation	Atrioventricular block, atrial fibrillation	Electrocardiography
Perampanel	Dizziness, headache, and sedation	Homicidal ideation	—

BMP = basic metabolic profile; CBC = complete blood count; IV, intravenously; PCOS = polycystic ovary syndrome.

[a]A serious and potentially fatal adverse effect that limits this drug's use (and requires close monitoring).

[b]A concern with all antiepileptic drugs, but especially levetiracetam.

TABLE 22. Key Pharmacologic Issues with Selected Antiepileptic Drugs

Inducers of Hepatic Enzymes[a,b]	Inhibitors of Hepatic Enzymes[a]	Requires Dose Adjustment in Kidney Dysfunction	Avoid in Hepatic Dysfunction	Highly Albumin Bound[c]	No Significant Drug-Drug Interactions
Carbamazepine	Valproate	Gabapentin	Carbamazepine	Phenytoin	Levetiracetam
Oxcarbazepine		Pregabalin	Phenytoin	Valproate	Lacosamide
Phenobarbital		Levetiracetam	Phenobarbital		Gabapentin
Phenytoin			Valproate		Pregabalin
Topiramate					Zonisamide

[a]May cause osteoporosis and interact with lamotrigine.

[b]May decrease statin and oral contraceptive efficacy.

[c]Warrants checking unbound (free) blood level, especially in kidney failure and hypoalbuminemia.

CONT.

supplementation of calcium and vitamin D are recommended with enzyme-inducing AEDs (and with valproic acid).

Phenytoin, carbamazepine, phenobarbital, and lamotrigine are AEDs that commonly cause rash, which usually resolves with discontinuation of the drug. AED-related rashes, however, are sometimes severe and life-threatening. For example, rapid titration of lamotrigine has been associated with the development of Stevens-Johnson syndrome, toxic epidermal necrolysis, and drug reaction with eosinophilia and systemic symptoms. These AEDs also should be avoided in patients of Asian heritage unless testing for genetic predisposition (presence of HLA-B*1502 allele) is negative. Nevertheless, lamotrigine is one of the most safe and effective AEDs used today, when titrated slowly.

All AEDs carry a warning about worsening depression and suicidality, and all patients must be screened and monitored for these symptoms. Levetiracetam may cause depression, anxiety, anger, or agitation. Perampanel may cause homicidal ideation. Topiramate may cause psychosis. Lamotrigine and valproic acid, on the other hand, are known to be mood stabilizing.

Monitoring and Discontinuing Antiepileptic Drugs

Measuring serum levels of certain AEDs (phenytoin, carbamazepine, valproic acid, phenobarbital, oxcarbazepine, lamotrigine) is useful, given their known therapeutic windows and predictable dose-related adverse effects. However, in a patient whose epilepsy is well-controlled without clinical adverse effects, dose reduction because of high levels usually is not warranted.

Generic AEDs are appropriate for most patients, given recent guidelines. Well-designed studies have not shown differences in AED bioequivalence (on the basis of FDA standards) when switching between generic drugs or switching from a brand to a generic drug for patients with epilepsy. Generic substitution reduces cost and does not compromise efficacy. Patients need to be informed of changes in the color and shape of pills.

In addition, phenytoin, carbamazepine, and valproic acid do not have a 1:1 conversion between immediate-release and extended-release formulations. Monitoring for AED toxicity and seizures is advised if a change is made.

Tapering of AEDs can be considered in patients remaining seizure free for at least 2 to 5 years. The best predictor of seizure freedom is time; a prolonged period of seizure freedom predicts further seizure freedom. Factors prohibiting AED weaning include the presence of JME, a history of difficulties in early seizure control, and the presence of significant epilepsy risk factors (see Table 19). Relevant MRI abnormalities, significant EEG abnormalities (especially when not taking AEDs), risk of physical injury, and loss of driving privileges (if unacceptable to the patient) are additional considerations. There are no accepted standards for tapering schedules for AEDs.

KEY POINTS

- Newer antiepileptic drugs (AEDs), although not more effective in controlling seizures than older AEDs, are often preferred because they have fewer adverse effects, fewer drug interactions, and a reduced need for laboratory monitoring.

- Epilepsy treatment usually is guided by the seizure type rather than drug mechanism or epilepsy cause.

- Enzyme-inducing antiepileptic drugs increase statin clearance and thus necessitate higher doses or alternative options; because they also can increase bone catabolism, bone density testing and supplemental calcium and vitamin D are recommended.

- Tapering of antiepileptic drugs can be considered in most patients who remain seizure free for 2 to 5 years; factors prohibiting weaning include the presence of juvenile myoclonic epilepsy, a history of difficulties in early seizure control, and the presence of significant epilepsy risk factors.

Counseling and Lifestyle Adjustments

All patients experiencing a seizure, even a single provoked seizure, must be instructed about seizure precautions, including driving restrictions. Most states restrict driving in patients with any episode of altered awareness or motor control, with the restriction varying by state from 3 to 12 months (see www.epilepsy.com/driving-laws). Additionally, patients should avoid common triggers and provoking factors (see Table 19). Most patients with epilepsy can work, even if they are not completely seizure free. Patients should avoid operating heavy machinery, using firearms, lifting more than 9 kg (20 lb), taking tub baths, swimming in unsupervised locations, and being near open flames or heights (such as rooftops).

Comorbidities and Complications of Epilepsy

Sudden Unexpected Death in Epilepsy Patients

Besides the risk of trauma, asphyxia, and death from a seizure or status epilepticus, epilepsy patients are at risk for unexplained death. This risk is approximately 1 in 1000 and increases to approximately 1 in 100 in patients with intractable seizures, especially those with uncontrolled GTCS and those taking multiple AEDs. Mechanisms are unknown and may involve cardiac, respiratory, and autonomic dysregulation. Studies show that patients prefer to discuss sudden unexplained death in epilepsy openly; doing so can encourage medication adherence and home safety planning (such as using webcams and bed monitors and sharing of bedrooms).

KEY POINT

- The risk of sudden unexpected death in epilepsy is approximately 1 in 1000 and increases to approximately 1 in 100 in patients with intractable seizures, especially those with uncontrolled generalized tonic-clonic seizures and those taking multiple antiepileptic drugs.

Intractable Epilepsy and Epilepsy Surgery

Any patient who does not achieve seizure freedom for at least 1 year after treatment with two adequately dosed, appropriately chosen AEDs is considered to have medically intractable (drug-resistant) epilepsy and should be referred to an epilepsy center to both confirm the diagnosis and evaluate the patient for surgical candidacy, starting with video EEG monitoring. The chance of achieving seizure control from additional medications (a regimen of three or more AEDs) is less than 10%; therefore, other treatment options must be considered. In appropriately chosen surgical candidates, especially those with temporal lobe epilepsy due to mesial temporal sclerosis, resection can lead to seizure freedom in 60% to 70% of patients.

Implantable vagus nerve stimulators and the ketogenic diet are available palliative therapies but do not result in complete seizure control.

KEY POINT

- Any patient who does not achieve seizure freedom after treatment with two adequately dosed, appropriately chosen antiepileptic drugs is considered to have medically intractable (drug-resistant) epilepsy and should be referred to an epilepsy center to both confirm the diagnosis and evaluate the patient for surgical candidacy.

Seizures and Epilepsy in Specific Populations

Older Adults

Incidence of new-onset epilepsy is highest in older adults (age > 60 years). Because recurrence after a new-onset seizure in this age group is more likely (50% to 60%) than in younger adults (40%), treatment after one seizure is sometimes considered. Major risk factors for seizure recurrence include stroke and dementia. Older adults usually require lower AED doses and are at increased risk of interactions and decreased drug clearance. Data suggest that levetiracetam, lamotrigine, and gabapentin are better tolerated and no less effective when compared with older AEDs. Valproic acid should be avoided because it can cause (reversible) parkinsonism and cognitive dysfunction.

KEY POINT

- In older patients, levetiracetam, lamotrigine, and gabapentin are better tolerated and no less effective when compared with older antiepileptic drugs.

Patients with Organ Failure

In patients with epilepsy and chronic kidney disease, dosages of levetiracetam, gabapentin, and pregabalin must be reduced because decreased clearance can lead to toxicity. Phenytoin is highly albumin bound; dosage should be reduced, and free (unbound) levels should be monitored. Gabapentin and pregabalin can cause encephalopathy and nonepileptic myoclonus, thus mimicking seizures. Valproic acid is typically avoided in patients with hepatic insufficiency. Because topiramate and zonisamide can cause acidosis and nephrolithiasis, they also should be avoided in patients with a predisposition to these disorders.

KEY POINT

- In patients with epilepsy and chronic kidney disease, dosages of levetiracetam, gabapentin, and pregabalin must be reduced, because decreased clearance can lead to toxicity.

Posttraumatic Epilepsy

AEDs are prophylactically given during the first week after severe head trauma (loss of consciousness > 12-24 hours, intracranial hemorrhage, depressed skull fracture, or brain contusion) to prevent acute seizure complications (hemorrhage, edema, or elevated intracranial pressure). As with acute stroke, such treatment does not reduce the risk of developing epilepsy later, and prophylaxis beyond 1 week is not recommended.

A single unprovoked seizure that occurs more than 1 month after a stroke or significant head trauma has a high enough recurrence risk to be considered epilepsy and requires treatment. Patients with a history of moderate or severe head trauma (skull fracture, penetrating head injury, or loss of consciousness > 30 minutes) are at increased risk of epilepsy.

Returning combat veterans who develop seizures require careful evaluation, often including video EEG monitoring. Many have had head trauma and are at increased risk for epilepsy, but many also have posttraumatic stress disorder and may have PNES. Assuming a diagnosis of epilepsy and empirically treating the patient can be detrimental, especially because veterans tend to have a delay in the diagnosis of PNES compared with the general population.

KEY POINTS

- Antiepileptic drugs are prophylactically given during the first week after severe head trauma (loss of consciousness > 12-24 hours, intracranial hemorrhage, depressed skull fracture, or brain contusion).

- A single unprovoked seizure that occurs more than 1 month after a stroke or significant head trauma has a high enough recurrence risk to be considered epilepsy and requires treatment.

Women with Epilepsy

Women with epilepsy may experience catamenial seizures (related to menstrual cycle), which may occur around menstruation or ovulation or because of an inadequate luteal phase. Some studies suggest adding progestin-containing oral contraceptives or acetazolamide to the AED regimen, but oophorectomy is not recommended to improve seizure control.

Reproductive Issues

Findings from various studies are contradictory about whether women with epilepsy have decreased fertility rates. Valproic acid, however, is associated with anovulation and polycystic ovary syndrome.

Pregnancy and Nursing

Most women with epilepsy have normal, healthy children. The rate of major congenital malformations (MCMs) in untreated women with epilepsy is likely similar to that of the general population. All women with epilepsy who are of childbearing age and are taking AEDs should receive preconception counseling and folate supplementation. Women with epilepsy who take AEDs are unlikely to have an increased risk of cesarean section, late-pregnancy bleeding, or premature delivery, unless they smoke; however, they may be at increased risk of having a newborn who is small for gestational age. The best predictor of seizure control during pregnancy is seizure frequency in the previous 9 to 12 months (especially for patients who have been seizure free).

In women with epilepsy who are of child-bearing age, levetiracetam and lamotrigine have minimal evidence of teratogenicity and are the preferred treatment options. Select patients, however, may need to continue potentially teratogenic medications, such as valproic acid, especially if seizures cannot be otherwise controlled. Discovery of pregnancy alone is not a sufficient reason to stop AEDs in women with epilepsy whose disease is well controlled. Women with epilepsy must balance risk of teratogenicity with risk of uncontrolled seizures, particularly GTCS, which can result in fetal anoxia and death.

Valproic acid, phenobarbital, and phenytoin are associated with MCMs and lower IQ in offspring; these drugs should be avoided if possible in pregnant women with epilepsy. Topiramate, carbamazepine, and AED polypharmacy also should also be avoided because of increased MCM risk. Valproic acid is associated with neural tube defects, and topiramate with cleft lip and palate.

Serum levels of lamotrigine, oxcarbazepine, and levetiracetam are known to decrease significantly during pregnancy. For lamotrigine, a dose escalation of approximately 50% is needed to maintain therapeutic levels and prevent seizures; levels should be followed at least monthly during pregnancy. Once delivery occurs, the lamotrigine dose should be rapidly decreased to avoid a sudden increase in serum levels, which would increase toxicity and risk of Stevens-Johnson syndrome.

Because the benefits of breastfeeding most often outweigh the risks, breastfeeding is recommended in most women with epilepsy who take AEDs. Sedation of the infant is a potential complication, but AED exposure through breast milk is usually minimal and probably less than that in utero.

Contraception

Enzyme-inducing AEDs (see Table 22) increase the metabolism of oral contraceptives, which decreases their effectiveness and thus increases chances of pregnancy occurring (while taking potentially teratogenic medications). Alternate methods of contraception, such as intrauterine devices or barrier methods, are thus recommended. Oral contraceptives also increase lamotrigine metabolism, which necessitates dosage increases.

KEY POINTS

- In women with epilepsy who are of child-bearing age, levetiracetam and lamotrigine have minimal evidence of teratogenicity and are the preferred treatment options.

- Discovery of pregnancy alone is not a sufficient reason to stop antiepileptic drugs in women with epilepsy whose disease is well controlled; women with epilepsy must balance risk of teratogenicity with risk of uncontrolled seizures, particularly generalized tonic-clonic seizures, which can result in fetal anoxia and death.

- Valproic acid, phenobarbital, phenytoin, topiramate, carbamazepine, and antiepileptic drug polypharmacy are associated with major congenital malformations and, if possible, should be avoided in pregnant women with epilepsy.

Status Epilepticus

Not all seizures require emergent treatment. Most GTCS will cease spontaneously within 2 to 3 minutes, and, if the patient has stopped shaking, treatment is not necessarily indicated. Treatment also differs depending on the type of status epilepticus. Convulsive status epilepticus (CSE) is analogous to ventricular fibrillation (that is, a true medical emergency). Nonconvulsive status epilepticus (NCSE) is analogous to atrial fibrillation with or without rapid ventricular response (management varies with symptom severity). The cause of a seizure most often determines the outcome; thus, evaluation for serious causes (meningitis, intracranial hemorrhage) must occur emergently and in parallel with treatment.

Convulsive Status Epilepticus

CSE is defined as a generalized tonic-clonic seizure lasting more than 5 minutes, or two GTCS occurring within 5 minutes of each other without a return to baseline mental status. CSE is diagnosed clinically and presents as continuous generalized clonic jerking of the entire body. Unless PNES is strongly suspected, empiric therapy is indicated without awaiting results of EEG, imaging, serum studies, or lumbar puncture because a longer duration of CSE is strongly linked to worse outcomes.

Securing the airway and obtaining intravenous (IV) access are the first steps in CSE management (**Figure 9**). If point-of-care glucose testing is not available, thiamine should be given, followed by IV glucose. First-line treatment is IV lorazepam, IV diazepam, or intramuscular midazolam. If IV access is not available, diazepam may be given rectally or intramuscularly, although absorption is erratic; intranasal and buccal midazolam also are available in some centers. Fear of respiratory depression should not limit treatment; there is clear evidence that respiratory depression is less common when CSE is treated with benzodiazepines than with placebo.

In a patient who is not already on AEDs, benzodiazepines should be followed by an IV AED to avoid seizure recurrence when the initial treatment wears off. Fosphenytoin is preferred over phenytoin because it can be infused more rapidly and has a lower incidence of skin necrosis (such as purple glove

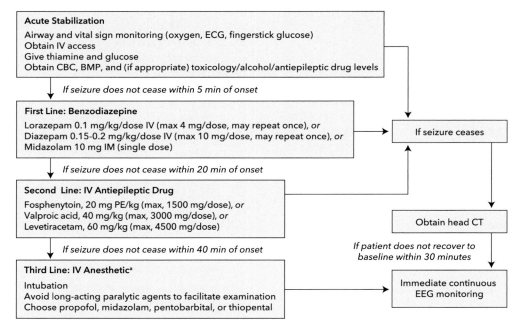

FIGURE 9. Management guidelines for convulsive status epilepticus. BMP = basic metabolic panel; CBC = complete blood count; ECG = electrocardiology; EEG = electroencephalographic; IM = intramuscularly; IV = intravenous(ly); max = maximum; PE = phenytoin equivalents.

^aOr choose an appropriate second-line agent.

syndrome due to drug extravasation). However, both fosphenytoin and phenytoin can cause acute bradycardia and hypotension. Alternative second-line therapies include IV valproic acid (especially in generalized epilepsy) or IV levetiracetam. There is not enough evidence to support the use of lacosamide as a standard treatment in CSE.

Simultaneously with treatment, emergent evaluation for the cause of CSE should be underway, including provoking factors and triggers. A complete blood count, comprehensive metabolic profile, and evaluation for infection (with urinalysis, chest radiography, and lumbar puncture) should be considered. Head CT is usually indicated before lumbar puncture, but no test should delay the administration of antibiotics if meningitis is suspected.

If convulsions stop but the patient does not either improve within 10 minutes or return to baseline within 30 minutes, immediate continuous EEG is required to diagnose NCSE. NCSE after CSE is still a medical emergency and should be treated aggressively. If convulsive seizure activity does not cease, intubation is typically required, and third-line therapy with IV anesthesia should be initiated. IV anesthesia carries considerable risk, including prolonged ICU hospitalization and associated morbidity (infection, deep venous thrombosis) because patients are typically placed in a drug-induced coma for 24 to 48 hours. Therefore, concomitant continuous EEG monitoring is mandatory. Infusion of propofol, midazolam, or pentobarbital may be considered for NCSE that follows CSE. Hypotension is most common with pentobarbital, which may accumulate in tissues and require many days for clearance. Midazolam is least likely to cause hypotension but often leads to tolerance and tachyphylaxis. Because risk is determined by dose and duration of drug therapy, treatment should be limited to less than 48 hours.

KEY POINTS

- In patients with likely convulsive status epilepticus (CSE), empiric therapy is indicated without awaiting results of electroencephalography, imaging, serum studies, or lumbar puncture because a longer duration of CSE is strongly linked to worse outcomes.

- First-line treatment of convulsive status epilepticus is intravenous benzodiazepines typically followed by an intravenous antiepileptic drug to avoid seizure recurrence when the initial treatment wears off.

Nonconvulsive Status Epilepticus

NCSE refers to episodes of electrical seizure activity without clinically evident seizure activity. It should be suspected when a patient, particularly a critically ill patient, has altered mental status with an unclear cause. NCSE may occur in as many as 48% (more typically, 15% to 25%) of patients with encephalopathy who are in the ICU. Certain situations should prompt consideration of NCSE and immediate continuous EEG monitoring (see Table 18). Although EEG is required for diagnosis of NCSE,

appropriate clinical correlation of EEG findings is necessary to confirm NCSE and guide treatment. EEG of a few hours duration typically is inadequate because many patients experience intermittent rather than continuous seizures. At least 24 hours of monitoring is recommended in noncomatose patients, and at least 48 hours is recommended in comatose patients.

NCSE that does not occur directly after GTCS or CSE may not necessarily carry as high a risk to the patient as NCSE that follows these seizure types, but evidence is lacking. Treatment is based on clinical examination and not on EEG alone. If the patient is not comatose, initiating aggressive therapy with intubation and an IV anesthetic–induced coma is usually avoided because risks may outweigh benefits. Outcome is typically based more on cause and less on severity or duration of seizures.

Absence status epilepticus is a form of NCSE that typically occurs in patients with a history of generalized epilepsy but sometimes is seen in healthy older patients. Patients with this condition have days to weeks of mild confusion, despite being able to speak and walk ("walking wounded"); EEG confirms the presence of continuous generalized spike-and-wave discharges. Prognosis is excellent because treatment with IV benzodiazepines, valproic acid, or levetiracetam will usually resolve the problem, even in patients with days or weeks of seizing.

KEY POINTS

- Nonconvulsive status epilepticus should be suspected when a patient, particularly a critically ill patient, has altered mental status with an unclear cause.

- Although electroencephalography is required for diagnosis of nonconvulsive status epilepticus (NCSE), appropriate clinical correlation of electroencephalographic findings is necessary to confirm NCSE and guide treatment.

- Nonconvulsive status epilepticus is diagnosed by continuous electroencephalographic monitoring; at least 24 hours of monitoring is recommended in noncomatose patients, and at least 48 hours is recommended in comatose patients.

Stroke

Definition of Stroke

Stroke is the leading cause of serious disability among adults and the fifth leading cause of death in the United States. Its incidence increases with each decade of life. The World Health Organization defines stroke as a disease of sudden-onset focal neurologic deficits associated with dysfunction in the brain, retina, or spinal cord due to occlusion or rupture of a cerebral or spinal artery. Ischemic stroke, which results from occlusion of an artery, is the most common type of stroke and can be further subclassified on the basis of its underlying cause. Transient ischemic attack (TIA) was formerly defined as a neurologic impairment lasting less than 24 hours but now is recognized as a transient neurologic deficit without the presence of infarction on neuroimaging. Hemorrhagic strokes comprise a small proportion of all strokes but are associated with higher short-term mortality. Intracerebral hemorrhage (ICH) presents with focal neurologic deficits and may also include headache or impairment in consciousness. Subarachnoid hemorrhage (SAH) commonly presents with sudden onset severe headache and impairment in consciousness without focal neurologic deficits. Although their clinical manifestations often overlap with stroke, subdural and epidural hematomas are not considered to be strokes and are discussed in Head Injury. Determining the exact subtype of stroke a patient experiences has important implications for acute therapeutics, prevention strategies, and prognosis. **H**

KEY POINT

- Determining the exact subtype of stroke (ischemic or hemorrhagic) has important implications for acute therapeutics, prevention strategies, and prognosis.

Diagnosis of Stroke

Stroke is a clinical diagnosis supported by neuroimaging. The clinical manifestations of stroke are highly variable. Although most strokes commonly manifest as rapid onset of specific neurologic symptoms, such as weakness, aphasia, dysphagia, and sensory changes, stroke also may present with more nonspecific symptoms, such as dizziness, altered mental status, or sudden unexplained coma. Examination will often show focal neurologic deficits. In the acute setting, rapid assessment is required to inform treatment, and validated scales, such as the National Institutes of Health Stroke Scale (NIHSS), are commonly used (**Table 23**). The neurologic examination, however, is not reliable enough to distinguish ischemic from hemorrhagic stroke, and neuroimaging is required before initiation of treatment. Noncontrast head CT is the most widely used test, given its rapid acquisition, low cost, wide availability, and high sensitivity for diagnosing hemorrhagic stroke (**Figure 10**). In ischemic stroke, the initial

TABLE 23. National Institutes of Health Stroke Scale	
Parameter (Testing Method)	**Scores[a]**
1a. Level of consciousness	0 = normal
	1 = not alert but arousable by minor stimulation
	2 = not alert and requires constant verbal or painful stimuli to remain interactive
	3 = unresponsive or responds with only reflexive movements
1b. Level of consciousness questions (state month and age)	0 = answers both correctly
	1 = answers one correctly
	2 = answers neither correctly
1c. Level of consciousness commands (close and open eyes; make fist or close one hand)	0 = performs both tasks correctly
	1 = performs one task correctly
	2 = performs neither task correctly
2. Best gaze (track a finger in a horizontal plane)	0 = normal
	1 = partial gaze palsy or isolated cranial nerve paresis
	2 = forced gaze deviation or total gaze paresis
3. Visual fields (each eye tested individually)	0 = no visual loss
	1 = partial hemianopia
	2 = complete hemianopia
	3 = bilateral hemianopia
4. Facial palsy (show teeth, raise eyebrows, close eyes)	0 = normal
	1 = minor paralysis (flattening of the nasolabial fold or asymmetry on smiling)
	2 = partial paralysis (paralysis of the lower face only)
	3 = complete paralysis (upper and lower face)
5. Arm strength (hold arm with palms down or lift arm for 10 s; each arm scored separately)	0 = no drift
	1 = some drift but does not hit bed
	2 = drifts down to bed
	3 = no effort against gravity
	4 = no movement
6. Leg strength (hold leg at 30 degrees for 5 s; each leg scored separately)	0 = no drift
	1 = some drift but does not hit bed
	2 = drifts down to bed
	3 = no effort against gravity
	4 = no movement
	(Continued on the next page)

TABLE 23. National Institutes of Health Stroke Scale *(Continued)*

Parameter (Testing Method)	Scores[a]
7. Limb ataxia (finger-nose-finger test, heel-knee-shin slide)	0 = absent 1 = present in one limb 2 = present in two limbs
8. Sensation (pinch/pinprick tested in face, arm, and leg)	0 = normal 1 = mild to moderate sensory loss or loss of sensation in only one limb 2 = complete sensory loss
9. Best language (describe a picture, name six objects, and read five sentences)	0 = no aphasia 1 = mild to moderate aphasia (difficulty with fluency and comprehension; meaning can be identified) 2 = severe aphasia (fragmentary language, meaning cannot be clearly identified) 3 = global aphasia or mute
10. Dysarthria (repeat or read words)	0 = normal 1 = mild to moderate 2 = severe (speech not understandable)
11. Extinction/inattention (visual and tactile stimuli applied on right and left sides)	0 = normal 1 = visual or tactile extinction or mild hemispatial neglect 2 = profound hemi-inattention or extinction to more than one modality

[a]Score interpretation (based on total score): 0 = no stoke; 1-4 = minor stroke; 5-15 = moderate stroke; 16-20 = moderate to severe stroke; 21-42 = severe stroke (maximum score, 42).

Adapted from www.ninds.nih.gov/sites/default/files/NIH_Stroke_Scale_Booklet.pdf. Accessed January 17, 2018.

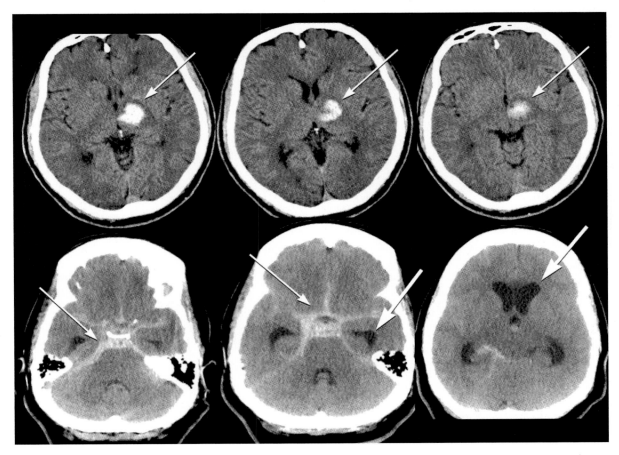

FIGURE 10. Noncontrast CT scans of the head. *Top panel*, an acute left thalamic intracerebral hemorrhage (*arrows*) without hydrocephalus or intraventricular extension is shown. *Bottom panel*, an acute subarachnoid hemorrhage is shown that involves the basal cisterns (*thinner arrows*) with associated enlargement of the lateral horn of the lateral ventricles, consistent with obstructive hydrocephalus and elevated intracranial pressure (*thicker arrows*).

noncontrast head CT scan is often normal, especially in patients seen within 3 hours of symptom onset (although some patients with larger deficits can exhibit early findings) (**Figure 11**). Even 24 hours after onset, a noncontrast head CT scan may not show evidence of infarction, given the poor resolution of small infarcts and those located in the brainstem. CT of the head with contrast rarely is indicated in the initial evaluation of a patient with stroke. CT angiography (CTA) of the head and neck, however, may be performed acutely if endovascular therapy is considered or in otherwise unexplained acute coma to rule out basilar artery thrombosis.

MRI is more sensitive than CT for acute infarction, with changes on the diffusion-weighted imaging sequence apparent within minutes from onset (**Figure 12**). The advantages of MRI include the ability to visualize small strokes, multifocal or bilateral infarcts that may suggest an embolic cause, and the presence of microbleeding. MRI, however, is never the initial test of choice in acute suspected stroke because of its longer acquisition time; if indicated, it is obtained after the initial noncontrast head CT.

Among patients with ICH seen on a noncontrast head CT scan, MRI or CTA is considered if clinical factors are present that raise the suspicion of a cause of hemorrhage other than hypertension or amyloid angiopathy, such as arteriovenous malformation. Likewise, if a patient has symptoms suggestive of SAH and noncontrast head CT findings are normal, lumbar puncture is required to evaluate for the presence of blood or xanthochromia (yellow color stemming from erythrocyte breakdown). If SAH is confirmed,

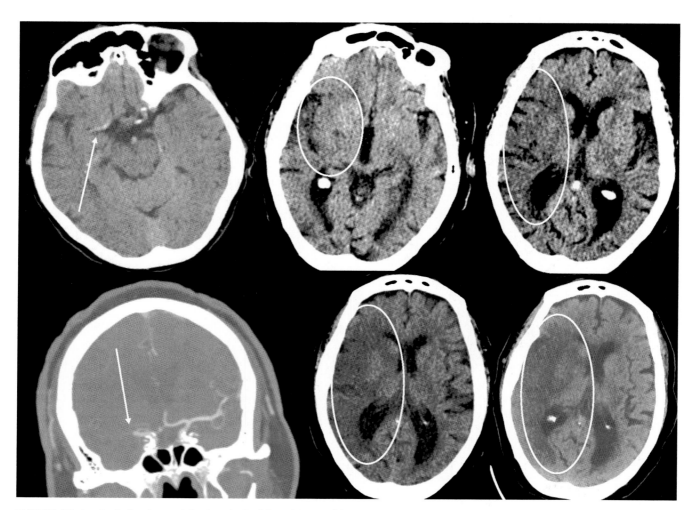

FIGURE 11. Imaging findings in acute ischemic stroke. *Top left panel*, CT scan of the head without contrast obtained 4 hours after acute onset of left-sided weakness and hemiparesis. The *arrow* points to a dense middle cerebral artery sign suggestive of a thrombus. *Top middle panel*, CT scan of the head showing hypodensity in the right insula (*oval*). *Top right panel*, CT scan of the head from the same patient showing early loss of the gray-white matter differentiation in the right middle cerebral artery territory distribution (*oval*). *Bottom left panel*, CT angiogram of the head showing abrupt cessation of filling in the right middle cerebral artery *(arrow)*. *Bottom middle and right panels*, CT scans of the head from the same patient as above 36 hours after symptom onset showing more prominent hypodensity (*middle panel, oval*) and cerebral edema (*right panel, oval*).

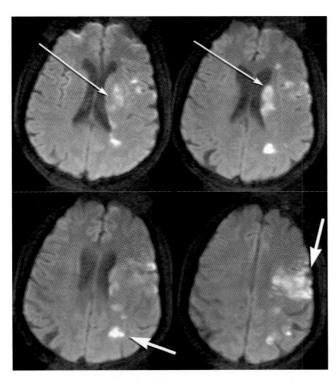

FIGURE 12. Diffusion-weighted MRIs from a patient with symptomatic atherosclerosis of the left middle cerebral artery reveal an acute infarction in deep (*thinner arrows*) and superficial (*thicker arrows*) structures in the left cerebral hemisphere.

H CONT. catheter-based angiography is required to diagnose, and potentially treat, a cerebral aneurysm.

Results of the physical and neurologic examination most likely will suggest the cause of ischemic stroke, such as the presence of atrial fibrillation or a carotid bruit. Further evaluation with cardiac testing or vessel imaging is required to confirm these causes. **H**

KEY POINTS

- Neuroimaging, preferably noncontrast head CT, is required before initiating treatment for stroke.

- Although MRI is more sensitive than CT for diagnosing acute infraction, it is not the initial test of choice to exclude hemorrhagic stroke or to make treatment decisions about thrombolysis for ischemic stroke because of its longer acquisition time.

H Stroke Subtypes

Transient Ischemic Attack

TIA is characterized by a temporary focal neurologic deficit with an absence of infarction on neurologic imaging. Similar to those of acute ischemic stroke, symptoms of TIA include hemiparesis, mono-ocular or visual field loss, dysarthria,

aphasia, and sensory loss. The presence of paresthesia, isolated dizziness or vertigo, or memory loss is more consistent with migraine or seizure. Patients with TIA are at high risk of stroke within the first 48 hours after symptom onset and should be evaluated promptly.

Several post-TIA stroke prediction scoring systems have been developed, with the most widely used being the ABCD[2] score, which is based on Age, Blood pressure, Clinical presentation, Duration of symptoms, and the presence of Diabetes mellitus (**Table 24**). TIA scoring systems, however, do not identify with sufficient sensitivity the highest-risk patients for whom treatment can ameliorate the risk of stroke. Patients with high-grade extracranial internal carotid artery (ICA) stenosis who have a TIA in a downstream neurologic territory have the greatest short-term risk of stroke. This risk is highest within 2 weeks of TIA for those with greater than 70% stenosis, although 50% to 70% stenosis also carries significant associated risk. In the long term, the risk of stroke is high among patients with atrial fibrillation or other cardioembolic sources requiring anticoagulation.

Expedited vascular imaging of the ICA and cardiac evaluation for atrial fibrillation are required for all patients with TIA. The initial test of choice for evaluating ICA stenosis is duplex ultrasonography because of its wide availability, low cost, and low risk; if high-grade ICA stenosis is detected and the patient is a candidate for surgery or stenting, confirmatory testing is required before intervention. Cardiac evaluation should include electrocardiography for atrial fibrillation, which may be followed by longer-term monitoring. Echocardiography is performed if there is a clinical suspicion of a cardioembolic source or structural heart disease. **H**

TABLE 24. ABCD Score[a]	
Patient Characteristics	**Score[b]**
Age ≥60 y	1
Blood pressure ≥140/90 mm Hg	1
Clinical symptoms	
Focal weakness with the TIA	2
Speech impairment without weakness	1
Duration of TIA	
≥60 min	2
10-59 min	1
Diabetes mellitus present	1

TIA = transient ischemic attack.

[a]Based on Age, Blood pressure, Clinical presentation, Duration of symptoms, and the presence of Diabetes mellitus.

[b]The 48-hour stroke risk based on total score: 0-1 = 0%; 2-3 = 1.3%; 4-5 = 4.1%; 6-7 = 8.1%.

Data from Johnston SC, Rothwell PM, Nguyen-Huynh MN, Giles MF, Elkins JS, Bernstein AL, et al. Validation and refinement of scores to predict very early stroke risk after transient ischaemic attack. Lancet. 2007;369:283-92. [PMID: 17258668]

Ischemic Stroke

Large Artery Atherosclerosis

The main mechanism of stroke due to large-artery atherosclerosis is plaque rupture with artery-to-artery embolism. The extracranial carotid artery is frequently involved; the intracranial arteries most commonly affected are the intracranial ICA, middle cerebral arteries, vertebral-basilar arterial junction, and midbasilar artery. Patients with stenoses of the extracranial ICA and the intracranial arteries are at high short-term risk for recurrent stroke and require prompt evaluation. As with TIAs, the extracranial carotid arteries are best evaluated with duplex ultrasonography. Magnetic resonance angiography (MRA) and CTA are both appropriate confirmatory tests after ultrasonography to inform intervention or if duplex examination is not available (**Figure 13**). Transcranial Doppler ultrasonography may help diagnose large-vessel intracranial atherosclerosis, although MRA and CTA are more sensitive tests and can help confirm the diagnosis. Catheter-based angiography is rarely used to diagnose either extracranial or intracranial vessel disease and is associated with a small risk of stroke.

Cardioembolic Stroke

A cardioembolic cause is suggested by clinical and radiologic factors, including infarcts that occur in multiple arterial territories or are located near the cortical surface of the brain with normal arterial imaging. Atrial fibrillation is the most common cardioembolic cause of stroke. Other potential

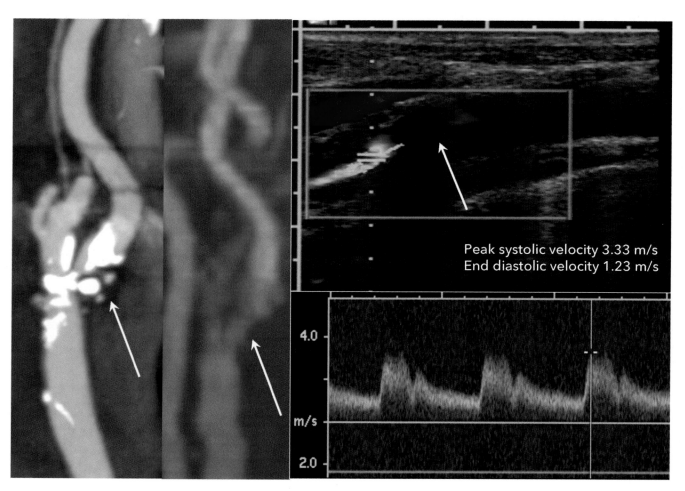

FIGURE 13. Diagnostic imaging modalities in a patient with a symptomatic extracranial internal carotid artery atherosclerotic plaque and associated 90% stenosis. The CT angiogram (*left panel*) and magnetic resonance angiogram (*middle panel*) show high grade stenosis at the origin of the internal carotid artery (*arrows*). Carotid ultrasounds (*right panel*) of the extracranial proximal internal carotid artery show a large plaque at the origin (*arrow*) of the artery, with associated elevated systolic (3.33 m/s) and diastolic (1.23 m/s) velocities consistent with 80% to 99% stenosis.

CONT.

cardioembolic sources include new ventricular thrombus after myocardial infarction and severe valvular disease (for example, rheumatic disease, infective endocarditis, and bioprosthetic and mechanical heart valves).

Radiographic findings suggestive of a cardioembolic source, however, are insufficient grounds for initiating anticoagulation. Patients admitted to the hospital with ischemic stroke should have telemetry monitoring to assess for atrial fibrillation. Similarly, when a clinical suspicion of structural heart disease or embolic stroke exists, transthoracic echocardiography is indicated to evaluate for a cardiac source that may require anticoagulation. Echocardiography also may reveal other findings suggesting the cause of stroke, such as a reduced ejection fraction or patent foramen ovale (PFO), although anticoagulation is not routinely indicated for patients with these conditions. The use of transesophageal echocardiography to evaluate for an intracardiac source of stroke is not routinely indicated, given the low yield for findings that require anticoagulation or surgery. In younger patients without stroke risk factors or in whom suspicion of endocarditis or an intracardiac tumor (such as myxoma or fibroelastoma) exists, transesophageal echocardiography may be considered on a case-by-case basis. For further details on anticoagulation criteria, see MKSAP 18 Cardiovascular Disease.

Small Subcortical Infarcts (Lacunar Infarcts)
Lacunar infarcts commonly lead to isolated motor or sensory syndromes; they rarely affect cognition or mental status. These infarcts (which are < 1.5 cm in diameter) involve the deep white matter, basal ganglia, or brainstem. Pathologically, these infarcts are due to occlusion of small penetrating arteries arising from ICAs (most commonly the middle cerebral and basilar arteries). The main risk factor is hypertension, which leads to local damage at the level of the penetrating artery with subsequent occlusion. Other stroke sources include artery-to-artery embolic thrombi from more proximal sources. Patients with lacunar infarcts still require vessel imaging of the extracranial ICAs to inform secondary prevention.

Cryptogenic Causes of Stroke
In many patients with ischemic stroke, a clear cause is not apparent: there is no lacunar infarct, arterial imaging is normal, and no clear cardioembolic source of stroke (such as atrial fibrillation) is found. When this occurs, the patient's clinical syndrome, underlying medical comorbidities, and neuroimaging characteristics can inform which additional diagnostic testing should be considered.

In a younger patient without risk factors for cardiovascular disease, an evaluation for autoimmune and hypercoagulable disorders should be considered, particularly with nonneurologic systemic findings. Hypercoagulable disorders, PFO, and other rare cardioembolic causes may present with an infarct pattern similar to that of atrial fibrillation. A PFO with a right-to-left shunt (diagnosed with a bubble study on transthoracic echocardiography) may explain stroke in a younger patient but is associated with a low risk of recurrent stroke.

For further information, including recent recommendations regarding percutaneous PFO closure to prevent a secondary stroke, see MKSAP 18 Cardiovascular Disease. Cerebral vasculitis is an extremely rare cause of stroke and presents with numerous infarcts affecting multiple arterial distributions.

Many patients with cryptogenic stroke may have undiagnosed paroxysmal atrial fibrillation. Neuroimaging findings are similar to those of atrial fibrillation without abnormalities on telemetry or electrocardiography. Prolonged cardiac monitoring with either surface electrodes or an implantable monitor can reveal paroxysmal atrial fibrillation in approximately one third of these patients. In patients with an implantable pacemaker, interrogation of the device may also reveal episodes consistent with atrial fibrillation. The benefit of anticoagulation for stroke prevention if atrial fibrillation is not found on monitoring is unclear.

KEY POINTS
- Carotid and transcranial Doppler ultrasonography may help diagnose large vessel atherosclerosis in a patient with ischemic stroke, although magnetic resonance angiography and CT angiography may provide additional information; catheter-based angiography is rarely used to diagnose either extracranial or intracranial vessel disease and is associated with a small risk of stroke.
- Atrial fibrillation is the most common cardioembolic cause of stroke, and anticoagulation is indicated; radiographic findings suggestive of a cardioembolic source, however, are insufficient grounds for initiating anticoagulation.
- The use of transesophageal echocardiography to evaluate for an intracardiac source of stroke is not routinely indicated, given the low yield for findings that require anticoagulation or surgery. **HVC**
- Lacunar (or small subcortical) infarcts resulting in isolated motor or sensory syndromes are caused by occlusion of the small penetrating arteries arising from intracranial arteries; the main risk factor for lacunar infarcts is hypertension.
- Many patients with cryptogenic stroke may have undiagnosed paroxysmal atrial fibrillation, and prolonged cardiac monitoring should be considered.

Hemorrhagic Stroke

Subarachnoid Hemorrhage
Examination findings suggestive of SAH include altered mental status, nuchal rigidity, pupillary dilation from compression of the occulomotor nerve (cranial nerve III) by a posterior communicating artery aneurysm, or subhyaloid hemorrhages on funduscopy. The most common cause of subarachnoid hemorrhage is saccular (berry) aneurysm rupture, with intracranial arterial dissection and mycotic aneurysm rupture occurring less commonly. Other rare causes of SAH are the reversible cerebral vasoconstriction syndromes, dural

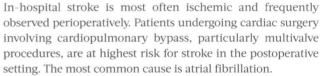

sinus thrombosis, vascular malformations, and cerebral amyloid angiopathy. Saccular aneurysms often can be visualized with CTA or MRA, although the resolution is not sufficient to detect smaller aneurysms; catheter-based angiography is necessary for the definitive diagnosis of aneurysms and other causes of SAH.

Elevated intracranial pressure from obstructive hydrocephalus and/or global cerebral edema is a common consequence of SAH. Examination findings that raise concern for elevated intracranial pressure include impairment in consciousness, loss of brainstem reflexes, and stereotyped posturing movements to painful stimuli. The presence of hydrocephalus on neuroimaging is associated with high mortality and should prompt neurosurgical placement of an external ventricular drain to relieve (and measure) elevated intracranial pressure. Impaired consciousness due to nonconvulsive status epilepticus also may occur and requires electroencephalographic monitoring for diagnosis.

Intracerebral Hemorrhage

ICH can present similarly to ischemic stroke, with headache and impaired consciousness as distinguishing characteristics. The most common cause of ICH that affects deep structures of the brain (thalamus, basal ganglia, pons, cerebellum) is hypertension. Lobar hemorrhages near the cortical surface may have various causes, including hypertension, hemorrhagic tumors, and cortical vein thrombosis. In patients older than 55 years, especially in those without hypertension, lobar ICH may be due to cerebral amyloid angiopathy. In this syndrome, amyloid protein similar to that seen pathologically in Alzheimer disease deposits in cerebral arterioles near the cortical surface, thereby weakening the arterial wall and making it prone to rupture.

The mainstay of acute treatment and prevention is control of blood pressure. Clinical and radiologic features can be used to calculate a patient's ICH score, which informs 30-day mortality and is recommended in the assessment of patients with ICH (**Table 25**). The main cause of early neurologic deterioration is hematoma expansion. Another leading cause of death is early withdrawal of care. Guidelines caution against termination of care within the first 48 hours. **H**

KEY POINTS

- Catheter-based angiography is necessary for the definitive diagnosis of aneurysms and other causes of subarachnoid hemorrhage.

- In subarachnoid hemorrhage, the presence of hydrocephalus on neuroimaging is associated with high mortality and should prompt neurosurgical placement of an external ventricular drain to relieve elevated intracranial pressure.

- The most common cause of intracerebral hemorrhage that affects deep structures of the brain (thalamus, basal ganglia, pons, cerebellum) is hypertension; the mainstay of prevention is control of blood pressure.

TABLE 25. Intracerebral Hemorrhage Score[a,b]

Clinical and Imaging Findings		Points
Glasgow Coma Scale score	3-4	2
	5-12	1
	13-15	0
Age	80 y or older	1
	Younger than 80 y	0
Infratentorial (brainstem, cerebellum)	Yes	1
	No	0
Volume	Greater than 30 mL	1
	Less than 30 mL	0
Intraventricular hemorrhage	Yes	1
	No	0

[a]30-Day mortality based on total score: 0 = 0%; 1 = 13%; 2 = 26%; 3 = 72%; 4 = 97%; 5 and 6 = 100%.

Adapted with permission from: Hemphill JC 3rd, Bonovich DC, Besmertis L, Manley GT, Johnston SC. The ICH score: a simple, reliable grading scale for intracerebral hemorrhage. Stroke. 2001;32:891-7. [PMID: 11283388]

In-Hospital Stroke Considerations

In-hospital stroke is most often ischemic and frequently observed perioperatively. Patients undergoing cardiac surgery involving cardiopulmonary bypass, particularly multivalve procedures, are at highest risk for stroke in the postoperative setting. The most common cause is atrial fibrillation.

The modifiable preoperative risk factors for in-hospital stroke are similar to those causing stroke in the short term without surgery, including symptomatic extracranial ICA stenosis of greater than 70%. Patients with a recent stroke secondary to ICA stenosis who are undergoing nonemergent surgery are likely to benefit from revascularization beforehand. The presence of asymptomatic ICA stenosis, however, is not clearly associated with perioperative stroke, and routine prophylactic ICA revascularization is not indicated.

Stroke within 30 days of surgery, regardless of cause, increases the risk of perioperative stroke; elective surgeries within this time period should be avoided. Patients with stroke involving a large brain volume or with a recent hemorrhagic stroke also are at risk of cerebral hemorrhage if placed on cardiopulmonary bypass and/or anticoagulation. If possible, nonemergency major cardiac procedures should be avoided. **H**

KEY POINTS

- Patients undergoing cardiac surgery involving cardiopulmonary bypass, particularly multivalve procedures, are at highest risk for stroke in the postoperative setting, most commonly from atrial fibrillation.

- Stroke within 30 days of surgery, regardless of cause, increases the risk of perioperative stroke, and elective surgeries within this time period should be avoided.

Acute Stroke Therapy

Ischemic Stroke Treatment

Thrombolysis and Endovascular Therapy

Intravenous recombinant tissue plasminogen activator (alteplase) is the only thrombolytic agent approved for use in acute ischemic stroke. Alteplase is most effective when administered early, and treatment within 3 hours of ischemic stroke onset with disabling symptoms is associated with a significant reduction in disability at 3 months. Although treatment within 4.5 hours also may have clinical benefit, treatment beyond 3 hours is not approved by the FDA. Because of the associated delays, obtaining advanced imaging or laboratory values should be avoided before treatment unless coagulopathy or thrombocytopenia is suspected. Treatment should start within 60 minutes of arrival at the emergency department or detection of in-hospital stroke, with best practices recommending treatment within 45 minutes. Contraindications for treatment with alteplase have evolved over the years, with the latest guidelines clarifying relative exclusion criteria and defining nondisabling symptoms (**Table 26**).

The main complication of alteplase treatment is symptomatic ICH, which can present with headache or worsening of NIHSS score or level of consciousness. Symptomatic hemorrhage occurs in up to 6% of treated patients, and mortality can be as high as 50% when present. The main risk factors for symptomatic hemorrhage are treatment after 4.5 hours and hypertension before and after treatment. Accordingly, before treatment with alteplase, the patient's blood pressure should be less than 185/110 mm Hg. Higher readings should prompt administration of intravenous labetalol or nicardipine before alteplase. Nitrates should be avoided because of their potential to increase intracranial pressure.

After treatment with alteplase, frequent monitoring of neurologic status and vital signs is required in the first 24 hours. Neurologic worsening should prompt urgent neuroimaging. Blood pressure should be maintained below 180/105 mm Hg, and both antiplatelet and anticoagulant agents should be held for the first 24 hours after alteplase administration. After 24 hours, antiplatelet agents for stroke prevention and anticoagulant agents for deep venous thrombosis prevention can be started if hemorrhage is absent on imaging.

Endovascular therapy (primarily with intra-arterial mechanical thrombectomy) within 24 hours of stroke onset can be considered for select patients with a clinically suspected large-vessel occlusion and specific examination and radiologic findings, such as a measurable neurologic deficit and small but radiographically evident ischemic changes. In patients for whom endovascular therapy is considered, prompt noninvasive vessel imaging with CT or MRA is recommended. The evaluation for endovascular stroke therapy with vessel imaging, however, should not replace or delay the administration of

TABLE 26. Contraindications to Intravenous Alteplase in Adults With Acute Ischemic Stroke

Absolute Exclusion Criteria	Relative Exclusion Criteria
Significant head trauma or prior stroke in the previous 3 months	Minor or rapidly improving nondisabling symptoms[a]
Suspicion of subarachnoid hemorrhage	Pregnancy
Noncompressible site arterial puncture within 7 days	Seizure at onset
Intracranial neoplasm, arteriovenous malformation, aneurysm	Major surgery or serious trauma within 14 days
Recent intracranial or spinal surgery	Recent gastrointestinal or genitourinary bleeding within 21 days
Blood pressure ≥185/110 mmHg despite treatment	Recent acute myocardial infarction
Active internal bleeding	
Active bleeding diathesis	
Platelet count <100,000/μL (100 × 10^9/L)	
Heparin within 48 hours with an activated partial thromboplastin time above normal range	
Current use of anticoagulant with INR >1.7	
Current use of non–vitamin K antagonist anticoagulants (within 48 hours) with associated elevated relevant laboratory tests	
Blood glucose less 50 mg/dL (2.8 mmol/L)	
Noncontrast head CT demonstrated multi-lobar infarction with >1/3 of the hemisphere involved	

[a]Disabling symptoms are defined as complete hemianopia (score of 2-3 on National Institutes of Health Stroke Scale [NIHSS] question 3), visual or sensory extinction (score of 1-2 on NIHSS question 11), any weakness against gravity (score of 2-4 on NIHSS question 6 or 7), and total NIHSS score >5.

Adapted with permission from: Demaerschalk BM, Kleindorfer DO, Adeoye OM, Demchuk AM, Fugate JE, Grotta JC, et al; American Heart Association Stroke Council and Council on Epidemiology and Prevention. Scientific Rationale for the Inclusion and Exclusion Criteria for Intravenous Alteplase in Acute Ischemic Stroke: A Statement for Healthcare Professionals From the American Heart Association/American Stroke Association. Stroke. 2016;47:581-641. [PMID: 26696642] doi:10.1161/STR.0000000000000086

CONT.

alteplase in otherwise eligible patients. A treatment algorithm for stroke within 6 hours of onset is provided in **Figure 14**.

Antiplatelet Therapy, Anticoagulation, and Medical Management

For the many patients with acute ischemic stroke who are not eligible for thrombolysis or endovascular stroke therapy, antiplatelet therapy is the mainstay of acute treatment. When administered either orally or rectally within 48 hours of stoke, aspirin reduces the short-term risk of recurrent stroke, and its use in the acute setting is a stroke-specific quality-of-care core measure. Monotherapy with clopidogrel, however, has no established benefit in the acute stroke setting.

The patient with TIA or minor stroke, usually defined as an NIHSS score of 5 or less, has been the focus of recent trials of antiplatelet therapy because of the high short-term risk of recurrent events. In one recent trial, aspirin was compared to ticagrelor within 24 hours of stroke onset, and no difference between the two medications in the risk of recurrent stroke during 90 days of treatment was noted. Another study compared aspirin monotherapy for 90 days with aspirin and clopidogrel combined for 21 days followed by clopidogrel monotherapy as long as 69 days. The combination arm had a

3% absolute reduction in recurrent ischemic stroke at 90 days, with no difference in hemorrhagic stroke. Further clinical trials are ongoing to evaluate the safety and efficacy of dual antiplatelet agents in the settings of acute minor stroke and TIA.

Acute administration of anticoagulation in ischemic strokes (whether related to atrial fibrillation or not) does not reduce the short-term risk of recurrent stroke and increases the risk of hemorrhage into the territory of cerebral infarction (hemorrhagic conversion).

Management of acute hypertension in ischemic stroke differs when thrombolysis is not involved. Blood pressure should not be treated within the first 48 hours unless it is greater than 220/120 mm Hg or there is evidence of end-organ dysfunction. Acute antihypertensive therapy has been associated with neurologic worsening in patients with ischemic stroke and should be started slowly after the first 48 hours until secondary prevention targets are reached. Statins have not been shown to reduce the risk of recurrent stroke when administered within 30 days but can be considered after a dysphagia evaluation has been completed, especially in those patients with an atherosclerotic stroke subtype. See Dyslipidemia section in MKSAP 18 General Internal Medicine. ⊞

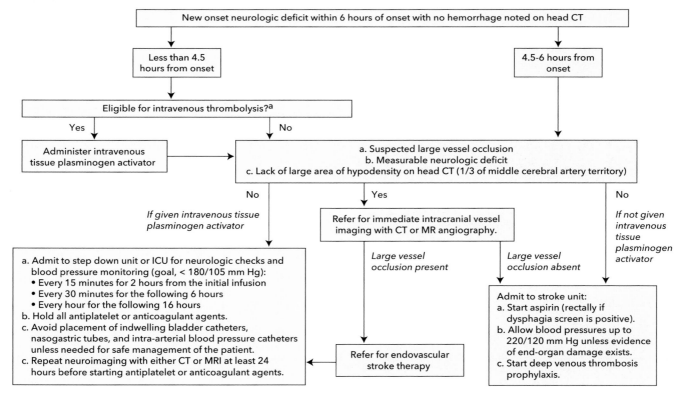

FIGURE 14. Proposed pathway for the evaluation and treatment of an acute stroke within 6 hours of onset.

aSee Table 26 for exclusion criteria for alteplase (tissue plasminogen activator).

- Treatment with intravenous recombinant tissue plasminogen activator (alteplase) within 3 hours of ischemic stroke onset is associated with a significant reduction in disability at 3 months after stroke; treatment within 4.5 hours of onset also may have clinical benefit but is not FDA approved.

- Endovascular therapy within 24 hours of stroke onset can be considered for select patients with a clinically suspected large-vessel occlusion and specific examination and radiologic findings, such as a measurable neurologic deficit and small but radiographically evident ischemic changes.

- When administered within 48 hours of ischemic stroke that is not eligible for thrombolysis, aspirin reduces the short-term risk of recurrent stroke; its use in the acute setting is a stroke-specific quality-of-care core measure.

- Acute administration of anticoagulation for ischemic stroke (whether related to atrial fibrillation or not) does not reduce the short-term risk of recurrent stroke and increases the risk of hemorrhage into the territory of cerebral infarction (hemorrhagic conversion).

Hemorrhagic Stroke Treatment

CONT.

Intracerebral Hemorrhage Treatment

Treatment of acute ICH is centered on preventing hematoma expansion. The primary predictor of early hematoma expansion is elevated blood pressure. Treatment of blood pressure is recommended for patients with ICH who have a systolic blood pressure greater than 180 mm Hg, although the most appropriate agent for the blood pressure control in this circumstance is not well established. Parenteral medications delivered by intravenous infusion with frequent blood pressure monitoring have the benefit of close titration to the intended target. Intravenous nitrates (such as nitroglycerin) and nitroprusside may raise intracranial pressure and reduce blood flow to the ischemic region and should be avoided in patients with ICH. Guidelines for the treatment of ICH indicate that acutely treating the systolic blood pressure in a specialized intensive care unit until it is 140 mm Hg is reasonable if the presenting systolic pressure is 150 to 220 mm Hg.

A recently completed trial compared a goal systolic blood pressure of 110 to 140 mm Hg with one of 140 to 180 mm Hg in patients with a systolic blood pressure of greater than 180 mm Hg who were seen within 4.5 hours of ICH onset. The more intensive control arm achieved a mean systolic blood pressure of 128 mm Hg versus 141 mm Hg in the usual care arm. No difference in mortality or neurologic outcomes was seen, but a significantly higher rate of adverse renal events occurred with intensive control. Treating systolic blood pressure if greater than 180 mm Hg is still advised but should be performed cautiously, and systolic blood pressure goals of less 140 mm Hg should be avoided.

Another risk factor for hematoma expansion is coagulopathy due to either antiplatelet agent use or anticoagulation. The use of platelet transfusion has been specifically studied in ICH in the setting of antiplatelet agent use, and no clinical benefit has been shown. Guidelines advise against its routine use. Anticoagulation should be reversed, although this incurs an increased risk of thrombotic events. For patients without coagulopathy, recombinant factor VII has no neurologic benefit and is associated with high rates of venous thromboembolic events.

Another source of neurologic decline in patients with ICH is nonconvulsive status epilepticus, which may present with impaired consciousness. Use of prophylactic antiepileptic medications in patients with ICH is not recommended, however, unless there are definitive clinical or electroencephalographic seizures.

Elevated intracranial pressure is a major determinant of morbidity and mortality in ICH. Osmotherapy with mannitol or hypertonic saline may temporarily reduce intracranial pressure in ICH; glucocorticoids are ineffective in reducing cerebral edema in ICH and should not be routinely administered. External ventricular drainage is indicated with hydrocephalus and impaired consciousness; other surgical measures are not routinely indicated unless as life-saving measures in rapidly deteriorating patients. Cerebellar hemorrhages greater than 3 centimeters in diameter are the exception because early surgical evacuation is necessary to prevent hydrocephalus, brainstem compression, and neurologic deterioration. H

- Treatment of blood pressure is recommended for patients with intracerebral hemorrhage whose systolic blood pressure is greater than 180 mm Hg; intravenous nitrates should be avoided.

- Routine use of platelet transfusion in patients with intracerebral hemorrhage who are being treated with antiplatelet agents is not indicated.

- Osmotherapy with mannitol or hypertonic saline may temporarily reduce intracranial pressure in patients with intracerebral hemorrhage; glucocorticoids are ineffective and should not be routinely administered.

- In patients with intracerebral hemorrhage, early surgical evacuation of cerebellar hemorrhages greater than 3 cm in diameter is necessary to prevent hydrocephalus, brainstem compression, and neurologic deterioration.

HVC

Subarachnoid Hemorrhage Treatment

Treatment of SAH focuses on prevention of early (≤48 hours) and late neurologic complications. Within the first 48 hours, a major cause of morbidity is aneurysmal rebleeding; early surgical exclusion of the ruptured aneurysm and maintenance of a blood pressure of less than 140/80 mm Hg is required. Elevated intracranial pressure from obstructive hydrocephalus, cerebral edema, seizures, and cerebral vasospasm are other leading causes of poor outcomes.

CONT.

Cerebral vasospasm with resultant cerebral ischemia and neurologic worsening may develop beginning near day 5. The degree of hemorrhage on a head CT may predict the risk of vasospasm, but frequent monitoring and daily transcranial Doppler imaging is recommended in all patients. Nimodipine should be started as early as possible to improve neurologic outcomes. The drug is continued for 21 days or until hospital discharge. If there is a high clinical suspicion of vasospasm, CTA or catheter-based angiography may be needed to establish vasospasm as the cause of neurologic worsening. The latter has the added benefit of potential endovascular treatment, including use of intra-arterial vasodilators and angioplasty. Another treatment option for vasospasm in patients with a treated aneurysm is induced hypertension, although the exact treatment targets are not well established.

Medical complications are a significant source of morbidity and mortality in patients with SAH. Patients with impaired consciousness and coma at presentation are at highest risk for stunned myocardium (with a decrease in left ventricular ejection fraction) and pulmonary edema due to the large sympathetic surge in SAH. Other medical complications include pulmonary and urinary tract infections, dysphagia, the syndrome of inappropriate antidiuretic hormone secretion, and cerebral salt wasting. Because of these possible medical and neurologic complications, patients with SAH require care in a specialized ICU with experience in treating SAH.

KEY POINTS

- Within the first 48 hours of a subarachnoid hemorrhage, aneurysmal rebleeding is a major cause of morbidity; early surgical exclusion of the ruptured aneurysm and maintaining a blood pressure of less than 140/80 mm Hg is required.

- In aneurysmal subarachnoid hemorrhage, cerebral vasospasm with resultant cerebral ischemia and neurologic worsening may develop beginning near day 5, and all patients should be treated with nimodipine to prevent poor neurological outcomes.

Stroke Prevention

Primary Prevention

MKSAP 18 General Internal Medicine provides information on the treatment of cardiovascular risk factors related to primary prevention of stroke. Patients with asymptomatic ICA stenosis require primary prevention strategies similar to those used for patients with asymptomatic atherosclerotic disease. Contemporary best medical therapy, including high-intensity statin therapy, is associated with a low risk of first stroke, likely less than 2% per year. ICA revascularization may reduce the risk of stroke further, but the risk of the procedure itself must be weighed against the potential benefit. ICA revascularization for primary prevention is not warranted unless high-risk

stroke features are present, such as stenosis greater than 80% or rapid progression of stenosis. For patients with high-risk predictors, the decision to refer for revascularization should be made on an individual basis. Ongoing clinical trials may provide more information on the relative advantages of revascularization and medical therapy.

The main modifiable risk factors for intracranial arterial aneurysm growth and rupture are hypertension and active tobacco use. Treatment of both is indicated. Surgical treatment of aneurysms with either endovascular therapy or craniotomy is associated with sufficiently high neurologic morbidity that treatment is reserved for patients at high risk of rupture and low surgical risk. The location and size of the aneurysm are the primary determinants of rupture risk, and both MRA and CTA can show these features noninvasively. Aneurysms less than 7 millimeters in diameter in the posterior circulation and less than 12 millimeters in the anterior circulation have a low risk of rupture and can be managed conservatively. Patients with these aneurysms should undergo annual noninvasive imaging because aneurysmal growth is a risk factor for rupture and may be an indication for surgery. Patients with two or more relatives with intracranial aneurysms or SAH also should be offered screening with noninvasive neuroimaging. Other predictors of aneurysmal rupture that should prompt surgical consideration include a previous aneurysmal SAH or the presence of cranial nerve palsy.

KEY POINTS

- Routine internal carotid artery revascularization for primary prevention of stroke is not warranted unless high-risk stroke features are present, such as stenosis greater than 80% or rapid progression of stenosis. **HVC**

- Aneurysms less than 7 millimeters in diameter in the posterior circulation and less than 12 millimeters in the anterior circulation have a low risk of rupture and can be managed conservatively with annual noninvasive neuroimaging. **HVC**

Secondary Prevention

Lifestyle Modifications and Medical Management

The risk factors for a second stroke are similar to those for ischemic heart disease and other atherosclerotic disease. Patients with stroke benefit from diet and exercise changes to maintain cardiometabolic health. Patients with ICH are at high risk for recurrent stroke due to hypertension; after the acute in-hospital setting, a target blood pressure of less than 130/80 mm Hg is advised. Similarly, patients with small subcortical infarcts in whom hypertension is the primary risk factor may also benefit from a systolic blood pressure of less than 130 mm Hg. High-intensity statin therapy reduces the risk of stroke among patients with ischemic stroke or TIA presumed to be of atherosclerotic origin and an LDL-cholesterol level greater than 100 mg/dL (2.6 mmol/L).

The choice of an antiplatelet agent for long-term (>90 days from stroke) secondary stroke prevention in the absence of atrial fibrillation has been the subject of several clinical trials. Consistent across trials is the finding that long-term use of aspirin and clopidogrel combined, versus a single antiplatelet agent, is associated with no reduction in risk of stroke but an increased risk of hemorrhage and death. Aspirin monotherapy is a reasonable first-line antiplatelet regimen for secondary stroke prevention, although clopidogrel or aspirin-dipyridamole is often prescribed because of their small absolute risk benefits over aspirin. Clopidogrel monotherapy, when compared with aspirin monotherapy in a trial involving ischemic stroke, peripheral arterial disease, and myocardial infarction, was associated with a 0.9% per year absolute benefit; however, the results of this trial were driven by peripheral arterial disease outcomes, with no clear difference in recurrent stroke. The combination of aspirin and dipyridamole versus aspirin alone has been associated with a modestly lower risk of recurrent stroke in the long term, although the combination is associated with high risk of discontinuation because of headache and other adverse effects. Clopidogrel has been compared with the aspirin-dipyridamole combination in one large clinical trial, with both having similar efficacy in stroke prevention. Cilostazol has been compared to aspirin in clinical trials in Japan and China; it has had similar efficacy in reducing ischemic stroke and resulted in slightly lower hemorrhagic complications, although its use is limited by adverse effects. Other antiplatelet agents, such as ticagrelor or prasugrel, have not been examined in long-term trials of secondary stroke prevention, although prasugrel is associated with a high risk of hemorrhage when used in patients with coronary artery disease who have a history of stroke. No data are available on blood assays examining a lack of response to antiplatelet agents in secondary stroke prevention or on the choice of antiplatelet agent after an additional clinical event.

Warfarin also has been compared to aspirin for secondary stroke prevention in the absence of atrial fibrillation, with no difference in stroke outcomes reported. In a trial of patients with intracranial atherosclerosis, warfarin was associated with increased mortality compared with aspirin. Non–vitamin K antagonist anticoagulants have not been tested in clinical trials of stroke not involving atrial fibrillation and are not routinely indicated in this setting. For a review of anticoagulation in atrial fibrillation–related stroke, see MKSAP 18 Cardiovascular Medicine.

Whether to start antithrombotic agents after hemorrhagic stroke has not been as well studied. Patients with cerebral amyloid angiopathy are at particularly high risk of recurrent lobar ICH, and the use of antiplatelet agents should only be considered in those with clear secondary prevention indications, such as coronary stents. Similarly, anticoagulation-related lobar ICH has a high risk of recurrence, and further anticoagulation should be avoided in patients with this type of hemorrhage. Anticoagulation also should be avoided in most patients with indications of low thromboembolic risk, such as atrial fibrillation with a low CHA_2DS_2-Vasc score (with one point each given for heart failure, hypertension, diabetes, vascular disease [previous myocardial infarction, peripheral arterial disease, aortic plaque], female sex, and age 65 to 74 years and two points each for previous stroke/transient ischemic attack/thromboembolic disease and for age ≥75 years), and used with caution in higher-risk scenarios (such as pulmonary emboli). Finally, with adequate control of hypertension, anticoagulation and antiplatelet treatment can be considered for appropriate indications 4 weeks after a deep ICH secondary to hypertension.

Surgical Management

The use of surgical approaches for secondary stroke prevention has been examined in patients with extracranial ICA stenosis, ICA occlusion, intracranial atherosclerosis, and PFO–related stroke. In extracranial ICA disease, patients with nondisabling stroke or TIA due to ICA stenosis of greater than 70% are at high risk for recurrent stroke and may benefit from early revascularization. The choice of endarterectomy or angioplasty with stenting is dictated by several patient-specific factors and by local surgical experience. A consistent finding in trials has been a higher risk of perioperative stroke with stenting and a higher risk of perioperative myocardial infarction with endarterectomy. In patients with a complete symptomatic occlusion of the ICA, however, direct revascularization is not feasible, and external carotid–to–internal carotid bypass is not effective for stroke prevention.

Symptomatic intracranial arterial stenosis of greater than 70% is associated with a high risk of recurrent stroke and should be treated with a statin. Stenting of the affected artery, however, is associated with a high risk of procedural stroke and should be avoided. Endovascular closure of a PFO for secondary stroke prevention may be considered in select patients (see MKSAP 18 Cardiovascular Disease).

KEY POINTS

- Long-term use of combination aspirin-clopidogrel is associated with no reduction in risk of stroke but an increased risk of hemorrhage and death when compared with single-agent antiplatelet use; aspirin monotherapy is a reasonable first line antiplatelet regimen for secondary stroke prevention. **HVC**

- Patients with nondisabling stroke or TIA due to greater than 70% stenosis of the internal carotid artery (ICA) may benefit from early revascularization; in those with a complete symptomatic occlusion of the ICA, however, direct revascularization is not feasible. **HVC**

- Symptomatic high-grade intracranial arterial stenosis is associated with a high risk of recurrent stroke, but stenting of the affected artery is associated with a high risk of procedural stroke and should be avoided. **HVC**

Standardized Discharge Orders

Adherence to secondary stroke prevention guidelines is inconsistent after hospital discharge. Standardized discharge orders, aligned with recommended core measures for patients with ischemic stroke, can reduce the risk of both hospital readmission and recurrent stroke. These standardized orders ensure that appropriate antiplatelet or anticoagulation agents and high-intensity statin therapy are started on hospital discharge. They include the essential component of patient education about diet, exercise, smoking cessation, and other healthy lifestyle choices to reduce the risk of recurrent events. Lastly, these discharge orders allow for stroke-specific education regarding typical stroke symptoms and the importance of rapid return to care if symptoms occur so that acute stroke therapeutics can be initiated. ⊞

Prognosis and Recovery

Neurologic Complications

Patients with stroke are at high risk for developing in-hospital and long-term neurologic complications beyond those previously outlined. Patients with ischemic stroke may develop worsening deficits from hemorrhagic conversion of the infarct, usually within 48 hours. Antiplatelet agents should be held for at least 1 week in most patients with hemorrhagic conversion (for example, a hematoma seen on brain imaging that is associated with mass effect or edema). Patients with hemorrhagic conversion not involving a hematoma and with stable repeat imaging can be started on antiplatelet agents within 48 hours. Patients with a large hemispheric ischemic stroke are at risk for neurologic deterioration from cerebral edema starting on day 2 after a stroke. Patients with significant symptomatic cerebral edema and increased intracranial pressure after an ischemic stroke have a survival advantage with decompressive hemicraniectomy, although neurologic compromise may be significant. Finally, patients with ischemic and hemorrhagic stroke may show neurologic worsening from seizures and systemic infections. ⊞

KEY POINTS

- Patients with ischemic stroke may develop worsening deficits from hemorrhagic conversion of the infarct, usually within 48 hours; antiplatelet agents should be held in the setting of hemorrhagic conversion involving a hematoma for at least 1 week and for a shorter period of time if there is no hematoma seen on imaging and repeat imaging is stable.

- Patients with significant symptomatic cerebral edema and increased intracranial pressure after an ischemic stroke have a survival advantage with decompressive hemicraniectomy, although neurologic compromise may be significant.

Medical Complications and Stroke Units

In-hospital medical complications are a leading cause of morbidity and mortality in patients with stroke. Admission to a specialized stroke unit is associated with a reduced long-term risk of all-cause mortality. Specialized stroke units are effective because they use multidisciplinary care teams focused on early mobilization and adherence to protocols, such as removing indwelling catheters to prevent urinary tract infection, preventing aspiration pneumonia by addressing/preventing dysphagia, and instituting oral hygiene protocols. Care protocols in stroke units also emphasize early initiation of pharmacologic prophylaxis of deep venous thrombosis in patients with ischemic stroke and prophylaxis initiation within 48 hours in patients with hemorrhagic stroke who have no evidence of active bleeding. ⊞

Long-Term Prognosis and Recovery

Long-term survivors of stroke are at high risk for delayed neurologic complications. Cognitive impairment, vascular dementia, and seizures all may occur. Most stroke survivors exhibit neurologic impairment and disability 1 year poststroke and beyond. Fatigue can arise from a high prevalence of sleep-disordered breathing. Depression is highly prevalent in stroke survivors and is one of the leading modifiable risk factors for long-term disability. Many stroke survivors require ongoing rehabilitative care to improve mobility, prevent falls, and treat spasticity.

KEY POINT

- Most stroke survivors exhibit neurologic impairment and disability 1 year poststroke and beyond; depression is highly prevalent in stroke survivors and is one of the leading modifiable risk factors for long-term disability.

Cognitive Impairment
Definition

Cognitive impairment is the progressive loss of cognitive function in at least one major category: memory, language, executive function, visuospatial function, or behavior. When the level of cognitive impairment is progressive, involves more than one cognitive function, and results in a loss of independent function, it is considered a dementia syndrome. Fixed cognitive disorders occurring after a brain lesion, such as stroke or traumatic brain injury, are excluded from the dementia category.

General Approach to the Patient With Cognitive Impairment

Dementia syndromes are chronic disorders that typically develop over years; intervention when dementia is well established is likely too late to have a meaningful effect on the disorder. Although definitive evidence that earlier diagnosis improves patient outcomes is lacking, screening for dementia has become the subject of increased interest. At this time, however, there are no accepted standards for dementia screening. The U.S. Preventive Services Task Force does not endorse screening, but the Association of Gerontology and Geriatrics recommends that some form (objective or subjective) of cognitive screening be performed annually in patients age 70 and older.

In the absence of screening, certain signs and behaviors may raise clinical suspicion of a cognitive disorder and provoke evaluation in a primary care setting. Examples include concerns expressed by family members or caregivers, frequent missed (or late arrival to) appointments, changes in medication adherence, unexplained weight loss, presence of a partner or family member at patient appointments when the patient previously was seen alone, and withdrawal from previously enjoyed hobbies.

Many bedside cognitive evaluation tools have demonstrated adequate sensitivity and specificity for detecting cognitive impairment in population-based settings. The most common are the Mini–Mental State Examination, the Montreal Cognitive Assessment, the Ascertain Dementia 8 questionnaire, the Mini-Cog test, and the five-word memory test. Each of these tests can be performed in less than 5 to 10 minutes; no compelling data support the superiority of one test over another. These tests are increasingly used to justify billing and medication-authorization decisions by insurers.

After cognitive impairment is diagnosed, determining whether it is reversible or nonreversible is imperative in the initial evaluation of the patient. Essential elements in this determination are the time course of symptom onset and progression, the principal cognitive domain or function affected and its functional impact, and other associated neurologic and nonneurologic symptoms (**Figure 15**). Access to a reliable informant familiar with the patient's condition is critical in the evaluation of the cognitive disorder. The signs and symptoms of a cognitive disorder also may have an anatomic correlate that can be used to help guide the diagnosis and treatment. For example, a progressive loss of language function localizes to a different anatomic location than does a primary memory problem, which may be helpful in determining the underlying cause of the impaired function. The age of the patient also is an important consideration; for example, both atypical presentations of typical dementia syndromes and nonneurodegenerative causes are more common in younger patients.

For a slowly progressive dementia syndrome in an older patient, the American Neurological Association recommends that a minimum evaluation include the following elements:

- General neurologic examination, including a cognitive screening evaluation
- Evaluation for depression, sleep disorders, alcohol use, and family history of dementia
- Detailed medication review
- Serum chemistries, including plasma glucose level
- Complete blood count
- Determination of vitamin B$_{12}$ and thyroid-stimulating hormone levels
- A rapid plasmin reagent test to evaluate for syphilis in high-risk populations
- Basic neuroimaging (MRI or CT without contrast)

In the older population, increasing evidence also suggests that chronic vitamin D deficiency increases the odds of developing dementia. Therefore, measuring serum 25-hydroxyvitamin D levels is a recommended part of the evaluation. When patient age, disease progression, or other associated symptoms

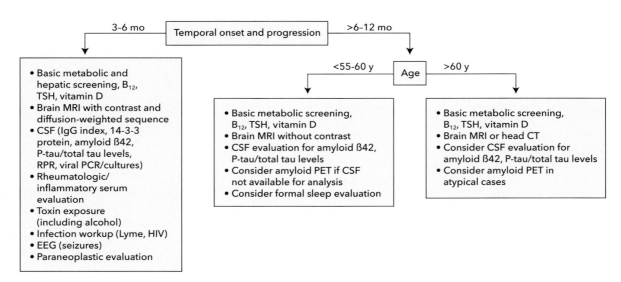

FIGURE 15. Diagnostic test consideration in patient with a dementia syndrome. CSF = cerebrospinal fluid; EEG = electroencephalography; PCR = polymerase chain reaction; PET = positron emission tomography; P-tau = phosphorylated tau; RPR = rapid plasma reagin test; TSH = thyroid-stimulating hormone.

raise the possibility of a more uncommon type of dementia, additional diagnostic tests and early referral to a specialist should be considered (see Figure 15).

Several more specialized testing modalities are available. These tests should be reserved for patients with an uncertain diagnosis (for example, to distinguish dementia from pseudo-dementia), for an atypical progression of a previously established diagnosis (such as an excessively slow course of Alzheimer disease), and for discriminating between two types of dementia with overlapping features (such as the detection of Alzheimer disease–specific biomarkers). These tests, if required, are typically ordered by a dementia specialist.

These specialized diagnostic tests fall into two categories:

1. Disease-specific tests: measurement cerebrospinal fluid (CSF) levels of the tau protein and 42-residue form of amyloid-β peptide ($A\beta_{42}$) in patients with Alzheimer disease; prion-specific PET (using ^{18}F-fluorodeoxyglucose [FDG]) to detect amyloid plaques in Alzheimer disease; and dopamine-transporter single-photon emission CT (SPECT) in patients with cognitive impairment and symptoms of parkinsonism (see Movement Disorder chapter).

2. Disease-nonspecific tests: FDG-PET to measure cerebral metabolism; SPECT measuring cerebral blood flow to detect disease-relevant patterns; MRI to detect and measure brain atrophy; and CSF analysis to detect inflammation, infection, neuronal injury, and paraneoplastic antibodies.

KEY POINTS

- Many bedside cognitive evaluation tools have demonstrated adequate sensitivity and specificity for detecting cognitive impairment in population-based settings; no compelling data support the superiority of one test over another.

- The minimum evaluation in slowly progressive dementia syndrome in an older patient includes assessment for a reversible cause with a general neurologic examination; evaluation for depression, sleep disorders, alcohol use, and a family history of dementia; a detailed medication review; basic laboratory studies, including vitamin B_{12} and thyroid-stimulating hormone measurement; and basic neuroimaging (MRI or CT without contrast).

HVC • Specialized tests for dementia—including cerebrospinal fluid tests, single-photon emission CT and PET scans—should be reserved for uncertain diagnoses or atypical presentations; they are usually ordered in conjunction with dementia specialists.

Dementias

Dementia syndromes can be divided into neurodegenerative and nonneurodegenerative categories. Neurodegenerative dementias involve a progressive loss of the underlying brain tissue related to a pathologically identifiable pattern of protein accumulation. Distinction between syndromes typically can be made through careful consideration of the temporal onset and progression, the core cognitive dysfunction, and the associated neurologic and nonneurologic signs and symptoms.

Neurodegenerative Diseases
Mild Cognitive Impairment

Within the framework of early detection of dementia, the diagnosis of mild cognitive impairment (MCI) is a commonly used measure to identify patients with clear symptoms of cognitive decline who do not meet criteria for dementia. The formal criteria for MCI are a subjective report (from either the patient or a witness) of a decline in cognitive abilities with relative preservation of day-to-day function and evidence of cognitive impairment on cognitive testing.

The annual risk of MCI progressing to dementia ranges from 5% to 15%, but a significant percentage of patients (as many as 20%) have normal findings on subsequent examinations. The risk of progression depends on the number of cognitive domains affected and the presence of markers of an underlying neurodegenerative process. Because of wide variability in the risk of progression, steps should be taken to confirm the underlying cause of the symptoms. The initial diagnostic approach should follow that used in patients with dementia, and specialized testing (CSF analysis, PET) is not recommended unless a specific dementia syndrome is suspected. Abnormalities on these studies may help more accurately predict the risk of progression.

Treatment

No specific treatments are currently approved for MCI, and no medications have been shown to prevent progression to dementia. All conditions that can contribute to cognitive impairment, however, should be aggressively treated.

KEY POINT

- No specific treatments are currently approved for mild   HVC
cognitive impairment, and no medications have been
shown to prevent progression to dementia.

Alzheimer Disease

The most common memory-predominant dementia is Alzheimer disease, which likely accounts for 60% to 80% of neurodegenerative dementias. Age is the greatest risk factor; after age 65 years, the prevalence doubles every 5 years. A second major risk factor is the presence of one or two copies of the apolipoprotein-E ε4 (APOE ε4) allele. Additional risk factors include a family history of dementia, female sex, history of stroke, and (to a lesser extent) head injury and cardiovascular disease. Evidence suggests that education, regular exercise, a Mediterranean diet, and cognitively stimulating leisure activities provide protection against developing Alzheimer disease.

The pathophysiology of Alzheimer disease is unclear. The principal pathologic findings, however, include brain volume loss, extracellular fibrillar Aβ plaques, and intracellular neurofibrillary tau tangles. Notably, the development of Aβ pathologic features begins as early as 15 to 20 years before symptom onset.

The typical presentation of Alzheimer disease is that of an insidious worsening of memory, language, and visuospatial abilities. Manifestations include forgetfulness (misplacing objects, missing appointments, frequently repeating questions or statements, missing bill payments), word-finding difficulties, hesitation in speech, and navigational problems (difficulty with directions while driving, even to familiar places, or disorientation in unfamiliar places). These symptoms are often followed by problems with executive function (organizational abilities and multitasking), problems with calculations (managing finances), and behavioral and mood symptoms (apathy, depression, anxiety, irritability, and agitation). In most instances, the patient's insight remains well preserved early in the disease. As the disease progresses, behavioral symptoms, including delusions, become more common. In contrast to dementia with Lewy bodies, however, hallucinations are rare. Motor symptoms and gait problems also do not typically occur until well into the moderate stages of the disease when daily function is significantly impaired. Early hallucinations and motor problems suggest the presence of a disorder other than Alzheimer disease (**Table 27**).

In younger-onset Alzheimer disease, nonmemory symptoms are more frequently the predominant pattern and include language-predominant, executive function–predominant (impaired organizational abilities, disorganized thoughts, poor attention span), and visual/perceptive–predominant (impaired depth perception, navigational problems, problems with coordination) forms. Memory impairment is initially minimal.

Evaluation

MRI of the brain supports the diagnosis of Alzheimer disease when it shows evidence of decreased volume of the

TABLE 27. Features That Distinguish Alzheimer Disease From Other Dementias	
Dementia Type	**Clinical Features**
Alzheimer disease	Impaired memory or forgetfulness as prominent early symptom
	Minimal motor symptoms until disease reaches moderate severity (that is, at the point of significant impairment of activities of daily living)
	Rare visual hallucinations
	Delusions not common at early stages of disease (that is, at the point of relatively preserved activities of daily living)
Dementia with Lewy bodies	Severe autonomic symptoms (such as orthostatic hypotension, constipation, and erectile dysfunction)
	Sleep disorders (such as rapid eye movement sleep behavior disorder and daytime hypersomnia)
	Severe fluctuations in mental status or seizure-like activity
	Early visual hallucinations
	Syncopal events or unexplained episodes of severe alteration in mentation
	Repeated falls
	Severe sensitivity to medications that act on the central nervous system
Frontotemporal dementia	Poor insight into impairment or denial of impairment, especially when cognitive impairment is mild
	New-onset obsessive-compulsive behaviors
	Criminal behaviors
	Gluttonous eating behaviors or adoption of bizarre food restrictions or fads
	Motor neuron disease (such as muscle wasting)
Vascular cognitive impairment	Pronounced gait disorder and repeated falls, especially early in the disease course (at mild dementia stage)
	Emotional incontinence (explosive crying, laughter)
	Pronounced apathy
	Severe cognitive slowing
Normal pressure hydrocephalus	Pronounced gait disorder and repeated falls, especially early in the disease course (at mild dementia stage)
	Minimal cognitive impairment, compared with much greater gait disorder and non–memory-predominant pattern
	Pronounced bladder incontinence proximate to onset of gait changes

hippocampi (**Figure 16**), although this is a nonspecific finding. When seen in MCI, decreased hippocampal volume predicts a higher likelihood of progression to Alzheimer disease. When the MRI is normal and the diagnosis is in question or a non–Alzheimer disease process is being considered, functional brain scans (FDG-PET or perfusion SPECT) can be used to look for the Alzheimer disease pattern of decreased brain function in the bilateral parietal and temporal regions.

In situations involving an uncertain diagnosis or a younger patient, Alzheimer disease–specific biomarkers also can be sought. A CSF test for Alzheimer disease biomarkers is FDA approved and frequently covered by insurers. In the presence of dementia, a pattern of decreased $A\beta_{42}$ and increased tau and phosphorylated tau levels is highly specific for Alzheimer disease; conversely, a normal $A\beta_{42}$ level has a high negative-predictive probability for Alzheimer disease. Three $A\beta$ plaque PET scans are FDA approved for detecting these findings, but their role in the diagnosis of dementia is unclear. Trials are currently underway that may further delineate the role of amyloid scanning in the evaluation of dementia and Alzheimer disease.

Treatment

The nonpharmacologic management of Alzheimer disease includes aggressively treating possible factors contributing to disease progression, such as sleep disorders (including obstructive sleep apnea) and cardiovascular disease; risk factors for cardiovascular disease also should be addressed. Adhering to an exercise program should be encouraged. Dietary recommendations for slowing cognitive decline in Alzheimer disease or MCI remain uncertain. Given the links between cardiovascular disease risk factors and Alzheimer disease, it is generally recommended that affected patients follow a "heart-healthy" diet (a diet rich in whole grains, fruits, and vegetables and low in simple carbohydrates, polyunsaturated or trans-fatty acids, nitrates, and alcohol). The use of nutraceuticals (supplements enriched with nutrient precursors of many substrates for healthy brain function) has shown benefit in some, but not all, trials and remains controversial. If homocysteine levels are elevated, folic acid supplementation is recommended. There is moderate evidence showing a benefit of vitamin E (200-400 U/d) for moderate Alzheimer disease but not for MCI. No conclusive data have shown a link between statin use and development of Alzheimer disease, and meta-analyses of randomized controlled trials have shown no clear benefit or harm to cognition from statins. However, given the numerous case reports of cognitive decline after statin therapy, the FDA has issued a warning about possible worsening cognition after initiation of some statins. Clinicians should consider discontinuing statin therapy if there is a clear temporal link between starting this therapy and significant cognitive decline.

The acetylcholinesterase inhibitors donepezil, rivastigmine, and galantamine are approved for treating mild to moderate dementia in patients with Alzheimer disease and have demonstrated modest benefits in cognitive performance without clear improvements in daily functioning. These three drugs have differences in pharmacodynamics and pharmacokinetics but appear equally efficacious. Because of their possible adverse effects on conduction, acetylcholinesterase inhibitors should be used with caution or avoided in patients with bradycardia or other conduction abnormalities. A transdermal form of rivastigmine is available but should be used

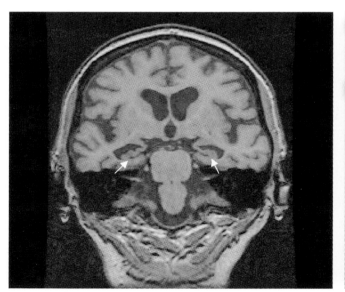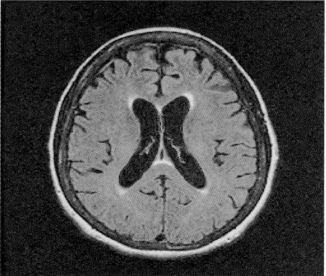

FIGURE 16. MRI findings showing bilateral hippocampal atrophy (*arrows*), which is a typical feature of Alzheimer disease, and diffuse cortical atrophy, which is recognized widening of the sulci and enlargement of the ventricles.

only after intolerance of oral forms has been established. The most common adverse effects are gastrointestinal issues, which result in discontinuation of the medication in nearly 20% of patients. Additional adverse effects include syncope, agitation, nocturnal cramps, and vivid dreams. Donepezil should be used with caution in patients with a history of seizures.

The N-methyl-D-aspartate receptor antagonist memantine is approved for moderate to severe dementia in patients with Alzheimer disease associated with significant functional impairment and is not associated with adverse cardiovascular effects. It has no established benefit in mild dementia. Some evidence suggests that combining an acetylcholinesterase inhibitor and N-methyl-D-aspartate receptor antagonist provides a synergistic benefit, but only when the latter is added at the moderate stage of dementia.

Antibodies targeting Aβ plaques represent another potential means of treatment and are the subject of current study. Preliminary clinical trials have shown that the antibody aducanumab reduces Aβ plaques in Alzheimer disease accompanied by a slowing of clinical decline.

KEY POINTS

- Evidence suggests that education, regular exercise, a Mediterranean diet, and cognitively stimulating leisure activities provide protection against developing Alzheimer disease.

- An MRI of the brain supports the diagnosis of Alzheimer disease when it shows evidence of decreased volume of the hippocampi.

- Acetylcholinesterase inhibitors have demonstrated modest benefits in cognitive performance in patients with mild to moderate Alzheimer disease without clear improvements in daily functioning; memantine is approved for moderate to severe dementia in patients with Alzheimer disease associated with significant functional impairment.

Frontotemporal Dementia

The frontotemporal dementias (FTDs), which comprise language-variant and behavioral-variant types, are the second most common cause of neurodegenerative dementia in patients younger than 65 years. The language-variant FTDs consist of the primary progressive aphasias and are discussed separately in Language-Predominant Dementias. In behavioral-variant FTD, there is a slight male predominance and shorter disease duration than in Alzheimer disease. As many as 10% of patients with behavior-variant FTD have a family history consistent with an autosomal-dominant inheritance of dementia, and as many as 30% to 40% have evidence of a family history of a dementia. Amyotrophic lateral sclerosis occurs in as many as 20% to 30% of patients with behavior-variant FTD and generally portends a much more rapid progression than other forms of FTD. The pathology underlying FTD involves

neurofibrillary tau tangles or transactive-response DNA-binding protein 43 inclusions.

The most prominent feature of behavioral-variant FTD is an alteration in personality and behavior that typically develops years before the onset of cognitive impairment. A clue to the diagnosis early in the disease is discordance between normal or near-normal performance on objective cognitive testing and a significant degree of functional impairment. Because these behaviors often manifest as obsessive-compulsive tendencies, impulsivity, apathy, and impaired judgment, patients with this disorder are often misdiagnosed as having bipolar disorder, obsessive-compulsive disorder, and depression. Other common symptoms are emotional coldness, disinhibition, excessive spending, and excessive eating, particularly of high-calorie foods. These behaviors occasionally result in legal troubles. Unlike patients with Alzheimer disease, those with behavioral-variant FTD often have poor insight into their disease.

Diagnostic criteria have been proposed, with the diagnosis of behavioral-variant FTD being established when three of the following six criteria are met: early behavioral disinhibition, early apathy or inertia, early loss of sympathy or empathy, perseverative or compulsive behaviors, hyperorality and dietary changes, and neuropsychological deficits in executive function with memory and visuospatial sparing.

Evaluation

Because cognitive testing results can be normal early in the disease course, Alzheimer disease screening tools are not helpful for evaluating FTD. When this diagnosis is suspected, detailed cognitive testing by a neuropsychologist is indicated.

Because structural lesions of the frontal lobes can result in a syndrome similar to behavioral-variant FTD, neuroimaging with MRI or CT is mandatory. Additionally, many patients with behavioral-variant FTD have frontotemporal lobe atrophy visible on imaging (**Figure 17**). If the MRI is normal, a functional brain scan (FDG-PET or perfusion SPECT) may show a pattern of prominent frontal lobe abnormalities.

A CSF evaluation also can be helpful in distinguishing FTD from Alzheimer disease because the $A\beta_{42}$ level is typically depressed in Alzheimer disease but normal in FTD.

Finally, because of the association with amyotrophic lateral sclerosis, all patients with a diagnosis of behavioral-variant FTD should be monitored closely for muscle weakness, cramping, or fasciculations.

Treatment

There are currently no approved therapies to treat behavioral-variant FTD, and clinical trials testing the effectiveness of acetylcholinesterase inhibitors and memantine have shown no benefit (and, in the case of memantine, possible detriment). Treatment is symptomatic and can involve collaboration with a psychiatrist.

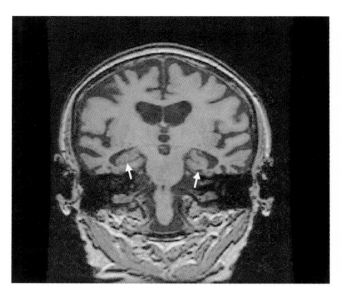
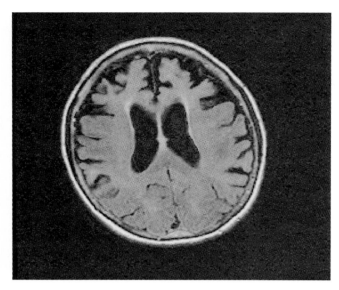

FIGURE 17. Brain MRI findings showing changes associated with frontotemporal dementia, including bilateral hippocampal atrophy (*arrows*) and more severe temporal and frontal cortical atrophy.

KEY POINT

- A clue to the diagnosis of behavioral-variant frontotemporal dementia early in the disease course is discordance between normal or near-normal performance on objective cognitive testing and a significant degree of functional impairment.

Language-Predominant Dementias

The primary progressive aphasias (PPA) are a group of neurodegenerative dementia syndromes in which a progressive impairment in language is the principal cognitive deficit and cause of functional impairment. PPAs can be subdivided into nonfluent and fluent (semantic) variants. In nonfluent PPA, patients predominantly have problems with language production; those with fluent PPA largely have problems with comprehension. Although language decline is common in many dementia syndromes, in PPA it is the symptom noted first, and language is often the only cognitive domain affected for years before the development of additional cognitive deterioration. Pathologically, the PPAs are related to FTD and Alzheimer disease but typically occur at a younger age. Because of the relationship to FTD, the fluent (semantic) variant of PPA often has significantly more behavioral symptoms than the nonfluent variant.

Evaluation

The language components of the cognitive screening evaluation are disproportionately affected in language-predominant dementias. Sentence or phrase repetition, timed word production, and object naming are all impaired. Because most cognitive tests are language based, patients with PPA often perform worse than expected given their level of day-to-day functioning (the opposite of what is seen in behavioral-variant FTD).

Structural imaging can be very helpful; attention should be paid to asymmetric involvement of the left temporal lobe, which controls language in most patients (**Figure 18**). Functional brain imaging (FDG-PET or perfusion SPECT) can identify a pattern of asymmetric hemispheric abnormality (left greater than right) in patients with inconclusive brain MRIs.

As with FTD, CSF evaluation can be helpful in diagnosing a language-predominant dementia if it identifies an Alzheimer disease pattern (decreased $A\beta_{42}$ with elevated levels of tau and phosphorylated tau), which may help with tailoring treatment.

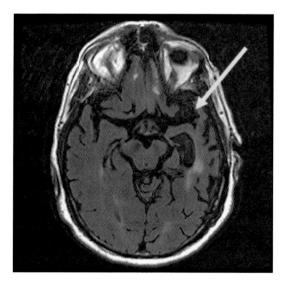

FIGURE 18. Brain MRI of a 64-year-old woman that shows severe left temporal lobe atrophy (*arrow*), consistent with fluent primary progressive aphasia.

Treatment

There are no pharmacologic therapies specifically approved for PPA. All affected patients should be assessed by a speech therapist. If language comprehension is an issue, assistive language devices can be helpful.

KEY POINT

- Because most cognitive tests are language based, patients with a primary progressive aphasia often perform worse than expected given their level of day-to-day functioning, in contrast to what is seen in behavioral-variant frontotemporal dementia.

Chronic Traumatic Encephalopathy

Chronic traumatic encephalopathy (CTE) is technically a pathologic diagnosis. Because of its relationship with a history of head injuries—most commonly, repeated head trauma—the term also is used clinically. The frontal and temporal lobes are most susceptible to damage from head trauma, and symptoms often reflect damage to these areas. CTE may develop over many years, which makes the diagnosis challenging, particularly when it occurs in patients in their sixties and seventies when the prevalence of other dementias also increases.

A major clinical feature of the disease is the greater frequency of somatic symptoms, particularly headache, that precede the onset of cognitive symptoms. Similarly, the behavioral and mood findings of apathy, irritability, impulsivity, emotional outbursts, and depression often occur before overt cognitive impairment. The cognitive pattern is often one of cognitive slowing and disorganized thought processing, with less involvement of memory and visuospatial function early in the disease course. As the disease progresses, symptoms of mild parkinsonism, such bradykinesia and gait changes, frequently occur.

Evaluation

A history of repeated head trauma is necessary for the diagnosis. Cognitive testing often will demonstrate a pattern of cognitive slowing (problems with timed tasks) as a prominent finding. In patients with more advanced disease, memory impairment may occur. No specific pattern of brain atrophy is seen on structural brain imaging, which can help differentiate CTE from FTD (which is associated with frontal lobe atrophy).

Treatment

No clinical trials comparing various treatments have been performed in CTE. Cholinergic deficits have been identified pathologically, which suggests that acetylcholinesterase inhibitors might be useful. As in behavioral-variant FTD, treatment is often symptom directed and includes Parkinson disease medications for motor symptoms, antidepressants, mood stabilizers, and (occasionally) stimulants for severe apathy. Close monitoring for suicidality also should be part of treatment strategy for patients with CTE.

KEY POINT

- The cognitive pattern typical of chronic traumatic encephalopathy is often one of cognitive slowing and disorganized thought processing, with less involvement of memory and visuospatial function early in the disease course; as the disease progresses, symptoms of mild parkinsonism, such as bradykinesia and gait changes, frequently occur.

Dementia with Lewy Bodies and Parkinson Disease Dementia

Because Parkinson disease is a progressive neurodegenerative disorder, cognitive symptoms frequently develop at some point in the disease course. When dementia occurs well after the motor symptoms, it is considered Parkinson disease dementia. When dementia and motor symptoms develop within 1 to 2 years of each other, it is classified as dementia with Lewy bodies (DLB).

DLB is the second most common neurodegenerative dementia after Alzheimer disease. α-Synuclein deposits, or Lewy bodies, are the chief pathologic feature of DLB and commonly coexist with pathologic features of Alzheimer disease. The prevalence of DLB significantly increases with age, and this dementia often progresses more rapidly than Alzheimer disease. The clinical diagnosis rests on the key features of dementia, parkinsonian motor features (particularly gait problems and slowness of movements), visual hallucinations, and frequent fluctuations in attention (**Table 28**). The latter may manifest as acute confusional episodes or brief, focal seizures with alteration of awareness (formerly known as complex partial seizures).

Distinguishing DLB from Alzheimer disease on the basis of cognition alone can be difficult, but other symptoms can help differentiate the two. Delusions and hallucinations are common and frequently occur at the mild stages of DLB. Additionally, significant sleep problems, especially daytime sleepiness, can be a debilitating feature of DLB, and rapid eye movement sleep behavior disorder is much more common.

TABLE 28. Diagnostic Features of Dementia With Lewy Bodies	
Features	**Specific Symptoms**
Central feature	Dementia
Core features	Parkinsonism, fluctuations in attention, and recurrent visual hallucinations
Suggestive features	Rapid eye movement sleep behavior disorder and (typically) severe neuroleptic sensitivity
Supportive features	Transient episodes of loss of consciousness, significant daytime somnolence, severe delusions (especially early in dementia course), apathy, repeated falls, and orthostatic hypotension

Making the diagnosis of DLB as early as possible is important because the behavioral problems associated with this condition frequently result in the use of antipsychotic agents. Many patients with DLB are extremely sensitive to neuroleptic medications, particularly first-generation agents, and are at high risk for developing a severe worsening of symptoms resembling neuroleptic malignant syndrome.

Evaluation

The evaluation of DLB is similar to that of the other dementia syndromes, and the cognitive impairment is often similar to that of Alzheimer disease. CSF evaluation is often inconclusive in DLB. The best diagnostic tools remain the clinical history and examination.

Treatment

Although not formally approved for DLB, acetylcholinesterase inhibitors can be effective in treating the cognitive symptoms of the disorder, according to expert opinion. Rivastigmine has been approved for treating Parkinson disease dementia but not DLB; there is no evidence that memantine is beneficial. The treatment of behavioral symptoms is often necessary, but first-generation antipsychotic agents are strongly contraindicated. In the case of severe hypersomnolence, stimulant-type medications can be considered.

KEY POINTS

- The clinical diagnosis of dementia with Lewy bodies rests on the key features of dementia, parkinsonian motor features (particularly gait problems and slowness of movements), visual hallucinations, and frequent fluctuations in attention.

- Many patients with dementia with Lewy bodies are extremely sensitive to neuroleptic medications, particularly first-generation agents, and are at high risk for developing a severe worsening of symptoms resembling neuroleptic malignant syndrome.

Treatment Approach to Neurobehavioral Symptoms of Dementia

Behavioral and psychiatric symptoms of dementia are a common problem in patients with dementia disorders and are among the most common reasons for admission to long-term care facilities. Nonpharmacologic environmental and behavioral treatments should be emphasized for these patients, although some pharmacologic therapies may improve function and patient safety. Antidepressant agents should be considered the first-line therapy for symptoms related to mood and anxiety. If appropriate, acetylcholinesterase inhibitors also may be tried early in the disease course. Benzodiazepines should be avoided, except in cases of extreme anxiety.

The use of antipsychotic agents to treat behavioral and psychiatric symptoms of dementia should be considered on an individual basis. Strong evidence links use of antipsychotic agents with increased mortality in older persons with dementia. At the same time, there is evidence of benefit for certain antipsychotic agents (such as risperidone, aripiprazole, and olanzapine). If antipsychotic agents are needed, newer-generation medications should be started at low doses with a regimented titration and a plan for regular follow-up evaluation and dose decreases. These drugs are associated with an increased risk of sudden death (likely cardiac), especially in the first 3 to 6 months of taking the medication; this risk should be clearly discussed with families before initiating the therapy and only after all other treatments have been tried. It is also advisable to obtain an electrocardiogram before the first dose to ensure that the patient's QT interval is normal; if the corrected QT interval is prolonged (>450 ms for men and >470 ms for women), antipsychotic agents should not be used.

Nonneurodegenerative Dementias

Two of the most common nonneurodegenerative dementias are normal pressure hydrocephalus (NPH) and vascular cognitive impairment. Both share the symptoms of prominent gait impairment and a pattern of cognitive slowing with less memory impairment.

Normal Pressure Hydrocephalus

NPH is characterized by the triad of gait changes, urinary incontinence, and cognitive impairment. Gait impairment, the most prominent feature, is characterized by a wide-based gait, short step length, and often problems with starting ambulation (hesitation).

Evaluation

Gait changes can occur for multiple reasons and in several neurodegenerative diseases, so recognition of the gait pattern specific for NPH is crucial. Similarly, alternative causes for urinary incontinence should be excluded. Cognitive testing typically reveals a pattern of slowing and executive cognitive impairment; some patients may require formal neuropsychological testing.

A brain MRI or CT scan should be obtained because NPH cannot be diagnosed without evidence of ventriculomegaly (**Figure 19**). Lumbar puncture with high-volume (30-50 mL) CSF removal and determination of opening pressure also is required. A timed gait evaluation should be performed just before CSF removal and within 60 minutes after removal. Objective improvement in gait after CSF removal is an accurate predictor of NPH improvement with shunting.

Treatment

CSF diversion through a ventriculoperitoneal shunt is the definitive treatment. Gait disturbance is the clinical symptom most amenable to ventricular shunting. The longer cognitive impairment has been present and the more pronounced the memory problem, the less certain is the response to shunting. If response to high-volume CSF removal is uncertain, referral to a neurosurgeon for a lumbar drain can be pursued. In the

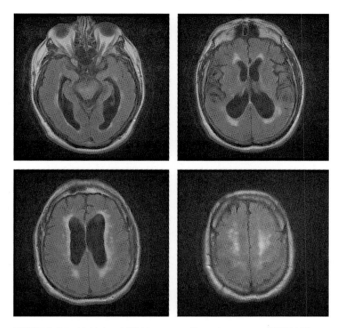

FIGURE 19. Multiple axial fluid-attenuated inversion recovery (FLAIR) MRIs of a 68-year-old man that show ventriculomegaly, little cortical atrophy, and mild periventricular FLAIR hyperintensities, all consistent with normal pressure hydrocephalus.

absence of a clear response to either high-volume CSF removal or lumbar drainage, a permanent ventricular shunt should not be pursued, and another diagnosis should be considered.

KEY POINTS

- Normal pressure hydrocephalus is characterized by the triad of gait changes, urinary incontinence, and cognitive impairment.

- Normal pressure hydrocephalus cannot be diagnosed without evidence of ventriculomegaly (enlarged cerebral ventricles) on a brain MRI or CT scan of the head; cerebrospinal fluid diversion through a ventriculoperitoneal shunt is the definitive treatment.

Vascular Cognitive Impairment

Vascular cognitive impairment encompasses a category of disorders in which the causal link between cerebrovascular disease and cognitive impairment is strong. In older populations, vascular cognitive impairment is likely second only to Alzheimer disease as the most common primary cause of dementia (but not of neurodegenerative dementia; see earlier discussion of dementia with Lewy bodies). This disorder may occur concurrently with Alzheimer disease in older patients.

The likelihood of vascular cognitive impairment increases with age and is associated with systemic vascular risk factors and a history of stroke (either clinically diagnosed or based on neuroimaging evidence). Several features distinguish vascular cognitive impairment from Alzheimer disease (see Table 27). Two major signs of vascular cognitive impairment are early

gait impairment and pseudobulbar affect ("emotional incontinence") that can manifest as excessive crying or laughter disproportionate to the context of the situation and is abrupt in onset and discontinuation.

Evaluation

Evaluation of vascular cognitive impairment relies on identification of vascular risk factors and, particularly, previous stroke. Abrupt changes in cognition and a cognitive pattern of disproportionate cognitive slowing compared with memory impairment are often noted.

As with NPH, brain imaging is a critical component supporting the diagnosis. In vascular cognitive impairment, MRIs typically display a pattern of diffuse and confluent changes in the white matter of the brain (**Figure 20**), cerebral microhemorrhages, and/or cortical infarcts beyond the mild periventricular hyperintensities commonly seen in older patients. The presence of severe extracranial or intracranial vascular disease also supports this diagnosis.

Treatment

Medications useful in treating Alzheimer disease are not approved for use in vascular cognitive impairment. However, some evidence suggests a modest benefit of the acetylcholinesterase inhibitors in vascular cognitive impairment, and treatment with this class of medications is generally recommended. Trials with memantine additionally indicated a modest cognitive benefit. However, aggressive treatment of vascular risk factors may be most beneficial.

KEY POINT

- Two major signs of vascular cognitive impairment are early gait impairment and pseudobulbar affect.

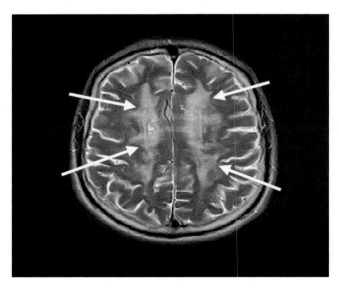

FIGURE 20. Axial T2-weighted MRI of the brain showing diffuse subcortical white matter hyperdensities (*arrows*) in the bilateral hemispheres. These findings are consistent with a severe microangiopathy seen in advanced vascular cognitive impairment.

Rapidly Progressive Dementia

Because of the many possibly treatable causes of rapidly progressive dementia, a systematic approach is required and can identify the underlying cause in most patients. The differential diagnosis includes Creutzfeldt-Jakob disease (CJD), paraneoplastic syndromes, autoimmune/inflammatory encephalopathy (lupus encephalopathy, Sjögren syndrome, Hashimoto encephalopathy, multiple sclerosis), granulomatous disease (central nervous system sarcoidosis, Behçet syndrome, neurosyphilis), vasculitis (primary or secondary), some infections (HIV, herpes simplex virus, *Borrelia burgdorferi*-caused disease), and toxicities (from alcohol or drug abuse, exposure to heavy metals).

CJD is a potentially transmissible prion-related disorder that often presents with rapidly progressive dementia. Time from disease onset to death is approximately 12 months in as many as 80% of patients with CJD. The rapid cognitive decline seen with this disorder is associated with myoclonus, gait problems, and interruption of the circadian rhythm. MRI is one of the most sensitive diagnostic tools for CJD, typically showing a pattern of increased intensity in the diffusion-weighted sequence in the basal ganglia and various cortical regions. Periodic sharp wave complexes are often seen on electroencephalography and are helpful but not necessary in making the diagnosis. CSF testing may establish the presence of 14-3-3 protein and an elevation in total tau protein levels.

Paraneoplastic syndromes can also present with rapidly progressive dementia, and many of these disorders are treatable if diagnosed early (see Neuro-oncology for further discussion of these syndromes).

KEY POINT

- MRI is one of the most sensitive diagnostic tools for Creutzfeldt-Jakob disease and typically shows a pattern of an increased intensity in the diffusion-weighted sequence in the basal ganglia and various cortical regions.

Delirium

Although rarely considered in the same light as acute dysfunction of other major organs, delirium is an acute alteration of brain function and should be approached with the same intent of alleviating the dysfunction as rapidly as possible. The clinical consequences of delirium are substantial because delirium is associated with greater hospital morbidity, more medical complications, longer lengths of stay, and a higher rate of discharge to long-term care facilities. The frequency of delirium depends on the setting and the patient population. Postsurgical and ICU patients, particularly older populations, have the highest prevalence of delirium. Risk also increases with the presence of baseline dementia, multiple medical problems, polypharmacy, and hypoxia.

Prevention of delirium is likely more effective than treatment of established delirium. In hospitalized patients, providing patients with assistive visual and hearing devices, adequately controlling pain, limiting psychoactive medications, frequent orientation, encouraging mobility, and enabling uninterrupted sleep on a normal sleep-wake cycle may help decrease the likelihood of developing delirium.

Delirium presents with numerous and variable symptoms and signs (**Table 29**). The core of delirium is an alteration in the arousal system (that is, in the ascending reticular activating system of the midbrain, thalamus, and hypothalamus that modulates sleep-wake transitions). Fluctuations in mental status, altered circadian rhythm, and poor attention are the hallmarks of the clinical syndrome. The Confusion Assessment Method is a useful tool with good sensitivity for diagnosing delirium. It includes assessment of onset and course, inattention, disorganized thinking, and level of consciousness.

Delirium also has a multitude of causes (**Table 30**), and almost any acute medical condition may provoke delirium in a susceptible patient. Evaluation for the underlying cause of delirium is mandatory but often difficult because the patient may not be able to direct the evaluation. Consideration should always be given to life-threatening causes of delirium, including vascular events and infection. Neuroimaging may be necessary, and in the appropriate setting, electroencephalography can be used to ensure that seizures are not the cause of the confusion.

Treatment

The primary treatment of delirium is identification and treatment of the underlying cause. Use of sedating medications, such as benzodiazepines and haloperidol, should be avoided because they may cause or worsen delirium. In severe cases, and especially when safety is a concern, newer-generation antipsychotic agents may help control behavior. Additionally, increasing evidence suggests that the melatonin receptor agonist ramelteon may be useful. The effectiveness of acetylcholinesterase inhibitors remains uncertain.

TABLE 29. Clinical Features of Delirium
Fluctuations in mentation
Hypervigilance more than hypovigilance
Disorganized thoughts
Delusions
Hallucinations
Poorly sustained attention
Altered circadian rhythm
Tremors (with occasional myoclonus)
Hyperreflexia
Motor restlessness more than stupor
Amnesia
Increased sympathetic tone (particularly with alcohol withdrawal)

TABLE 30.	Causes of Delirium

Drugs

  Prescription medications (such as psychotropic medications, opioids, sedative hypnotics, anticonvulsants, antiparkinsonian agents, glucocorticoids, immunosuppressants, antiarrhythmics, antihypertensive agents, skeletal muscle relaxants, antibiotics)

  Nonprescription medications (such as NSAIDs, antihistamines)

  General anesthesia

  Alcohol or drug withdrawal

Central nervous system diseases

  Seizure, including nonconvulsive status epilepticus

  Acute ischemic infarction

  Intracranial hemorrhage

  Head injury

Metabolic disorders

  Electrolyte disturbance

  Hyperglycemia or hypoglycemia

  Hypoxemia

  Hypercarbia

  Organ failure (such as cardiac failure, kidney impairment, liver failure)

  Endocrine (such as hypothyroidism, hyperthyroidism, hyperparathyroidism, Cushing syndrome, adrenal insufficiency)

  Nutritional (such as malnourishment, vitamin B_{12} deficiency, thiamine deficiency, niacin deficiency)

Cardiovascular disease

  Myocardial infarction

  Hypertensive emergency

  Dysrhythmias

Infections[a]

Surgery

Trauma

Environment

  Post-acute care setting

  ICU

Other

  Acute blood loss

  Uncontrolled pain

  Fecal impaction

  Urinary retention

[a]Such as urinary tract infections, respiratory infections, cellulitis, meningitis or encephalitis, and sepsis.

KEY POINT

- The confusion assessment method is a useful tool with good sensitivity for diagnosing delirium; treatment is identification and treatment of the underlying causes.

Movement Disorders

Overview of Movement Disorders

Movement disorders are characterized by hypokinetic and hyperkinetic patterns of motor output. The most typical hypokinetic pattern, parkinsonism, is characterized by paucity and slowness of movements. Hyperkinetic disorders are categorized on the basis of the type of involuntary excessive movements displayed (**Table 31**).

Neurologic examination of movement disorders should include detailed assessment of motor function and gait. The key features in the classification of movement disorders are the speed, amplitude, and fatigability of voluntary movements and the rhythmicity, suppressibility, randomness, and directionality of hyperkinetic movements. Muscle tone should be assessed for rigidity, which is an increase in resistance to passive movements that is independent of the velocity and direction of those movements. Gait examination should consider the base of standing, pace of ambulation, stride length, foot clearance off the ground, postural stability, and arm swing.

KEY POINT

- The key features in the classification of movement disorders are the speed, amplitude, and fatigability of voluntary movements and the rhythmicity, suppressibility, randomness, and directionality of hyperkinetic movements.

Hypokinetic Movement Disorders

The most common type of hypokinetic movement disorder is parkinsonism. Parkinson disease is the most common form of parkinsonism; Parkinson-plus syndromes combine features of parkinsonism with other features found in the patient's history or physical examination. Vascular parkinsonism results from microvascular disease or large strokes and is characterized by predominant gait impairment with relative sparing of upper extremities. Parkinsonism also may arise as an adverse effect of medication. Some patients with normal pressure hydrocephalus exhibit parkinsonism with gait instability, dementia, and urinary incontinence (see Cognitive Impairment).

Parkinson Disease

Parkinson disease is a slowly progressive neurodegenerative disorder involving the gradual loss of dopamine-producing neurons in the substantia nigra. Pathologic findings include the aggregation of α-synuclein protein and formation of Lewy body inclusions in the substantia nigra and other brain regions. Both genetic influences and exposure to certain environmental factors, including pesticides, can increase the risk for Parkinson disease. Aging is a major risk factor.

Clinical Features of Parkinson Disease

Parkinson disease has four cardinal signs: tremor at rest, bradykinesia, rigidity, and gait/balance impairment. Resting

TABLE 31. Classification of Movement Disorders

Movement Type	Clinical Features	Examples
Hypokinetic		
Parkinsonism	Cardinal features: bradykinesia/hypokinesia, rigidity, rest tremor, postural instability Additional features: freezing gait, stooped posture, masked face, hypophonia, micrographia	Parkinson disease, Parkinson-plus syndromes, dementia with Lewy bodies, vascular parkinsonism, hydrocephalus, medication-induced parkinsonism, Wilson disease, young-onset Huntington disease
Hyperkinetic		
Tremor	Rhythmic oscillations of a body part, can occur at rest or with action (including postural or kinetic) Intention tremor is characterized by marked increase in tremor amplitude near target	Rest tremor: parkinsonism Postural and kinetic tremor: essential tremor, enhanced physiologic tremor Intention tremor: cerebellar
Dystonia	Sustained or intermittent, stereotyped, and directional twisting and posturing movements of various body parts; can be associated with sensory trick ("geste antagoniste" or movement or touch that interrupts dystonia)	Primary: primary generalized dystonia (DYT1), dopa-responsive dystonia, torticollis, blepharospasm, writer's cramp Secondary: basal ganglia lesion, anoxic injury, postencephalitic, cerebral palsy, medications
Chorea	Random, nonrepetitive, quick, unsustained, purposeless movements with a flowing dance-like pattern	Huntington disease, neuroacanthocytosis, poststreptococcal, chorea gravidarum, autoimmune, metabolic, vascular, medications
Hemiballismus	Unilateral high-amplitude proximal flailing, ballistic, choreiform movements of limbs	Lesions of contralateral subthalamic or adjacent parts of basal ganglia (often stroke)
Athetosis	Slow convoluted writhing movements of digits and toes Pseudoathetosis similar but elicited by eye closure	Early-life damage to basal ganglia (hypoxia, kernicterus, vascular event) Pseudoathetosis caused by lesions of proprioceptive pathway
Tic	Stereotyped, brief, purposeless, rapid movements that break the flow of normal movements; can be simple or complex, motor or vocal; premonitory sensory urges, suggestibility, and suppressibility Stereotypy is a coordinated ritualistic and highly repetitive movement	Tourette syndrome, autism, developmental delay syndromes, Huntington disease, medications Stereotypy can be normal in young children or associated with developmental delay and neurometabolic syndromes
Myoclonus	Rapid, shock-like, jerky movement of isolated body parts or whole body	Metabolic, medications, infections, autoimmune, myoclonic epilepsies, benign essential myoclonus, corticobasal degeneration, Alzheimer disease, prion disease, sleep-related (hypnic jerks)
Akathisia	Inner restlessness associated with repetitive movements	Drug-induced, restless legs syndrome
Psychogenic	Highly variable, inconsistent, distractible, acute onset, episodic, with variable frequency of tremor, with fixed dystonia, with acrobatic uneconomic gait (astasia-abasia)	Conversion disorder (functional neurological symptom disorder), malingering, somatoform disorder

tremor is characteristically unilateral at onset and remains asymmetric. The tremor typically emerges after few seconds of outstretched posturing of the arms and during ambulation. Bradykinesia is characterized by slowness and gradual lessening of the amplitude of repetitive movements. This feature often is associated with reductions in facial expression and arm swing. Small handwriting (micrographia) is common, and patients may report difficulty with both fine and gross movements. Rigidity, manifesting as increased resistance to movement, is often asymmetric and may occur on the same side as tremor. It may be "cogwheel" with intermittent release of the rigidity with passive movement, resulting in a jerking or ratcheting quality of movement. As many as 30% of patients with Parkinson disease have a tremor-free akinetic rigid syndrome at presentation. Gait disturbance manifests as a slow, narrow-based, and shuffling gait with associated reduced arm swings, stooped posture, and imbalance when turning. As the disease progresses, severe freezing of gait and postural instability are noted. In contrast, cerebellar ataxic gait is characterized by a wide base, frequent truncal swaying and veering, and impaired tandem walking in a straight line. Additional cerebellar signs, such as nystagmus, scanning speech, and extremity dysmetria, also may be seen in cerebellar disorders. Early prominent postural instability with frequent falls suggests a Parkinson-plus condition.

Parkinson disease also is associated with various nonmotor symptoms, ranging from autonomic dysfunction to problems with sleep, mood, and cognition (**Table 32**). Premotor symptoms, including hyposmia (diminished sense

TABLE 32. Nonmotor Symptoms of Parkinson Disease

Category	Nonmotor Symptoms
Cognitive	Bradyphrenia (slow processing), mild subcortical cognitive impairment (slow processing speed, impaired short-term memory, and attention deficits with relative sparing of cortical functions, such as language and declarative memory), dementia possible at advanced stages
Affective and behavioral	Primary: depression, anxiety, apathy, pseudobulbar affect (emotional incontinence)
	Medication-induced: psychosis, impulse control disorder, punding (purposeless stereotyped behavior), dopamine dysregulation syndrome (craving for dopaminergic medications)
Sleep related	Sleep fragmentation, sleep-wake reversal, rapid eye movement sleep behavior disorder, restless legs syndrome, medication-related sedation and sleep attacks, fatigue
Autonomic	Constipation, postural hypotension, bladder and sexual dysfunction, sialorrhea, seborrhea, excessive sweating, hyposmia or anosmia
Musculoskeletal	Truncal and cervical stooped posturing, camptocormia (truncal flexion during standing and walking), frozen shoulder, dystonic joint deformities in hands and toes, and fall-related injuries
Pain related	Painful dystonia, painful rigidity, mechanical pain, central and visceral pain

of smell), constipation, and rapid eye movement (REM) sleep behavior disorder, may precede onset of motor symptoms by years.

Cognitive impairment in Parkinson disease is not uncommon and initially involves mild subcortical deficits, especially in processing speed, short-term memory, and attention domains. Cortical functions, such as language and declarative memory, are relatively spared. As many as a third of patients may develop dementia in the later stages of Parkinson disease,

but early cognitive impairment is a red flag pointing to other diagnoses, such as dementia with Lewy bodies (see Cognitive Impairment).

Diagnosis of Parkinson Disease

The diagnosis of Parkinson disease requires the presence of bradykinesia and at least one other cardinal feature and the absence of red flags for atypical forms of parkinsonism (**Table 33**). Brain imaging is recommended to rule out

TABLE 33. Red Flags for Atypical Forms of Parkinsonism

Red Flags	Features	Likely Alternative Diagnosis
Dysautonomia	Prominent orthostatic hypotension, urinary incontinence, impotence, inappropriate sweating (mild autonomic deficits can been seen in early Parkinson disease)	MSA
Abnormal eye movements	Supranuclear vertical gaze palsy (which can be overcome by oculocephalic maneuver), slowness of vertical saccades	PSP
Prominent early cognitive impairment	Dementia within first year of onset (mild cognitive impairment common in Parkinson disease; dementia may develop in a notable subgroup of patients in advanced stages)	DLB but sometimes PSP or vascular parkinsonism
Visual hallucinations	Early and not provoked by medications (levodopa-induced hallucinations can be seen in Parkinson disease, especially in later stages)	DLB
Early prominent postural instability and falls	Within first year of onset	MSA, PSP
Prominent gait ataxia	With or without additional cerebellar deficits (dysmetria, nystagmus)	MSA
Symmetric or markedly asymmetric involvement	In Parkinson disease, characteristically asymmetric at onset and throughout its course	
	Lack of asymmetry indicative of atypical parkinsonism	MSA, PSP
	Very severe asymmetric involvement, possibly suggestive of corticobasal degeneration, and usually associated with severe fixed dystonic posturing, myoclonus, apraxia, and sensory cortical deficits	CBD
Rapid onset and step-wise deterioration	More suggestive of vascular parkinsonism (Parkinson disease is associated with slow onset and gradual course)	Vascular parkinsonism
Lack of response to levodopa[a]	Most important red flag of atypical parkinsonism	MSA, PSP, CBD, vascular parkinsonism

CBD = corticobasal degeneration; DLB = dementia with Lewy bodies; MSA = multiple system atrophy; PSP = progressive supranuclear palsy.

[a]Must not be secondary to adverse effects or insufficient dosing of medication.

vascular disease and hydrocephalus. A dopamine transporter scan, such as a single-photon emission CT scan of the brain using ioflupane-123 ligand, can be used as a confirmatory test. Its use, however, should be limited to select patients in whom the differentiation between Parkinson disease and essential tremor or drug-induced parkinsonism is not possible on clinical grounds. The test cannot distinguish between Parkinson disease and Parkinson-plus conditions. A therapeutic trial of levodopa also can help when the diagnosis is in question; patients with Parkinson disease usually respond well, but other disorders rarely improve with levodopa.

Depression and Fall Screening

All patients with Parkinson disease should be screened for depression and be assessed for fall risk. Depression and anxiety are common nonmotor symptoms of Parkinson disease and can be detected by using common clinical mood and anxiety scales. Treatments include psychotherapy, antidepressants (excluding antipsychotic agents), and dopaminergic medications (when mood symptoms correlate with motor symptoms). Depression should be distinguished from apathy, a state of reduced motivation and goal-directed behavior that is not associated with emotional distress.

Falls in Parkinson disease may be related to postural imbalance, insufficient control of motor symptoms, or orthostatic hypotension. Detection of risk factors for falling and implementation of a multidisciplinary approach–including medications, therapy, supportive devices, and education–can reduce morbidity and costs related to falls. Postural stability can be best assessed by the pull test, in which an examiner throws the patient off balance by pulling backward on the shoulders. A positive test, characterized by toppling into examiner's arms or taking more than two corrective steps, is the most reliable predictor of a risk of backward falls.

Treatment of Parkinson Disease

Currently, no medication with established efficacy is available to slow the progression of Parkinson disease. Rigorous daily exercise can improve the quality of gait and balance and also may provide disease-modifying benefits.

Symptomatic treatments include medications (**Table 34**), surgical therapy, and supportive measures. Dopaminergic medications (various formulations of the dopamine precursor levodopa, pramipexole, ropinirole, and rotigotine) are the mainstay in the treatment of motor symptoms. Several other medications can supplement the dopaminergic agents and help reduce the medication-induced complications that may emerge over time as Parkinson disease progresses (see Table 34).

Dopamine agonists, such as pramipexole and ropinirole, are the preferred initial first-line dopaminergic

medications in patients younger than 65 years and may be used with levodopa as an adjunct treatment at any point in the disease course. Many experts encourage the use of dopamine agonists in younger patients to decrease long-term exposure to levodopa and to delay the onset of levodopa-related complications. Patients taking dopamine agonists should be warned about impulse control disorder, which manifests as a tendency to engage in out-of-character impulsive behaviors, such as excessive gambling, overspending, and hypersexuality. Other adverse effects include sleep attacks, dependent edema, nausea, hallucinations, and confusion.

Eventually, all patients with Parkinson disease will require levodopa. The drug should be started as initial therapy in older patients and as replacement or additional therapy in younger patients with insufficient response to dopamine agonists. Carbidopa, a peripheral decarboxylase inhibitor, blocks the adverse effects of levodopa outside the brain and is used in combination with levodopa. Motor fluctuations, such as the "wearing-off" phenomenon (loss of the beneficial effect of the medication before the next dose is administered) and medication-induced dyskinesia (involuntary choreic movements), are common problems with levodopa. These complications emerge in as many as 50% of patients treated for more than 5 years with levodopa and may reflect disease progression rather than duration of exposure to levodopa.

Several formulations of levodopa are commercially available, including oral immediate-release, extended-release, and rapidly disintegrating formulations; an enteral gel infusion also has recently become available (see Table 34). The immediate-release formulations of levodopa have a rapid peak dose effect that many patients find helpful. The newer extended-release formulations may provide a more sustained control of symptoms throughout the day, which can prove beneficial by reducing any wearing off between doses. Wearing off also can be lessened by frequent dosing of levodopa and by the addition of dopamine agonists, catechol-O-methyltransferase inhibitors, or monamine oxidase B inhibitors. Amantadine can be added to the treatment regimen to prevent dyskinesia. Anticholinergic medications also can be added to provide additional benefit in patients with prominent tremor or dystonia; adverse events, such as urinary retention, constipation, tachycardia, and memory impairment, are limiting factors, especially in older patients with dementia. Finally, droxidopa, a norepinephrine precursor, can improve neurogenic orthostatic hypotension.

Medication-induced psychosis, especially visual hallucinations, also can occur with use of dopaminergic medications. Treatment strategies include addressing any systemic trigger, simplifying the medication regimen (including removal of non-levodopa medications and decreasing the levodopa dosage), and, if needed, using antipsychotic agents. Pimavanserin, a selective serotonin 5-HT2b receptor inverse agonist, is the

TABLE 34. Medications for Parkinson Disease

Class	Forms	Clinical Indication
Dopamine precursor	Levodopa	Most effective treatment for motor deficits
		Initial therapy in patients older than 65 years or those with severe motor symptoms, freezing, or falls
		Second-line treatment in younger patients who have failed dopamine agonists
Oral	Immediate-release levodopa	Maintenance therapy during waking hours, peak effect provides good "on"-time benefit
	Continued-release levodopa	Nighttime therapy
	Extended-release carbidopa-levodopa	Maintenance therapy if immediate-release formulation causes motor fluctuations and dyskinesia
	Orally disintegrating levodopa	Rapid relief of sudden "off"-time
Enteral gel	Enteral levodopa	Maintenance therapy in advanced Parkinson disease associated with severe motor complications of immediate-release levodopa, provides sustained levodopa release, can cause a higher rate of gastrointestinal complications
Decarboxylase inhibitors	Carbidopa, benserazide[a]	Suppression of peripheral adverse effects of levodopa
Dopamine agonists		
Oral	Pramipexole, ropinirole, cabergoline[a]	First-line treatment in younger patients, adjuvant therapy to limit total dose of levodopa
Patch	Rotigotine	Similar to oral forms
Subcutaneous injection	Apomorphine	Rapid relief of sudden "off"-time
Catechol-O-methyltransferase inhibitors	Entacapone (often used), tolcapone (hepatic toxicity)	Counteracting of wearing-off phenomenon, prolongation of levodopa effect
Monoamine oxidase type B inhibitors	Selegiline, rasagiline, safinamide	Initial therapy in mild cases, potentiation of levodopa effect, tremor
Glutamate NMDA antagonist	Amantadine, rimantidine	Dyskinesia, tremor, fatigue
Anticholinergic agents	Trihexyphenidyl, benztropine	Tremor, mild benefit against parkinsonism, higher adverse effect profile in old age and dementia
Antipsychotic agents	Pimavanserin, quetiapine	Medication-induced psychosis, medication-reduction strategies should be prioritized, increased mortality risk in patients with dementia
Norepinephrine precursor	Droxidopa	Neurogenic orthostatic hypotension, requires coadministration with carbidopa; other measures (including liberal salt intake, fludrocortisone, and midodrine) also are effective

NMDA = N-methyl-D-aspartate.

[a]Available in Europe but not the United States.

only FDA-approved medication for Parkinson psychosis; quetiapine and clozapine also are often used as less expensive, albeit off-label, options.

In patients with severe motor complications, enteral infusion of carbidopa-levodopa gel through a jejunal tube with a portable pump can provide more sustained levodopa release and reduce motor complications. High rates of gastrointestinal and tube-related complications are limiting factors.

Deep brain stimulation (DBS) is a surgical therapy that involves the delivery of electrical stimulation to key brain targets, such as the subthalamic nucleus and the globus pallidus interna. The stimulation disrupts the abnormal neurophysiologic activity within the basal ganglia and simulates a patient's response to medications. This mode of treatment is indicated for patients who continue to benefit from levodopa but experience severe motor fluctuations or have a refractory tremor. An algorithm for selection of appropriate candidates for DBS surgery is shown in **Figure 21**. Given the evidence of improved quality of life after early implementation of DBS, the FDA has expanded the indication for this procedure to patients with Parkinson disease of 4 years' duration who experience early motor fluctuations.

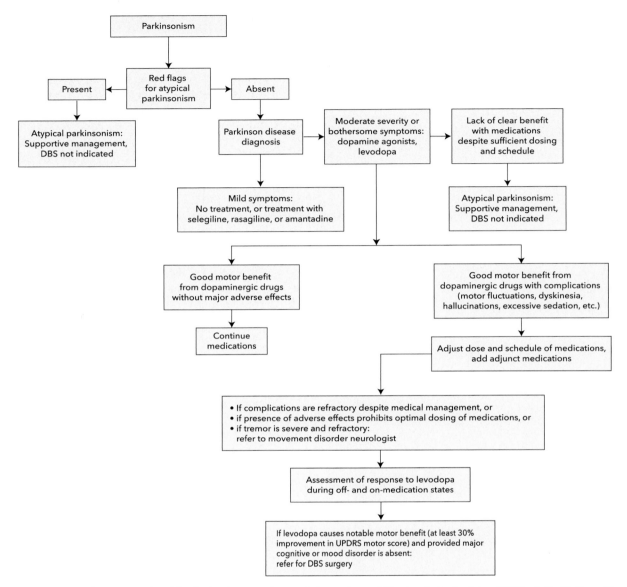

FIGURE 21. Algorithm for evaluation of candidacy for deep brain stimulation in Parkinson disease. DBS = deep brain stimulation; UPDRS = Unified Parkinson Disease Rating Scale.

KEY POINTS

- The diagnosis of Parkinson disease requires the presence of bradykinesia and at least one of the other cardinal features of the disorder (tremor at rest, cogwheel rigidity, and gait or balance impairment) and the absence of red flags for atypical forms of parkinsonism.

HVC • In Parkinson disease, a dopamine transporter scan, such as single-photon emission CT of the brain, is unnecessary except to differentiate between Parkinson disease and essential tremor or drug-induced parkinsonism if the distinction cannot be made on clinical grounds.

(Continued)

KEY POINTS (continued)

- Detection of risk factors for falling and implementation **HVC** of a multidisciplinary approach—including medications, therapy, supportive devices, and education—can reduce morbidity and costs related to falls; a positive pull test is the most reliable predictor of a risk of backward falls in Parkinson disease.

- Dopamine agonists are the preferred initial first-line medication in patients younger than 65 years and levodopa is the preferred initial therapy in older patients.

- Deep brain stimulation is indicated for patients who continue to benefit from levodopa but experience severe motor fluctuations or have a refractory tremor.

Parkinson-Plus Syndromes

Parkinson-plus syndromes typically present with a combination of parkinsonism and additional features that are atypical for idiopathic Parkinson disease. These conditions often are more rapidly progressive than Parkinson disease and less responsive to standard therapies, particularly levodopa. The primary syndromes include progressive supranuclear palsy, multiple system atrophy (formerly Shy-Drager syndrome, acquired olivopontocerebellar atrophy, and striatonigral degeneration), and corticobasal degeneration. Patients with progressive supranuclear palsy have parkinsonism, impairment in both ocular range of movement and saccades (very fast jumps from one eye position to another, particularly in the vertical direction), facial dystonia, axial rigidity, and prominent postural instability with early falls. Multiple system atrophy presents with a combination of parkinsonism, ataxia, and severe dysautonomia and also is associated with early falls. Corticobasal degeneration often presents with markedly asymmetric parkinsonism and frequently is associated with dystonia, myoclonus, cortical sensory deficits, cognitive deficits, and apraxia (impaired motor planning).

KEY POINT

- Parkinson-plus syndromes often are more rapidly progressive than Parkinson disease, have additional features that are atypical for idiopathic Parkinson disease, and are less responsive to standard antiparkinsonian therapies, particularly levodopa.

Drug-Induced Parkinsonism

A number of drugs, especially dopamine receptor–blocking antipsychotic agents, can cause parkinsonism (**Table 35**). Drug-induced parkinsonism is symmetric, lacks nonmotor features, and is reversible after removal of the causative agent. Several other extrapyramidal complications of dopamine-receptor blockers have also been described (**Table 36**).

TABLE 35. Medications Causing Drug-Induced Parkinsonism

Medication Class	Examples
Common	
Antipsychotics	Typical: haloperidol, chlorpromazine
	Atypical: risperidone, olanzapine, ziprasidone, aripiprazole
Antiemetics	Metoclopramide, prochlorperazine
Dopamine depleters	Tetrabenazine, reserpine
Uncommon	
Mood stabilizers, antiepileptic agents	Lithium, valproic acid
Other	Amiodarone, flunarizine, SSRIs (including fluoxetine)

SSRI = selective serotonin reuptake inhibitor.

TABLE 36. Extrapyramidal Complications of Dopamine Receptor Blockers

Type of Movement Disorder	Symptoms
Acute reactions (reversible)	
Acute dystonia	Immediate dystonic spasms; often involves neck, face, larynx, and eyes (oculogyric crisis); rapid reversal with intravenous diphenhydramine
Acute akathisia	Immediate sensation of restlessness with urge to constantly move and pace
Subacute or chronic syndromes (reversible)	
Parkinsonism	Similar to Parkinson disease, dose dependent, resolves within months after removal of the offending agent, symmetry and absence of nonmotor features favors a drug-induced over an idiopathic cause
Tardive syndromes (late onset, may be irreversible)	
Tardive dyskinesia	Repetitive stereotyped choreiform movements, oral-buccal-lingual predominance (tongue protrusion, lip smacking, puckering and chewing movements), also can affect the extremities (piano playing movements, foot tapping) and trunk (including respiratory muscles)
Tardive dystonia	Sustained dystonic posturing commonly affecting the face, neck, trunk, and arms; extensor cervical and axial dystonia
Tardive akathisia	Chronic sensation of inner restlessness with urge to constantly move and pace, leg crossing, body rocking
Tardive tics	Clinical presentation similar to Tourette syndrome but triggered after exposure to dopamine blockers
Other Disorders	
Withdrawal emergent syndrome (reversible)	Choreiform dyskinesia starting after sudden withdrawal from a neuroleptic agent and stopping with reinstitution of the causative agent (or another agent from same class) and a subsequent slow taper within a few months; differential diagnosis of tardive dyskinesia that may be masked by antipsychotic agents and only unmasked after their removal (and may become persistent)
Neuroleptic malignant syndrome (treatable emergency)	Idiosyncratic, rapid onset and progressive, rigidity, dystonia, hyperthermia, rhabdomyolysis, altered mental status

Hyperkinetic Movement Disorders

Essential Tremor

Tremor is an oscillatory movement of a body part that is classified on the basis of its presence at rest or with action (**Table 37**). Essential tremor is the most common movement disorder and often presents with a bilateral upper extremity postural and action tremor. This type of tremor also can involve the voice, head, or legs. Common features include a positive family history (50% of patients), slow progression, and onset at either adolescence or middle age. The tremor may be alleviated by alcohol and may be aggravated by stress, illness, fatigue, or the use of caffeine or other stimulants. A minority of affected patients experience substantial progression, leading to marked disability.

The differential diagnosis includes enhanced physiologic tremor, which is a low-amplitude tremor that is unnoticeable in most people but may become prominent because of physical and psychological stressors, medications, thyroid disease, or caffeine. Assessment of any form of action tremor should include thyroid function studies and review of medications (**Table 38**). Patients younger than 40 years should undergo screening for Wilson disease with serum ceruloplasmin and 24-hour urine copper measurements, and slit-lamp examination for Kayser-Fleischer rings should be considered. Other rare causes of action tremor include dystonic tremor, rubral tremor, and fragile X–associated tremor/ataxia syndrome (see Table 37).

The treatment of essential tremor is symptomatic. Weighted utensils and wrist weights can help reduce tremor amplitude during feeding. The most effective pharmacologic treatments for essential tremor are propranolol, primidone, and topiramate. Additional second-line options include atenolol, sotalol, clonazepam, gabapentin, and nimodipine.

TABLE 37. Classification of Tremors		
Tremor Type	**Disease Association**	**Features**
Resting tremor[a]		
Parkinsonian rest tremor	Parkinson disease	Reemergence of tremor after a short delay with outstretched posturing and during ambulation, associated with other parkinsonian signs (rigidity, bradykinesia, gait impairment)
	Atypical, drug-induced, and vascular parkinsonism	Similar to Parkinson disease; tremor sometimes symmetric; red flags for atypical parkinsonism sometimes present
Dystonic tremor	Dystonia	Associated with dystonic posturing; seen both at rest and with action; task specificity seen with action; position dependent, with a null point at which tremor stops
Action tremor		
Postural and kinetic tremor[b]	Essential tremor	Present in the outstretched arm position and with various actions; commonly (but not universally) associated with a positive family history and an improvement in symptoms with ethanol
	Enhanced physiologic tremor	Normal low-amplitude, high-frequency tremor seen in association with triggers, such as stress, drugs, and thyroid disease; similar to essential tremor but resolves with resolution of underlying physiologic stressor
Intention tremor[c]	Cerebellar disease	Tremor during movements that increases in amplitude as hand approaches target (also known as terminal tremor); possible association with other cerebellar symptoms, including dysmetria
	Severe essential tremor	Terminal tremor can be seen but often without prominent cerebellar dysmetria
	Fragile X-associated tremor/ataxia syndrome	Neurodegenerative disease seen in older men who are carriers of a premutation in the fragile X intellectual disability 1 gene; typically, there is a family history of intellectual disability in young males and premature ovarian failure in females; symptoms of (intention) tremor, ataxia, parkinsonism, neuropathy and dementia
Rubral tremor	Cerebellar outflow disorders (multiple sclerosis, stroke, traumatic brain injury)	Coarse proximal tremor present at rest, worse with posturing (especially large-amplitude and proximal tremors in the wing-beating position with elbows flexed), and most severe during movements
Task-specific tremor	Primary writing tremor	Only present with specific task
Orthostatic tremor	Orthostatic tremor	High-frequency tremor emerging in the legs only during standing (orthostatic position); resolving with sitting or action

[a]Tremor present with the affected extremity resting unsupported.

[b]Postural tremor is present with the arm in an outstretched position, and kinetic tremor is present during reaching, writing, and other movements.

[c]Intention tremor is a specific subtype of kinetic tremor that becomes very prominent near target, exhibiting a crescendo of increased severity at the terminal section of the movement path.

TABLE 38. Medications Causing Drug-Induced Action Tremor

Medication Class	Examples
β-Adrenergic agonists	Albuterol, terbutaline, theophylline
Stimulants	Amphetamines, methylphenidate, nicotine, caffeine
Mood stabilizers/ antiepileptic drugs	Lithium, valproic acid, carbamazepine
Neuroleptic agents	Haloperidol, olanzapine (postural and at rest)
Tricyclic antidepressants	Amitriptyline
Selective serotonin reuptake inhibitors	Fluoxetine
Immunosuppressant agents	Cyclosporine, tacrolimus
Other agents	Amiodarone, procainamide, mexiletine, levothyroxine, verapamil, atorvastatin, glucocorticoids

Botulinum toxin injection can help with some tremors, especially those involving the neck and voice, but its benefit for limb tremor is limited by local weakness. Medication-refractory tremor can be effectively treated by targeting the ventral intermediate nucleus of the thalamus with DBS or thalamotomy.

KEY POINTS

- Essential tremor is the most common movement disorder and often presents with a bilateral upper extremity postural and action tremor; common features include a positive family history, slow progression, and onset at either adolescence or middle age.

- The treatment of essential tremor is symptomatic; the most effective pharmacologic agents are propranolol, primidone, and topiramate.

Dystonia

Dystonia involves sustained or intermittent muscle contractions leading to stereotyped and directional twisting and posturing movements of various body parts. Dystonias are classified according to age of onset, body distribution, temporal pattern, associated features, and cause (**Table 39**). Generalized dystonias involve multiple body parts, including the trunk, whereas focal and segmental dystonias have a more restricted distribution and usually spare the lower extremities. Hemidystonia is limited to one side of the body. Generalized dystonias often start at a young age (<25 years) and have inherited, metabolic, or vascular causes. The most common type of generalized dystonia involves mutation in the dystonia 1 gene (*DYT1*). Patients with primary generalized dystonia should be challenged by a short trial of levodopa to screen for dopa-responsive dystonia, a rare but treatable cause of generalized dystonia. Young adults with progressive dystonia should be screened for Wilson disease, especially in the presence of other associated findings (such as tremor and parkinsonism).

Focal adult-onset dystonias include cervical dystonia (spasmodic torticollis), eyelid dystonia (blepharospasm), vocal cord spasmodic dysphonia, and task-specific hand dystonia (writer's cramp). Cervical dystonia often involves involuntary deviation of the head from midline, an irregular head tremor that lessens with positional changes (null point), and transient improvement of movements by specific sensory tricks (such as gently touching the face with the hand). Treatment includes anticholinergic agents, benzodiazepines, baclofen, and levodopa.

TABLE 39. Classification of Dystonia

Clinical Feature	Subtype
Age of onset	Infancy, childhood (<13 years), adolescence (13-18 years), young adulthood (18-40 years), late adulthood (>40 years)
Temporal pattern	Persistent, paroxysmal, action induced
Associated neurologic features	Isolated dystonia (no other deficits), dystonia plus (with parkinsonism or myoclonus)
Anatomic distribution	Focal, segmental (contiguous regions), multifocal (noncontiguous regions), hemidystonia, generalized (trunk plus two other regions)
Paroxysmal	Primary genetic paroxysmal dyskinesia (kinesigenic, nonkinesigenic, exercise induced, hypnogenic), secondary paroxysmal dyskinesia (stroke, demyelination)
Diurnal variation (better in morning)	Dopa-responsive dystonia
Cause	**Example**
Genetic	Autosomal dominant (DYT1, DYT6), autosomal recessive (Wilson disease), X-linked (Lesch-Nyhan syndrome), mitochondrial (Leigh syndrome)
Structural lesion	Hemidystonia secondary to stroke, vascular malformation or lesion in contralateral basal ganglia, postencephalitis, posttraumatic
Neurodegeneration	Parkinson disease, Parkinson-plus syndromes, Huntington disease
Perinatal brain injury	Dystonia associated with cerebral palsy, delayed-onset dystonia
Sporadic	Adult-onset focal dystonia (torticollis, blepharospasm, writer's cramp, musician's cramp, spasmodic dysphonia), Meige syndrome (facial and oromandibular segmental dystonia)
Psychological	Psychogenic dystonia
Medications	Neuroleptic-induced tardive dystonia, antiemetic-induced acute dystonic reaction, antiepileptic drug–induced dystonia

Injection with botulinum toxin targeting the most active muscles in focal dystonia also is beneficial. In genetic or idiopathic dystonia, DBS of the globus pallidus interna can markedly improve symptoms. The benefit of DBS is more variable in secondary dystonia with the exception of tardive dystonia, which responds well.

KEY POINTS

- Dystonia involves sustained or intermittent muscle contractions leading to stereotyped and directional twisting and posturing movements of various body parts.

- Treatment of cervical dystonia includes anticholinergic agents, benzodiazepines, baclofen, and levodopa; injection with botulinum toxin targeting the most active muscles in focal dystonia also is beneficial.

Choreiform Disorders and Huntington Disease

Chorea manifests as random, nonrepetitive, flowing dance-like movements and can be caused by medications, endocrine derangement, streptococcal infection (as in Sydenham chorea in rheumatic fever), autoimmune disease, pregnancy, and neurodegenerative disorders involving the basal ganglia (**Table 40**). The most common neurodegenerative cause of generalized chorea is Huntington disease, which involves symptoms of progressive parkinsonism, gait impairment, impulsiveness, psychiatric disease, and dementia. Substance abuse also has been associated with Huntington disease. An autosomal dominant condition, this disorder is caused by a trinucleotide repeat expansion in the *huntingtin* gene. Age of onset has a reverse correlation with length of repeat expansion and may be younger with paternal transmission (anticipation phenomenon). Huntington disease is invariably fatal. Symptomatic treatments of chorea include the dopamine depleters tetrabenazine and deutetrabenazine, antipsychotic agents, clonazepam, and antiepileptic drugs.

KEY POINT

- Huntington disease is an autosomal dominant condition marked by symptoms of progressive parkinsonism, gait impairment, impulsiveness, psychiatric disease, and dementia.

Myoclonus

Myoclonus is a brief, shock-like, jerky movement that can be physiologic (hiccups, hypnic jerks at sleep onset) or pathologic (caused by medications, toxins, or systemic or central disease) (**Table 41**). Myoclonus can originate from various parts of the nervous system, including the cortex, subcortical structures, the spine, or peripheral nerves. Cortical myoclonus is often epileptic. Negative myoclonus is caused by sudden loss of muscle tone, as seen in asterixis and in the legs after hypoxia (Lance-Adams syndrome). Treatment of myoclonus includes addressing the underlying systemic or toxic cause and administering antimyoclonic agents, such as clonazepam, valproic acid, levetiracetam, zonisamide, or topiramate.

KEY POINT

- Treatment of myoclonus includes addressing the underlying systemic or toxic cause and administering antimyoclonic agents, such as clonazepam, valproic acid, levetiracetam, zonisamide, or topiramate.

Tic Disorders and Tourette Syndrome

Tics are stereotyped, rapid movements interrupting the flow of normal movements. Tics may provide transient relief in response to premonitory unconformable sensations and are at least partially suppressible. Tics usually start during childhood and subside during adulthood, but they may persist in a minority of those affected.

Tourette syndrome is characterized by childhood-onset motor and phonic tics with a duration of at least 1 year. Phonic tics include vocalizations and, less commonly, echolalia (repetition of others' words) and coprolalia (utterance of obscenities). Tic severity may range from minimal to very disruptive. Tourette syndrome is considered a network disease in which basal ganglia and prefrontal cortex interactions are dysregulated. Common comorbidities include attention-deficit hyperactivity disorder, obsessive compulsive disorder, and mood disorders. Diagnosis is clinical. Treatment options include reassurance (often appropriate in mild disease), cognitive

TABLE 40.	Causes of Chorea
Cause	**Example**
Medications	Antipsychotic agents, estrogen-containing drugs, levodopa, amphetamines, methylphenidate, lithium, phenytoin
Pregnancy	Chorea gravidarum
Endocrine	Hyperglycemia (especially acute), thyrotoxicosis
Infection	Streptococcal (Sydenham chorea), prion disease, herpes encephalitis, HIV
Autoimmune	Systemic lupus erythematous, antiphospholipid syndrome, anti-GAD antibody
Paraneoplastic	Anti-CRMP5 antibody, anti-NMDA antibody, voltage-gated potassium channel antibody
Genetic	Benign hereditary chorea, neuroferritinopathy
Neurodegenerative	Huntington disease, Huntington-like disease 2, spinocerebellar ataxia 17 and 8, C9orf72 expansion syndrome, Friedreich ataxia, chorea-acanthocytosis, neurodegeneration with brain iron accumulation

CRMP5 = collapsin response mediator protein 5; GAD = glutamic acid decarboxylase; NMDA = N-methyl-D-aspartate

TABLE 41. Causes of Acquired Myoclonus

Cause	Example	Features
Metabolic	Kidney, hepatic or respiratory failure, sleep apnea, hyponatremia, hypocalcemia, hyperglycemia	Both positive and negative myoclonus (asterixis)
Endocrine	Hyperthyroidism	With tremor and ophthalmopathy
Toxic	Opioids, gabapentin, amiodarone, SSRIs	Prominent in serotonin syndrome
Infectious	Lyme disease, Whipple disease, viral encephalitis (especially herpes)	Oculomasticatory myorhythmia (rhythmic movements of eye convergence with chewing) in Whipple
Paraneoplastic	Opsoclonus-myoclonus syndrome	Anti-Ri antibody
Autoimmune	Celiac disease, associated with thyroid antibodies	With other symptoms, such as ataxia or encephalopathy
Cortical pathology	Epileptic myoclonus (primary and secondary myoclonic epilepsies), posthypoxic myoclonus (Lance-Adams syndrome), corticobasal degeneration, advanced Alzheimer disease	Epileptic activity on EEG, giant somatosensory evoked potentials
Basal ganglia pathology	Myoclonus dystonia	Genetic, associated with dystonia, ethanol-sensitive
Brainstem pathology	Brainstem reticular myoclonus	Stimulus-sensitive (noise or action) myoclonus, coordinated flexion of trunk and limbs
Cord pathology	Segmental spinal myoclonus, propriospinal myoclonus, multiple sclerosis, cord tumor or trauma	Jerks in limited myotomes (segmental) or spreading distally and proximally (propriospinal), associated with myelopathy signs
Peripheral nerve pathology	Hemifacial spasm	Focal compression or irritation of the facial nerve (cranial nerve VII)

EEG = electroencephalography; SSRI = selective serotonin reuptake inhibitor.

behavioral therapy (including tic diversion techniques), and addressing psychiatric comorbidities. Anti-tic medications are indicated when tics interfere with daily functioning, education, or work. First-line treatments are clonidine, guanfacine, topiramate, levetiracetam, and tetrabenazine. Antipsychotic agents (aripiprazole, pimozide, ziprasidone, risperidone, and haloperidol) can help in the treatment of refractory tics, but the risk of tardive dyskinesia should be considered in adults. Botulinum toxin may be useful for focal tics and severe refractory disease; DBS may also be beneficial in severe disease.

KEY POINTS

- Tics are stereotyped, rapid movements interrupting the flow of normal movements and may provide transient relief in response to premonitory unconformable sensations.

- Tourette syndrome is characterized by childhood-onset motor and phonic tics with a duration of at least 1 year.

Restless Legs Syndrome and Sleep-Related Movement Disorders

Restless legs syndrome (RLS) is a common movement disorder characterized by an urge to move the legs. Patients report an uncomfortable sensation that is worse at rest and at night and is transiently relieved by movement. Patients with RLS should be screened for iron deficiency because iron supplementation in the presence of low-normal ferritin levels

(15-75 ng/mL [15-75 µg/L]) may resolve the symptoms. Other risk factors for RLS include uremia, sleep apnea, pregnancy, and certain medications (including selective serotonin reuptake inhibitors, antipsychotic agents, and stimulant drugs). Nonpharmacological measures include improvement of sleep hygiene, exercise, and the use of a vibrational device. First-line pharmacologic treatments include dopamine agonists (especially pramipexole and the rotigotine patch). Additional options include ropinirole, gabapentin, pregabalin, levodopa, and opioid agonists (prolonged release oxycodone-naloxone and methadone). Chronic use of dopamine agonists, however effective, may lead to either augmentation (that is, symptoms start earlier in the day) or rebound (that is, symptoms return with greater severity after the medication wears off). Use of long-acting formulations can lessen both of these complications. Gabapentin enacarbil, an $\alpha_2 \delta$ calcium channel ligand, is a slow-release prodrug of gabapentin that is also FDA approved for the treatment of RLS.

Periodic limb movements of sleep are brief triple flexion movements of the legs that repeat in 20-second cycles during sleep. This disorder is very common and can occur independently of or be associated with RLS, sleep-disordered breathing, or narcolepsy. The diagnosis is made by using polysomnography. Treatment of this disorder is only required if it causes marked sleep fragmentation.

REM sleep behavior disorder is caused by loss of normal paralysis during the REM phase of sleep, leading to dream-enactment behavior. Patients with this condition tend to shout, kick, punch, and jump while dreaming. Diagnosis is based on either the report of a bed partner or polysomnography. The main differential diagnosis is nocturnal epilepsy. REM sleep behavior disorder responds well to clonazepam and melatonin. It is a strong predictor of future development of synuclein-related neurodegeneration, such as Parkinson disease, multiple system atrophy, or dementia with Lewy bodies.

> **KEY POINTS**
> - Patients with restless legs syndrome should be screened for iron deficiency because iron supplementation in the presence of low-normal ferritin levels may resolve the symptoms.
> - The diagnosis of periodic limb movements of sleep is made by using polysomnography; treatment is only required if the disorder causes marked sleep fragmentation.

Other Drug-Induced Movements
Tardive Dyskinesia
Tardive dyskinesia is an extrapyramidal complication of dopamine receptor–blocking medications (see Table 36). It is associated with characteristic choreiform and dystonic craniofacial movements, which often involve other body parts, such as the neck and trunk. Treatment involves removal of the offending medication. Symptoms of dyskinesia, however, can take months to resolve or become permanent. Longer duration and higher doses of medication exposure, older age, and female gender increase the risk of irreversibility. Risk is highest with typical antipsychotic agents, but many atypical antipsychotic and antiemetic agents also can cause tardive dyskinesia. All patients receiving these agents must be warned about the risk of this complication. Recently, valbenazine, a monoamine depleter, was the first medication to receive FDA approval for treatment of tardive dyskinesia. Other pharmacologic therapies include tetrabenazine, amantadine, clonazepam, and anticholinergic agents. In severe cases, DBS of the globus pallidus may be effective, although it lacks FDA approval for this indication.

Neuroleptic Malignant Syndrome
Neuroleptic malignant syndrome is an acute life-threatening disorder caused by an idiosyncratic reaction to therapeutic doses of dopamine-blocking agents. Its pathophysiology involves a sudden decrease in dopamine D_2 receptor activity. Patients present with fever, rhabdomyolysis, altered mental status, rigidity, and dystonia. The creatine kinase level often is remarkably elevated. The most effective treatment is removal of the offending agent and supportive management. Treatment options include dopamine agonists and the muscle relaxant dantrolene, although there is weak evidence supporting their effectiveness. Mortality may be as high as 10%. Patients who have dementia with Lewy bodies are particularly susceptible

to neuroleptic malignant syndrome. A similar syndrome can be triggered by rapid withdrawal of dopaminergic medication in patients with Parkinson disease, including when medications are stopped in the hospital before surgery. See MKSAP 18 Pulmonary and Critical Care Medicine for more information about neuroleptic malignant syndrome.

> **KEY POINTS**
> - Tardive dyskinesia is an extrapyramidal complication of dopamine receptor–blocking medications characterized by choreiform and dystonic craniofacial movements; symptoms can take months to resolve or become permanent.
> - Neuroleptic malignant syndrome is an acute life-threatening disorder caused by exposure to therapeutic doses of dopamine-blocking agents; it presents with fever, rhabdomyolysis, altered mental status, rigidity, and dystonia.

Multiple Sclerosis
Presenting Signs and Symptoms
Multiple sclerosis (MS) is an autoimmune disorder of the central nervous system (CNS) that causes inflammatory damage to the brain, spinal cord, and optic nerve. Most of the overt clinical symptoms of MS occur as a direct consequence of functional interruption of critical axonal pathways by inflammatory lesions. Relapses or flares involve development of neurologic symptoms over the course of hours to days and often peak in severity over the course of days to weeks. This is typically followed by a period of remission lasting weeks to months. Remyelination and recruitment of other brain regions to functionally substitute for the damaged area may result in clinical improvement during times of remission.

The most common clinical manifestations of MS are optic neuritis, myelitis, and brainstem/cerebellar syndromes. Patients with optic neuritis typically have subacute visual deficits in one eye that are occasionally associated with pain with eye movement and/or flashing lights (photopsia). Formal ophthalmologic examination shows a reduction in visual acuity, a scotoma or visual field deficit, difficulty with color discrimination, and an afferent pupillary defect. Papillitis (flared appearance of the optic disc caused by inflammatory changes; **Figure 22**) can sometimes be seen, although this finding only occurs with involvement of the head of the nerve. Optic disc pallor (**Figure 23**) is usually seen as a late consequence of optic neuritis and is secondary to atrophy of the optic nerve.

Spinal cord involvement or myelitis results in sensory and/or motor symptoms below the affected spinal level. Unlike other spinal cord processes, MS generally causes a partial myelitis, and symptoms of full-cord transection are rare; crossed sensory-motor symptoms may also occur (as in

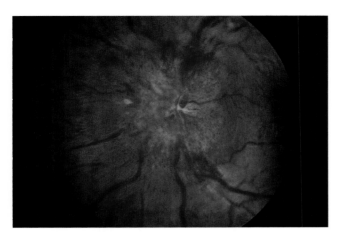

FIGURE 22. Optic nerve papillitis is characterized by hyperemia and swelling of the disk, blurring of disk margins, and distended veins. Papillitis is seen in one-third of patients with optic neuritis.

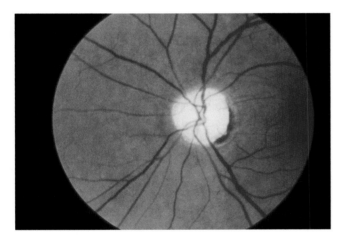

FIGURE 23. A pale, flat optic disk characteristic of optic nerve atrophy.

partial Brown-Séquard syndrome). Neurologic examination generally reveals focal weakness and/or reduced sensation below a specific spinal dermatome. Muscle tone can be reduced acutely, whereas spasticity and hyperreflexia often are delayed findings. During acute inflammation, some patients will also experience a tight, band-like sensation around the body involving the affected spinal level ("MS hug"). Lhermitte sign, which also can occur with upper cervical cord lesions from other causes, manifests as a shock-like sensation radiating down the spine or limbs with flexion of the neck. Urinary frequency, urgency, hesitancy, or retention also may be seen.

Brainstem syndromes often involve pathways for eye movement and result in diplopia or oscillopsia (a sensation of jerking of the visual field). Examination may reveal dysconjugate eye movements, nystagmus, and/or internuclear ophthalmoplegia (inability to adduct one eye and nystagmus in the abducting eye). Disruption of vestibular or cerebellar pathways may result in ataxia and/or vertigo. Neurologic examination will reveal appendicular or truncal ataxia, dysmetria on finger-to-nose testing, difficulty with rapid alternating movements, and impairment of tandem gait.

Most patients with MS also develop subtle, chronic symptoms that occur as a consequence of more widespread cortical demyelination and nonlesional axonal pathology. At least 50% of patients with MS experience cognitive deficits, typically in domains of short-term memory, visuospatial function, and processing speed. Many patients with MS also report fatigue, which can manifest as a feeling of exhaustion despite adequate sleep, a feeling of brain fog, and easy physical fatigability.

Many patients with MS also experience Uhthoff phenomenon, a transient worsening of baseline neurologic symptoms in the setting of hot weather, physical exertion, or fever. This worsening occurs because of a temporary reduction in neuronal electrical conductance at higher temperatures, which causes magnification of symptoms from previously demyelinated pathways. Any patient with a suspected relapse should be screened for causes of Uhthoff phenomenon masquerading as a relapse (or "pseudorelapse") to avoid unnecessary treatment. Patients often need reassurance and counseling that such events are not indicative of new inflammatory damage. **H**

KEY POINTS

- Most of the overt clinical symptoms of multiple sclerosis (MS) occur as a direct consequence of functional interruption of critical axonal pathways by inflammatory lesions; the most common clinical manifestations of MS are optic neuritis, myelitis, and brainstem/cerebellar syndromes.

- Any patient with a suspected relapse should be screened for causes of Uhthoff phenomenon (transient worsening of neurologic symptoms associated with increased body temperature) masquerading as a relapse (or "pseudorelapse") to avoid unnecessary treatment. **HVC**

Diagnosis of Multiple Sclerosis
Diagnostic Criteria and Testing

Because no specific genetic or serologic diagnostic biomarker is available for diagnosing MS, the diagnosis is made through rigorous application of diagnostic criteria that integrate clinical and radiologic findings. The McDonald criteria require symptoms of CNS demyelination separated in space and time from a series of clinical relapses or progression, signs on physical examination, distribution of lesions on MRI, and (if necessary) the presence of cerebrospinal fluid (CSF)-unique oligoclonal bands. Proper application of the diagnostic criteria can prevent unnecessary neurologic testing, referrals, and misdiagnoses. A standardized MRI brain protocol should be used for all diagnostic evaluations of potential MS. Spinal cord imaging also should be performed in patients with symptoms of myelitis, patients with insufficient features on a brain MRI to support the diagnosis, and patients older than 40 years with nonspecific brain MRI findings. Strict adherence to the McDonald criteria for MS-specific lesions is critical because many other disorders (migraine, head trauma, and cerebrovascular disease) also can cause brain (but not spinal) lesions on MRI. **Figure 24** shows examples of periventricular, juxtacortical, and infratentorial lesions that are specific to MS and satisfy the McDonald criteria; if visible, lesions in the cortex may substitute for juxtacortical lesions, according to the official diagnostic criteria. Ancillary testing can show objective clinical evidence of a demyelinating lesion. Demyelinating lesions of the optic nerve can be electrophysiologically confirmed with visual evoked potentials. Optic coherence tomography, which uses near-infrared light to quantify the thickness of the retinal nerve fiber layer and macula, also can confirm optic nerve damage in acute or previous optic neuritis. Conductance delay in brainstem auditory evoked potentials and somatosensory evoked potentials can act as surrogate markers of demyelination in brainstem and spinal cord pathways. Despite the usefulness of such testing for determining anatomic localization, however, MRI is the only objective measure that fulfills the diagnostic criteria.

CSF testing is not required for a diagnosis of MS if the McDonald criteria are otherwise met. However, CSF findings can be used to support the diagnosis when the MRI criteria are not fully met. The normally functioning blood-brain barrier excludes immunoglobulins from the CSF in healthy persons, which results in a blood to CSF IgG ratio of 500:1 or greater. Oligoclonal bands indicate elevations in oligoclonal immunoglobulin concentrations in the CSF and may result from disruption of the blood-brain barrier or intrathecal production of IgG. The presence of oligoclonal bands in the CSF that are absent in the serum occurs in 85% to 90% of persons with MS. An elevated IgG blood-to-CSF index and an elevated IgG synthesis rate also are possible. Nonspecific mild elevations in the CSF leukocyte count or protein level are sometimes seen.

KEY POINTS

- The McDonald criteria for diagnosing multiple sclerosis require symptoms of central nervous system demyelination separated in space and time from a series of clinical relapses or progression, signs on physical examination, distribution of lesions on MRI, and (if necessary) the presence of CSF-unique oligoclonal bands.

- Proper application of diagnostic criteria can prevent **HVC** unnecessary neurologic testing, referrals, and misdiagnoses in patients suspected of having multiple sclerosis.

Differential Diagnosis of Multiple Sclerosis

Knowledge of the various rheumatologic, inflammatory, infectious, and metabolic disorders with the potential to mimic the clinical signs/symptoms and radiologic changes of MS is important when considering the diagnosis (**Table 42**).

Clinical Course of Multiple Sclerosis

The clinical phenotypic definitions of MS recently have been modified to acknowledge that manifestations of MS are heterogeneous and can evolve over time (**Figure 25**). Approximately 85% of patients with MS experience an initial relapsing-remitting course. Those with a first demyelinating event that does not meet the definition of clinically definite MS are said to have a clinically isolated syndrome. Any future disease activity, defined as a clinical relapse or a new or contrast-enhancing lesion on MRI, results in conversion to a diagnosis of clinically definite relapsing-remitting MS. Because disease-modifying

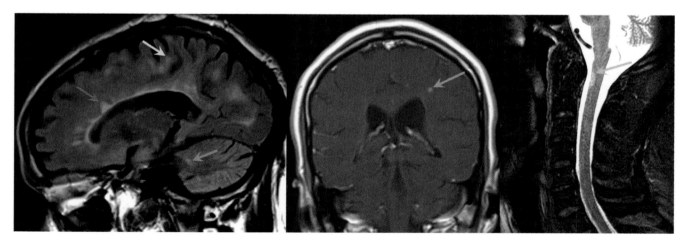

FIGURE 24. *Left,* fluid-attenuated inversion recovery brain MRI that shows periventricular (*red arrow*), juxtacortical (*yellow arrow*), and infratentorial (*green arrow*) lesions specific to multiple sclerosis (MS); if visible, lesions in the cortex can substitute for juxtacortical lesions, according to official diagnostic criteria. *Middle,* coronal T1-weighted postcontrast MRI of the brain showing a contrast-enhancing MS lesion (*blue arrow*). *Right,* sagittal T2-weighted MRI of the spinal cord showing an MS lesion (*gold arrow*).

TABLE 42. Differential Diagnosis of Multiple Sclerosis

Disorder	Notes
Other demyelinating diseases	
ADEM	Monophasic, often postinfectious syndrome causing large, diffuse areas of inflammatory CNS demyelination
	Characterized by fevers and encephalopathy, typically with focal neurologic symptoms, which differentiate ADEM from MS
	Rare in adults
Neuromyelitis optica (Devic disease)	Antibody-mediated inflammation directed at aquaporin-4 antibody channels in the CNS that results in inflammatory demyelination in the optic nerves and spinal cord
	Can be differentiated from MS by NMO IgG antibody testing and by its lack of significant brain involvement, large and longitudinally extensive spinal cord lesions, and profound cerebrospinal fluid leukocytosis
Idiopathic transverse myelitis	Monophasic, often postinfectious syndrome causing spinal cord inflammation
	Differentiated from MS by the presence of symptoms and findings unique to the underlying systemic disorder in addition to any neurologic symptoms[a]
Systemic inflammatory diseases	
SLE	White-matter changes on MRI and encephalopathy sometimes present
Sjögren syndrome	Can cause an NMO-like disorder (with optic neuritis and myelitis), multiple cranial neuropathies, and a small-fiber neuropathy
Sarcoidosis	Causes granulomatous inflammation in the parenchyma and meninges of the brain and spinal cord
	Occasionally associated with myelopathy
Metabolic disorders	
Adult-onset leukodystrophies (such as adrenoleukodystrophy and metachromatic leukodystrophy)	Rare
	May cause white-matter changes and progressive neurologic symptoms
	Family history typically present
Vitamin B_{12} deficiency	Can cause optic neuropathy, cognitive changes, and subacute combined degeneration of the spinal cord (spasticity, weakness, and vibratory and proprioceptive sensory loss)
Copper deficiency	Can cause a myelopathy identical to that of vitamin B_{12} deficiency; associated with bariatric gastric surgery, malabsorption syndromes, and excessive zinc ingestion
Infections	
HIV infection, Lyme disease, and syphilis	Can cause encephalopathy and myelopathy
	Can be diagnosed with appropriate serologic and spinal fluid analysis
HTLV	Causes a slowly progressive myelopathy with thoracic cord atrophy
	Sometimes termed tropical spastic paraparesis because more common in patients in equatorial latitudes
Vascular disorders	
Sporadic and genetic stroke syndromes (hypercoagulability and viscosity disorders, such as polycythemia and myeloma)	Microvascular ischemic diseases potentially causing nonspecific white-matter changes on MRI that are often confused with MS
	Distinguished from MS by age, other vascular risk factors, and findings on neurologic exam
CNS vasculitis	Primary type diagnosed by catheter angiography or tissue biopsy
	Can present with both stroke-like changes and meningeal contrast enhancement on MRI
Susac syndrome	Causes small-vessel arteriopathy that causes dysfunction of the retina and cochlea and corpus callosum lesions seen on MRI
	Subacute clinical progression, without remission or relapse
Migraine	Subcortical white-matter lesions sometimes present and often confused with MS lesions
	CADASIL a possible diagnosis in patients with a familial syndrome of migraine, subcortical strokes, mood disorders, and early dementia

(Continued on the next page)

TABLE 42. Differential Diagnosis of Multiple Sclerosis *(Continued)*

Disorder	Notes
Neoplasia (primary CNS neoplasm [gliomas or lymphomas] or metastatic disease)	Neoplasms with progressively worsening symptoms and neuroimaging findings
	Brain biopsy indicated when imaging cannot differentiate neoplasms from demyelinating disease
Paraneoplastic syndromes	May cause progressive cerebellar ataxia or myeloneuropathy (neuropathy affecting the spinal cord and peripheral nerves)
	Personality and mental status changes in addition to seizures and movement disorders possible with paraneoplastic limbic encephalitis
	Diagnosis often made on the basis of cancer screening and antibody testing
Somatoform disorders	Psychiatric disorders presenting with neurologic-like symptoms that are due to somatization, conversion, and similar conditions
	Neurologic evaluation findings entirely normal

ADEM = acute disseminated encephalomyelitis; CADASIL = cerebral autosomal dominant arteriopathy with subcortical infarcts and leukoencephalopathy; CNS = central nervous system; HTLV = human T-lymphotropic virus; MS = multiple sclerosis; NMO = neuromyelitis optica; SLE = systemic lupus erythematosus.

ªFor more information on idiopathic transverse myelitis, see Disorders of the Spinal Cord.

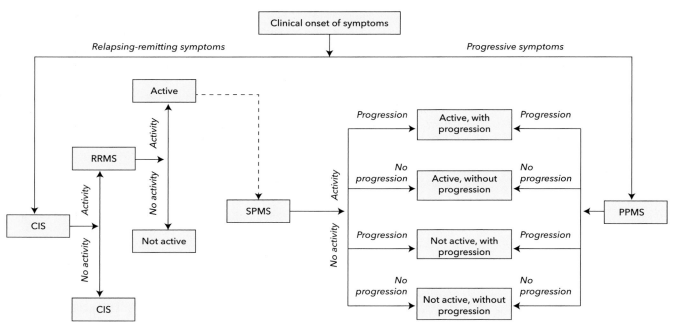

FIGURE 25. At clinical onset, multiple sclerosis (MS) can be either relapsing or progressive in nature. An initial, isolated demyelinating event results in a preliminary diagnosis of a clinically isolated syndrome. Any further activity (defined as a clinical relapse, new or enlarging T2-weighted lesion on MRI, or gadolinium-enhancing lesion on MRI) results in a diagnosis of relapsing-remitting MS (RRMS). Over time, RRMS can either be classified as active (if evidence of activity exists) or not active. Some patients with RRMS can later exhibit signs of progression (defined as slowly progressive accumulation of disability), and their condition can be reclassified as secondary progressive MS (SPMS). An initial clinical onset of progressive, nonrelapsing symptoms is diagnosed as primary progressive MS (PPMS). Any patients with progressive MS (PPMS or SPMS) can later exhibit signs of activity and/or progression, which allows for further stratification into four categories based on the presence or absence of these qualities.

CIS = clinically isolated syndrome; MS = multiple sclerosis; PPMS = primary progressive MS; RRMS = relapsing-remitting MS; SPMS = secondary progressive MS.

therapies reduce the risk of conversion from a clinically isolated syndrome to relapsing-remitting MS by approximately 50%, stratification of risk for conversion can inform treatment decisions. Patients with brain lesions on MRI at the time of their clinically isolated syndrome have a 10-year risk of conversion to relapsing-remitting MS of approximately 90%, whereas patients without brain lesions have a much lower risk (10%–20%).

Determination of activity status may also inform treatment decisions in relapsing-remitting MS. In the first few years that a patient has this type of MS, significant or complete recovery from relapse is common. Over time, however, postrelapse recovery generally diminishes, and permanent disability accumulates. Without treatment, half of patients with relapsing-remitting MS develop secondary progressive MS after a median of 10 to 15 years. Data now suggest that the introduction of disease-modifying therapies has decreased the proportion of patients converting to secondary progressive MS. In secondary progressive MS, relapses become infrequent or cease completely, but slowly progressive neurologic disability continues to accrue in multiple domains.

Approximately 15% of patients with MS have primary progressive MS at presentation. This subtype often develops later in life (in the fifth or sixth decade) compared with the younger age of onset (third or fourth decade of life) in typical relapsing-remitting MS. Because patients with both primary and secondary progressive MS can have periods of disability progression or stability (with some even having permanent halting of progression), adding the modifiers "with progression" and "without progression" to these diagnostic terms has been suggested. Occasionally, patients with these types of MS may meet criteria for relapsing activity (clinical relapses, new or contrast-enhancing lesions on MRI) and thus can be further stratified into "active" and "not active" categories.

Patients with a radiologically isolated syndrome have no clinical symptoms of MS but are found incidentally to have MRI findings that meet the radiologic criteria for MS. Although an MS diagnosis cannot be made in the absence of demyelinating signs and symptoms, it has been shown that patients with a radiologically isolated syndrome are at high risk for later conversion to clinically definite MS and should be monitored closely.

KEY POINTS

- Disease-modifying therapies reduce the risk of conversion from a clinically isolated syndrome to relapsing-remitting multiple sclerosis by approximately 50%.

- Approximately 85% of patients with multiple sclerosis (MS) experience an initial relapsing-remitting course; 15% have primary progressive MS at presentation.

- Without treatment, half the patients with relapsing-remitting multiple sclerosis (MS) develop secondary progressive MS after a median of 10 to 15 years; the proportion of patients converting to secondary progressive MS has decreased since the introduction of disease-modifying therapies.

Treatment of Multiple Sclerosis
Lifestyle Modifications and General Health Care

Although some patients with MS may avoid physical activity because of disability, fatigue, and the Uhthoff phenomenon, repeated studies have shown multiple benefits from both strengthening and aerobic exercise programs. Patients with significant Uhthoff phenomenon induced by exercise should be reassured that neurologic injury will not result from exercise; they also can be counseled on strategies to minimize discomfort, such as heat avoidance or external cooling (cold water, fans, body-cooling devices) during exercise.

Exercise also can help preserve bone health. Patients with MS have a three- to sixfold increased risk of reduced bone mineral density, most likely from a combination of reduced physical activity, repeated use of glucocorticoids, and vitamin D deficiency. Vitamin D deficiency is common in MS patients, and reduced serum levels of vitamin D are predictive of MS development and future accumulation of lesions on MRI. A randomized trial of vitamin D supplementation added to interferon beta treatment resulted in reduced accumulation of lesions seen on MRI compared with placebo. Vitamin D supplementation is now recommended for all patients, although the ideal dosing regimen and serum 25-hydroxyvitamin D level are still being investigated.

Measures to prevent infection are needed for patients receiving more aggressive, immunosuppressive MS treatments, especially given the increased risk of MS relapse at the time of systemic infection. Current MS treatment guidelines recommend vaccination against influenza (with inactivated vaccine) and maintenance of standard immunizations. Patients with MS-related bladder dysfunction are at higher risk of recurrent urinary tract infection, and thus strategies to reduce the frequency of bladder infections are necessary.

Smoking cessation is advised for all patients with MS because of the threefold risk of conversion from relapsing-remitting MS to secondary progressive MS and faster rates of disability accumulation in cigarette smokers.

Many patients with MS are women in their childbearing years. The estrogenic state of pregnancy has an immunomodulatory effect that tends to reduce MS disease activity during pregnancy, often precluding the need for treatment during this period. Although the risk of relapse is increased slightly in the first 3 months of pregnancy, this does not seem to contribute negatively to prognosis; multiple studies have shown that pregnancy does not result in additional permanent disability and that multiparous women have better long-term MS outcomes than nulliparous or uniparous women. Data on the effect of breastfeeding on MS relapse risk are inconclusive.

KEY POINTS

- Studies have shown multiple benefits from both strengthening and aerobic exercise programs in patients with multiple sclerosis. **HVC**

- Current multiple sclerosis (MS) treatment guidelines recommend vaccination against influenza and maintenance of standard immunizations; smoking cessation also is advised because of the threefold risk of conversion from relapsing-remitting MS to secondary progressive MS and faster rates of disability accumulation in cigarette smokers. **HVC**

Treatment of Acute Exacerbations

An MS relapse is defined as new or worsening neurologic symptoms lasting more than 24 hours. Symptoms lasting only minutes to hours should not be considered or treated as a relapse. The possibility of a pseudorelapse should always be considered before initiating treatment; suspicion of this condition should trigger clinical investigation for an underlying cause. The subsequent treatment of any infection or metabolic disturbance often results in improvement in neurologic symptoms.

The standard treatment for MS relapses is high-dose glucocorticoids, typically intravenous methylprednisolone (1 g/d for 3 to 5 days). Multiple trials have shown that bioequivalent doses of oral glucocorticoids (such as prednisone, 1250 mg/d) are equally effective and well tolerated, with reduced cost. Adverse effects of high-dose glucocorticoids include insomnia, hyperglycemia, metallic taste, gastritis, fluid retention, irritability, and (rarely) psychosis. These effects are typically short lived, given the brief duration of treatment. Frequent or prolonged glucocorticoid treatment should be avoided to minimize the risks of osteopenia and early cataracts.

MS relapses also can be treated with administration of a short course of intramuscular adrenocorticotropin hormone gel. This approach has a more favorable adverse-effect profile compared with external glucocorticoid administration. Use of this gel is limited by prohibitive pricing.

Patients not responding to glucocorticoid treatment may respond to plasmapheresis, administered as five consecutive exchanges.

KEY POINT

- The standard treatment for MS relapses is high-dose glucocorticoids, typically intravenous methylprednisolone; frequent or prolonged glucocorticoid treatment should be avoided to minimize the risks associated with long-term glucocorticoid use.

Disease-Modifying Therapies

Prevention of MS relapse is vital. Various immunomodulatory or immunosuppressive medications have been shown to reduce the risk of relapse, disability progression, and new MRI lesion formation. Currently, many disease-modifying therapies are approved and available for use in relapsing-remitting MS (**Table 43**), each differing in its route of administration, mechanism of action, and potential adverse effects. Interferon beta preparations, glatiramer acetate, and teriflunomide have additional utility in clinically isolated syndrome for prevention of conversion to clinically definite MS. Despite many options for those with relapsing disease, the options for patients with progressive forms of MS are limited. Mitoxantrone is currently the only FDA-approved therapy for secondary progressive MS, and ocrelizumab is the only FDA-approved therapy for primary progressive MS.

Clinical trials of interferon beta, glatiramer acetate, fingolimod, and natalizumab in progressive forms of MS have failed to show benefit, and thus prescribing these medications in progressive MS not only increases cost but burdens patients with unnecessary adverse effects.

Selection of an appropriate disease-modifying therapy involves consideration of comorbidities, patient tolerability, risk stratification, and disease activity. Treatment decisions often are made in consultation with a neurologist or MS specialist. There is no clear consensus about how to select the appropriate therapy, what defines treatment failure, or how to decide in what order medications should be introduced. Generally, most physicians recommend self-injection medications (an interferon beta or glatiramer acetate) as first-line agents, given their favorable risk profiles. Patients who exhibit disease breakthrough on these medications or who are unable to tolerate their adverse effects are often switched to agents with better efficacy profiles. Although the oral therapies and monoclonal antibodies provide greater efficacy, they are associated with greater risk and the need for more intensive monitoring.

Interferon beta (available as interferon beta-1a and interferon beta-1b) is an immunomodulatory cytokine treatment that shifts immune responses away from autoimmunity and increase the integrity of the blood-brain barrier. Interferons beta-1a and beta-1b are available in multiple formulations and are administered via subcutaneous or intramuscular injection on schedules varying from every other day to twice monthly. They reduce relapse rates by approximately one-third compared with placebo and have positive effects on disability progression and MRI findings. Head-to-head studies show general equivalence of the formulations, although those requiring frequent injections have slightly higher efficacy in some studies. Interferon beta may exacerbate depression, and care should be taken when administering it to patients with a history of psychiatric disease.

Glatiramer acetate exerts its immunomodulatory effect through modification of the nonbinding sites of major histocompatibility complex molecules. Structurally similar to myelin basic protein, it also may work through molecular mimicry. Glatiramer acetate is available for daily or three times weekly subcutaneous injection. Reduction in relapse rates is similar to that of the interferon beta formulations. Combining glatiramer acetate with interferon beta provides no added benefit.

Fingolimod is an oral agent that results in sequestration of activated lymphocytes within lymph nodes. Fingolimod reduces relapse rates by approximately one-half compared with placebo and also reduces the risk of disability progression and the development of new MRI lesions. However, intensive monitoring is mandatory with fingolimod because of its rare adverse effects, including infection and heart block.

TABLE 43. Disease-Modifying Therapies for Relapsing-Remitting Multiple Sclerosis

Medication	Route of Administration	Potential Adverse Effects	Recommended Monitoring	Pregnancy Category[a]
Interferon beta-1a (three formulations) and interferon beta-1b (two formulations)	Intramuscular or subcutaneous injection	Flu-like symptoms, fatigue, depression, increased spasticity, transaminitis, rare autoimmune hepatitis, and injection-site reactions	CBC and liver enzymes every 3-6 months	C
Glatiramer acetate (three formulations)	Subcutaneous injection	Injection-site reactions, lipoatrophy of skin at injection sites, and rare systemic panic attack–like syndrome	None	B
Fingolimod	Oral	Transaminitis, lymphopenia, increased risk of serious herpesvirus infection, hypertension, bradycardia (usually only with the first dose), macular edema, basal cell carcinoma, PML	Cardiac monitoring (for bradycardia) after administration of first dose, ophthalmologic screening (for macular edema), liver enzymes, CBC monitoring (for excessive lymphopenia), yearly skin examination (for basal cell carcinoma)	C
Dimethyl fumarate	Oral	Diarrhea, nausea, abdominal cramping, flushing, lymphopenia, PML	Frequent monitoring of CBC in first 6 months after administration and then every 6 months thereafter	C
Teriflunomide	Oral	Alopecia, gastrointestinal distress, respiratory infections, transaminitis, lymphopenia, hypertension, and peripheral neuropathy	Monitoring of CBC for lymphopenia, liver enzymes, and blood pressure frequently in the first 6 months, every 6 months thereafter	X
Natalizumab	Intravenous	Black-box warning of increased risk of PML, common adverse effects of headache and chest discomfort, and rare hepatotoxicity, infusion reactions, and anaphylactic reactions	Rigorous, regimented, industry-sponsored monitoring (TOUCH program) and JC virus antibody testing (both screening and intermittent monitoring)	C
Alemtuzumab	Intravenous	Infusion reactions (including anaphylaxis), infections (especially herpes virus and fungal), autoimmune thyroiditis, ITP, glomerular nephropathy, increased risk of dermatologic malignancy	Rigorous, regimented, industry-sponsored monitoring program (Lemtrada REMS); monthly CBC, serum creatinine measurement, and urinalysis; quarterly thyroid function for 48 months after first infusion; yearly skin examination	C
Ocrelizumab	Intravenous	Allergic infusion reactions (such as urticaria, pruritus, anaphylaxis), infections (especially herpesvirus or hepatitis B virus reactivations); possible increased risks for PML and cancer	Preinfusion screening with CBC and hepatitis B serologies; consider preinfusion vaccinations (against, for example, zoster, streptococcal pneumonia, hepatitis B)	No assigned category, with some risk seen in animal studies; contraception suggested for 6 months after each infusion
Mitoxantrone	Intravenous	Black-box warnings for cardiotoxicity and acute myelogenous leukemia; other adverse effects of infection, nausea, oral sores, alopecia, menstrual irregularities, and blue discoloration of urine	Required monitoring of cardiac function by echocardiography or multigated radionucleotide angiography before each infusion and regular CBC	D

CBC = complete blood count; HYP = high-yield process; ITP = immune thrombocytopenic purpura; PML = progressive multifocal leukoencephalopathy; REMS = risk evaluation and migraine strategy.

[a]Pregnancy categories: A, no disclosed fetal effects; B, animal studies failed to demonstrate fetal risk; C, animal studies suggest adverse fetal effects; D, evidence of human fetal risk; X = documented fetal abnormalities. The FDA is no longer using these letter categories for newly approved drugs; for prescription drugs that were previously approved, these changes will be phased in gradually.

Dimethyl fumarate is an oral agent that activates the nuclear factor–like 2 transcriptional pathway and results in immunomodulation. It reduces relapse rates by slightly less than half and reduces the risk of disability progression and MRI lesion development. Infectious risks of dimethyl fumarate correlate with prolonged lymphopenia, and frequent blood-count monitoring is required.

Teriflunomide is an oral medication that inhibits a mitochondrial enzyme involved in pyrimidine synthesis in rapidly dividing cells. This drug reduces relapse rates by a third compared with placebo and also reduces the risk of disability progression and new MRI lesion development. Dual-method contraception is recommended with teriflunomide because of its known teratogenic effects.

Natalizumab is a monoclonal antibody targeting a cellular adhesion molecule on activated T-cells required for transmigration into the CNS. Administered intravenously once monthly, natalizumab is a highly effective treatment, resulting in a two-thirds reduction in relapse rates, slowing of disability progression by approximately 40%, and a reduction in MRI activity of approximately 90% compared with placebo. Despite this high efficacy, natalizumab is typically limited to use as a second-line agent because of the risk of progressive multifocal leukoencephalopathy (PML), a CNS demyelinating infection caused by reactivation of the JC virus. Duration of treatment, seropositivity for the JC virus, and previous exposure to chemotherapy or immunosuppressants increase PML risk. PML is uncommon in time-limited treatment in patients without other risk factors.

Alemtuzumab is an anti-CD52 monoclonal antibody that causes complement-mediated lysis of circulating lymphocytes. It is administered as an intravenous infusion with an initial course of once daily for 5 days, followed by 3 consecutive days 1 year later. Alemtuzumab reduces relapse rates and disability progression by approximately half and reduces new lesions and brain atrophy on MRI compared with interferon beta. Despite high efficacy, use of this drug also is limited due to significant safety concerns (see Table 43), all of which require intensive safety monitoring and potential prophylaxis.

Ocrelizumab is a monoclonal antibody against the CD20 antigen that causes lysis of circulating B cells. This drug is administered through intravenous infusion, initially as two infusions 2 weeks apart followed by a one-time infusion every 6 months. Ocrelizumab is the first medication to show benefit for patients with both relapsing-remitting MS (reductions in relapse rates, MRI disease burden, and disability accumulation) and primary progressive MS (reduced chance of disability progression). Safety concerns include allergic infusion reactions and increased risk for treatment-related infections.

Mitoxantrone is an anthracenedione chemotherapy drug that exerts an immunosuppressive effect by reducing lymphocyte proliferation. Although mitoxantrone is highly effective for relapsing-remitting MS and is the only drug approved for use in secondary progressive MS, it has fallen out of favor given its significant risks of cardiac toxicity and treatment-related leukemia.

KEY POINTS

- Generally, self-injection medications (interferon beta or glatiramer acetate) are recommended as first-line agents for relapsing-remitting multiple sclerosis because of their favorable risk profiles.

- Ocrelizumab is the only available therapy for primary progressive multiple sclerosis (MS), and mitoxantrone is the only FDA-approved therapy for secondary progressive MS; given the lack of benefit of other MS therapies in these disease subtypes, using agents other than ocrelizumab and mitoxantrone in patients with progressive forms of MS not only increases cost but burdens patients with unnecessary risk. **HVC**

- Natalizumab is a highly effective treatment in multiple sclerosis that causes a two-thirds reduction in relapse rates, slowing of disability progression by approximately 40%, and a reduction in MRI activity of approximately 90% compared with placebo; it is typically limited to use as a second-line agent because of the risk of progressive multifocal leukoencephalopathy.

Symptomatic Management

Despite the use of disease-modifying therapies, many patients still experience both chronic and intermittent neurologic symptoms. Proper management of these symptoms with pharmacologic and nonpharmacologic approaches can increase quality of life for patients with MS.

MS spasticity is due to corticospinal tract damage, resulting in increased muscle tone, painful muscle cramps, spasms, and contractures. The use of muscle relaxants, such as baclofen, tizanidine, cyclobenzaprine, and the benzodiazepines may be helpful. Gabapentin, medical marijuana, synthetic tetrahydrocannabinol compounds, and cannabis extract are beneficial in reducing painful spasms. Strategic use of botulinum toxin and intrathecal baclofen pumps may help in patients whose disease is refractory to oral therapies. Physical therapy, stretching, and massage therapy can be used as nonpharmacologic alternatives or additions to therapy.

Neuropathic pain is a common MS-related symptom and can be addressed with many of the same pharmacologic agents used to treat painful diabetic neuropathy (see MKSAP 18 Endocrinology and Metabolism). Nonpharmacologic approaches, such as transcutaneous electrical nerve stimulation, also can be integrated into the management plan.

Chronic fatigue is a common and life-impairing symptom in MS. Although fatigue is sometimes related to concurrent depression, insomnia, or other comorbid conditions, patients with MS without any of these issues also can experience disabling fatigue. Improved sleep hygiene, regular exercise, and treatment of underlying depression can be beneficial. The stimulant medications modafinil, armodafinil, amantadine, and amphetamines may be helpful. Complementary and alternative medicine approaches, such as magnetic therapy and ginkgo biloba, also have shown efficacy in some studies.

Depression is far more common in MS patients than in those without the disorder. Furthermore, the suicide rate for patients with MS and depression is elevated compared with that of patients with depression only. MS-related depression is likely multifactorial, involving the emotional response to dealing with a chronic disease, the consequence of demyelinating lesions and inflammatory cytokines on neurotransmitter function, and the adverse effects of treatments (such as interferon beta). Clinicians should be vigilant for the signs of depression, screen for suicidality if present, and have a low threshold for initiating antidepressants and offering referrals to psychiatry or psychology for counseling.

Cognitive dysfunction occurs in at least half of patients with MS, affecting employability and quality of life. Typical findings include deficits in short-term memory and processing speed, although almost any domain can be impaired. Trials of pharmacologic therapy, such as memantine, donepezil, and methylphenidate, have not shown efficacy. Exercise, formal neuropsychological testing, and cognitive rehabilitative and accommodative strategies (such as creating checklists to overcome memory deficits) are sometimes beneficial.

Maintenance of mobility in MS patients is essential to maintaining quality of life. An active healthy lifestyle is necessary to help stave off future disability. Physical and occupational therapy can provide gait safety training and improve balance and endurance. Assistive devices, such as braces, canes, walkers, and electrostimulatory walk-assist devices, can provide additional benefit. Pharmacologic therapy with dalfampridine, a voltage-gated potassium channel antagonist, can improve walking speed, leg strength, and gait in patients with MS and baseline gait impairment. Dalfampridine has a rare risk of seizures and should not be used in patients with known epilepsy or with kidney impairment.

Bladder dysfunction occurs in many patients with MS. Urinary frequency and urgency can be ameliorated with abstinence from caffeine, timed voids, and anticholinergic medications (solifenacin, oxybutynin, tolterodine). Patients with urinary hesitancy or retention can be more difficult to treat. Anticholinergic agents can worsen retention and increase the risk of urinary tract infection. Patients with a mixed pattern of bladder symptoms should be evaluated by a urologist; intermittent catheterization or an indwelling catheter may be necessary.

Limb tremor can occur in patients with MS and is often difficult to treat. Occupational therapy and botulinum toxin may be helpful.

Pseudobulbar affect is a rare complication of MS that can be a significant impediment to social interaction for affected patients. This symptom manifests as uncontrolled fits of laughter or crying that occur without distinct or appropriate triggers. Dextromethorphan-quinidine can help reduce this symptom.

KEY POINTS

- Muscle relaxants, such as baclofen, tizanidine, cyclobenzaprine, and the benzodiazepines, can help treat multiple sclerosis–associated spasticity due to corticospinal tract damage.

- Clinicians should be vigilant for the signs of depression in patients with multiple sclerosis; if present, they should screen for suicidality and have a low threshold for offering therapy and referrals to psychiatry.

Disorders of the Spinal Cord

Presenting Symptoms and Signs of Myelopathy

Myelopathy (any disorder involving the spinal cord) arises from extrinsic (external compression) and intrinsic (intramedullary) pathologic causes. Recognition and treatment of spinal cord injury in a timely manner is crucial, given the vital anatomy contained within this small-diameter structure.

Determining the location and mechanism of injury is crucial for rapidly deciding on the accurate site and type of neuroimaging required and the kind of specialty consultation (such as neurosurgical) needed. Spinal cord injury often presents with symptoms and signs at or below the site of a lesion. Corticospinal tract injury results in spastic paresis or paralysis, with weakness, hyperreflexia, muscle spasticity, and extensor plantar responses. There is often loss of sensation at or below the site of injury. Performance of a detailed sensory examination, with ascending pinprick testing throughout the entire torso and neck, is essential. Gait is abnormal in most patients with myelopathy; a sensory ataxia or spastic gait sometimes can be an isolated presenting sign. Involvement of the distal spinal cord and lower roots (cauda equina syndrome) results in decreased muscle tone, areflexia, and loss of perianal sensation.

Many patients with myelopathy report pain at the level of the compressive disease. Squeezing or banding sensations around the chest or abdomen near the level of spinal cord compression may be reported. Focal tenderness to percussion over the spinal column may be elicited. Disruptions in bowel and bladder function and loss of sphincter tone also are often noted. These varied symptoms may lead to unnecessary cardiac, pulmonary, gastrointestinal, or urinary tract evaluations and to a delayed diagnosis.

KEY POINTS

- Corticospinal tract injury results in spastic paresis or paralysis, with weakness, hyperreflexia, muscle spasticity, and extensor plantar responses; there is often loss of sensation at or below the site of injury.
- Injury to the distal spinal cord and lower roots (cauda equina syndrome) results in decreased muscle tone, areflexia, and loss of perianal sensation.

Compressive Myelopathy
Clinical Presentation

Spinal cord compression often presents with neck or back pain, followed by weakness, sensory changes, and bladder or bowel dysfunction. Examination typically reveals upper motor neuron signs (weakness, spasticity, hyperreflexia, and extensor planar responses), but lower motor neuron signs (atrophy, hyporeflexia) sometimes can occur near the level of compression. Specific signs and symptoms can provide clues as to the cause of compression. The presence of fever and focal back pain and tenderness, especially in patients who have had recent back instrumentation or have a history of intravenous drug use, may indicate an epidural abscess (see MKSAP 18 Infectious Diseases for more information on cranial and spinal epidural abscesses). A history of neoplasia and focal back pain should raise concern for metastatic disease (**Figure 26**) or pathologic vertebral fracture. Anticoagulant use raises the risk of compression from an epidural hematoma, particularly in the setting of recent back instrumentation.

Patients with chronic spinal stenosis due to osteoarthritic degenerative spinal disease frequently present with chronic myelopathic symptoms. Compressive myelopathy should thus be considered in older patients with gait dysfunction or weakness. Degenerative spinal disease often affects the cervical and lumbar regions, but thoracic cord involvement is quite rare. Most patients with chronic compressive myelopathy initially report progressive leg weakness, spasticity, distal numbness, and bladder impairment. Some with lumbar stenosis describe symptoms similar to vascular claudication (pseudoclaudication), with exertional groin, thigh, or buttock pain, and possibly also of weakness or numbness.

Diagnosis

Initial MRI of the spinal cord at the suspected region of injury is the preferred means of diagnosing compressive myelopathy and will often reveal the cause. Imaging should be performed

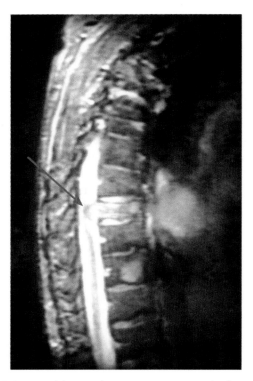

FIGURE 26. MRI of the spine showing metastatic cancer with collapse of the vertebral body and compression of the spinal cord from the posteriorly displaced bony fragments (*red arrow*).

emergently in cord compression thought to be secondary to abscess or malignancy because neurologic compromise can progress rapidly. CT myelography can show compressive myelopathy when MRI is not feasible but often does not reveal the cause of compression. Additionally, this type of imaging may be difficult to arrange emergently and is problematic in patients with allergies to contrast dyes or impaired kidney function.

KEY POINTS

- In patients with compressive myelopathy, a history of neoplasia and focal back pain should arouse concern for metastatic disease; the presence of fever and focal back pain and tenderness may indicate an epidural abscess.
- An initial MRI of the spinal cord at the suspected region of injury is the preferred means of diagnosing compressive myelopathy and will often reveal the cause.

Treatment
Surgical decompression is typically required to treat spinal cord compression, but medical therapies can complement surgical treatment, depending on the underlying cause. Emergent treatment usually is indicated because the most important indicator of long-term neurologic function is the neurologic function at the time of decompression. Neurologic

CONT.

function is rarely regained as a result of therapy, but further deterioration may be prevented.

Adjunctive therapy is important; an epidural hematoma may first require management of the bleeding diathesis, and cord compression caused by epidural abscess requires antibiotics. The use of glucocorticoids in traumatic spinal cord compression is controversial. They generally are not indicated with hematoma and abscess. A joint panel of the American Association of Neurological Surgeons and the Congress of Neurological Surgeons has argued against the use of high-dose glucocorticoids in acute spinal cord trauma, given the lack of definitive evidence of benefit and some evidence of potential harm. Despite these recommendations, this issue remains controversial, and many physicians still offer glucocorticoid treatment for this select patient population because of the lack of alternative beneficial strategies.

Spinal cord compression from metastatic disease requires emergent use of high-dose glucocorticoids and urgent surgical decompression, followed by radiation for most tumor types. Clinical trials have shown the superiority of surgical decompression in optimizing ambulation. Certain radiosensitive tumor types, such as leukemia, lymphoma, myeloma, and germ cell tumors, may not require initial surgical decompression and instead may be treated urgently with radiation therapy. Surgical intervention also is sometimes deferred in patients with a completed neurologic deficit, patients with a poor prognosis or functional status, and patients without a distinct neurologic deficit. For more information on spinal cord compression due to metastatic disease, see MKSAP18 Hematology and Oncology.

For chronic cervical or lumbar stenosis or acute disk herniation, symptomatic management can control symptoms in most patients. Surgical decompression may be required for patients with myelopathy refractory to medical management. See MKSAP 18 General Internal Medicine for more information about treating musculoskeletal pain.

KEY POINT

- Spinal cord compression from metastatic disease requires emergent use of high-dose glucocorticoids and urgent surgical decompression, followed by radiation for most tumor types.

Noncompressive Myelopathy

Noncompressive myelopathy can be caused by many inflammatory, infectious, metabolic, vascular, and genetic disorders. Inflammatory causes are most common, including multiple sclerosis (see Multiple Sclerosis), neuromyelitis optica, and sarcoidosis.

Idiopathic Transverse Myelitis

Idiopathic transverse myelitis (ITM) (**Figure 27**) is a monophasic, inflammatory, and demyelinating disorder of the spinal

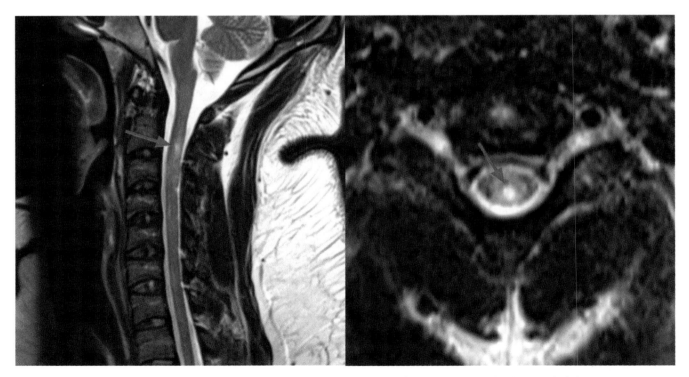

FIGURE 27. MRI of the cervical spine in a patient with transverse myelitis. Sagittal T2-weighted (*left*) and axial T2-weighted (*right*) images both demonstrate hyperintensity within the parenchyma of the spinal cord (*red arrows*).

cord. ITM typically affects only one region of the spinal cord and is considered to be a para- or postinfectious inflammatory response. Affected patients frequently experience subacute weakness, sensory changes, and bladder or bowel dysfunction. Some patients experience an initial prodrome of back pain or a thoracic banding sensation.

The diagnostic criteria for ITM require presence of clinical features of the syndrome, evidence of inflammation (either cerebrospinal fluid leukocytosis or contrast enhancement on spinal cord MRI), and exclusion of other potential causes. Those with complete myelitis (symptoms referable to complete rather than partial cord transection), a lack of elevated oligoclonal bands or IgG index in the cerebrospinal fluid, and no lesions on brain MRI are much more likely to have ITM than other disorders, such as multiple sclerosis. This is a crucial distinction because ITM is not a recurrent disorder and does not require long-term immunomodulatory therapy. Recurrence of symptoms or new symptoms beyond a 30-day period should arouse suspicion for multiple sclerosis or other recurrent disorders.

The consensus-based treatment of ITM is intravenous methylprednisolone, 1 g/d for 3 to 7 days. This therapy is intended to stop inflammatory damage of the spinal cord and allow for recovery of neurologic function. Patients whose disease is refractory to glucocorticoids may benefit from plasmapheresis or cyclophosphamide.

Infectious causes of transverse myelitis should always be considered when evaluating patients for possible ITM. Herpes simplex virus, varicella zoster virus, West Nile virus, human T-lymphotropic virus, Lyme disease, and neurosyphilis infections can affect the spinal cord. HIV infection can cause a transverse myelitis–like syndrome at the time of seroconversion or result in a chronic degenerative vacuolar myelopathy in patients with chronic low CD4 cell counts. Mycobacterium tuberculosis can infect the meninges and spinal cord and present with a transverse myelitis-like syndrome. Treatment should be directed against a particular infection if present. The addition of glucocorticoids to treat these disorders is controversial but may be indicated when infections are associated with significant spinal cord edema.

KEY POINTS

- Patients with complete myelitis, no oligoclonal bands or IgG index in the cerebrospinal fluid, and no lesions on brain MRI are much more likely to have idiopathic transverse myelitis than multiple sclerosis.
- Treatment of idiopathic transverse myelitis is intravenous methylprednisolone; secondary causes of transverse myelitis, including infection, should first be excluded.

Subacute Combined Degeneration

Severe and prolonged vitamin B_{12} deficiency can result in subacute combined degeneration, which refers to a dysfunction of the corticospinal and dorsal sensory tracts of the spinal cord that manifests as spastic paresis with reduced vibration and position sense and ataxia. MRI can show increased signal in the affected white-matter pathways without associated inflammatory changes. Laboratory study results show a low serum vitamin B_{12} level with elevated levels of serum methylmalonic acid and homocysteine. Macrocytic anemia may be present, but the neurologic manifestations of B_{12} deficiency may precede development of anemia. The clinical symptoms of vitamin B_{12} deficiency can sometimes occur with low-normal serum B_{12} levels, and thus supportive laboratory studies should be performed in patients with a high index of clinical suspicion. Vitamin B_{12} replacement usually halts progression of the disease but may not necessarily reverse existing symptoms.

Nitrous oxide abuse also can cause a relative vitamin B_{12} deficiency that results in subacute combined degeneration. Supplementation of vitamin B_{12} in those circumstances without cessation of the drug may impede improvement in symptoms.

Copper deficiency (due to malabsorption, nutritional deficiency, or zinc toxicity) can also cause subacute combined degeneration. This entity should be considered in patients with suggestive symptoms who have normal vitamin B_{12} levels. Myelopathy from such nutritional deficiencies should specifically be considered in patients with previous bariatric surgical procedures.

KEY POINT

- Severe and prolonged vitamin B_{12} deficiency can result in subacute combined degeneration; in patients with suggestive symptoms of this disorder and normal vitamin B_{12} levels, copper deficiency should be considered.

Vascular Disorders

Infarcts in the territory of the anterior spinal artery typically present as sudden-onset flaccid paralysis with preservation of vibration and position sense because of the lack of dorsal column involvement. Prolonged hypotension during cardiovascular or aortic surgery can also sometimes result in lack of perfusion to watershed regions of the spinal cord, especially in the area where the anterior spinal artery meets the most prominent radicular artery (artery of Adamkiewicz) in the upper thoracic cord. ■

Dural arteriovenous fistulas of the spinal vascular supply can either result in chronic myelopathy due to venous congestion or cause infarction of the cord due to altered vascular dynamics or thromboses. Fistulas are most common in men older than 50 years and in persons with previous spinal surgery. Abnormal vascular flow voids often are seen on careful review of spinal MRIs. Diagnosis is often challenging and typically requires digital subtraction angiography of all radicular vessels along the entire spine.

Genetic Disorders

Although rare, several genetic disorders can result in chronic myelopathy. Some of these disorders have clear familial inheritance, but others may result from de novo mutations. Hereditary spastic paraplegia comprises hereditary disorders that result in chronic, progressive, ascending weakness and spasticity, often beginning in childhood or adolescence. Genetic screening is available, but no treatment currently exists. Female carriers of X-lined adrenoleukodystrophy sometimes develop adrenomyeloneuropathy, a degenerative condition of the spinal cord and peripheral nerves. These patients can be diagnosed through alterations in the serum very-long-chain fatty acid profiles or genetic testing. Genetic counseling is indicated in such settings.

Neuromuscular Disorders
Overview
Peripheral and central nervous system disorders can be differentiated on the basis of history and neurologic examination findings (**Table 44**). Neuromuscular disorders include myopathies, neuromuscular junction disorders, peripheral neuropathies, plexopathies, radiculopathies, and motor neuron diseases (**Table 45** and **Table 46**).

Peripheral Neuropathies
Classification, Findings, and Diagnosis
Symptoms of peripheral neuropathy include negative (sensory loss) or positive (paresthesia, dysesthesia, and pain) sensory symptoms, weakness, or autonomic dysfunction. Neuropathies are classified on the basis of distribution of sensorimotor deficits (symmetry, distal versus proximal, focal versus generalized), pathology (demyelinating versus axonal), family history, and autonomic involvement (**Figure 28**, on page 78).

For all patients with a suspected peripheral neuropathy, a complete blood count, an erythrocyte sedimentation rate determination, serum protein electrophoresis with immune fixation, thyroid function tests, hemoglobin A_{1c}/fasting plasma glucose determination, and vitamin B_{12} measurement are necessary. In specific clinical settings, additional

TABLE 44. Features Distinguishing Peripheral From Central Nervous System Disorders

Features	PNS Disorder	CNS Disorder
Onset	Subacute or insidious	Sudden (stroke) or gradual (mass lesions)
Pattern of weakness	Focal or multifocal (in the territory of the affected nerve, plexus, or root) or generalized	Entire limb, unilateral, or a pyramidal pattern of weakness[a]
Atrophy	Yes (at times prominent)	No (or mild, and related to disuse)
Fasciculations	Yes	No
Tone	Decreased or normal	Increased (spasticity or rigidity[b]) or normal
Pattern of sensory symptoms	Focal or multifocal (in the territory of the affected nerve, plexus, or root) or stocking-glove in distribution	Entire limb or unilateral
Type of sensory symptoms	Positive symptoms (paresthesia, dysesthesia, or allodynia[c]) more frequent, but negative symptoms (numbness) possible	Negative symptoms more frequent, but positive symptoms possible
Dissociated sensory loss	Pain/temperature and vibration/proprioception deficits travel together	Dissociation of pain/temperature and vibration/proprioception deficits possible with spinal and brainstem lesions
Deep tendon reflexes	Diminished or normal	Increased
Pathologic reflexes	Absent	Present, including extensor plantar response, Hoffman sign,[d] knee cross adduction, jaw jerk, snout, and clonus
Additional localizing symptoms	Cramps	Headache, seizures, and visual and language-related symptoms
EMG	Abnormal	Normal

CNS = central nervous system; EMG = electromyography; PNS = peripheral nervous system

[a]Pyramidal weakness is caused by upper motor neuron lesions and affects extensors more than flexors in the upper limbs and flexors more than extensors in the lower limbs.

[b]Spasticity is a direction- and velocity-dependent increase in tone and is associated with pyramidal lesions; rigidity is an increase in tone that is independent of velocity and direction and is associated with extrapyramidal lesions.

[c]Paresthesia is an abnormal spontaneous sensation, such as tingling, burning, or electrical sensation. Dysesthesia is an unpleasant sensation provoked by neutral stimuli, such as light touch or contact of clothes. Allodynia is pain provoked by nonnoxious stimuli.

[d]Hoffman sign is positive if the thumb is flexed in response to a flicking or snapping of the distal phalanx of the middle finger.

TABLE 45. Classification of Neuromuscular Disorders

Type	Features	Examples
Myopathy		
Acquired	Proximal greater than distal weakness, absence of sensory and autonomic symptoms, symmetric, late hyporeflexia after atrophy, adult onset	Inflammatory, toxic, systemic, and endocrine myopathies
Inherited	Similar to acquired myopathy, onset in childhood or early adulthood, positive family history, some possibly associated with distal or multifocal (scapuloperoneal, oculopharyngeal) weakness and atrophy, myotonia, exercise-induced pain	Muscular dystrophies; mitochondrial, metabolic, and congenital myopathies
Neuromuscular junction disorder	Fluctuating weakness; fatigue; absence of sensory and autonomic symptoms; symmetric, bulbar, and respiratory involvement	Myasthenia gravis, Lambert-Eaton myasthenic syndrome
Peripheral neuropathy		
Axonal	Symmetric distal sensory and sensorimotor impairment, possible involvement of autonomic nerves, early or late hyporeflexia	Diabetic, toxic, hypothyroid, uremic, nutritional polyneuropathy
Demyelinating	Proximal and distal symmetric or multifocal weakness with variable sensory loss, early areflexia, low back radicular pain; hereditary forms associated with foot deformities and slow progression	GBS, CIDP, hereditary (CMT1)
Mononeuropathy	Sensory and motor deficits within the distribution of a single nerve, symptoms distal to site of compression	Carpal tunnel syndrome, ulnar neuropathy, peroneal neuropathy
Plexopathy	Motor and sensory deficits in multiple contiguous nerves in upper or lower extremities, asymmetric, severe pain at onset with autoimmune and diabetic types	Idiopathic brachial plexitis, idiopathic lumbosacral radiculoplexus neuropathy, diabetic amyotrophy, postradiation and carcinomatous plexopathy
Radiculopathy	Motor, sensory, and reflex deficits in the area innervated by affected nerve root, radicular pain and paresthesia, neck or low back pain	Cervical and lumbar radiculopathy
Ganglionopathy	Severe loss of vibration and joint position sense in single limb, no motor deficit	Paraneoplastic and autoimmune ganglionopathy
Motor neuron disease	Concomitant signs of upper motor neuron (hyperreflexia, pyramidal signs, and spasticity) and lower motor neuron (weakness, atrophy, and fasciculation) dysfunction, no sensory deficit, asymmetric onset, bulbar and respiratory involvement	ALS
Myelopathy[a]	Lower motor neuron signs at the level of compression and upper motor neuron signs below it, sphincter dysfunction, sensory symptoms present, sensory level	Cervical cord compression

ALS = amyotrophic lateral sclerosis; CIDP = chronic inflammatory demyelinating polyradiculoneuropathy; CMT1 = Charcot-Marie-Tooth disease type 1; GBS = Guillain-Barré syndrome.

[a]Myelopathy is a key differential diagnosis for neuromuscular disorders.

tests, including CSF analysis, genetic testing, and other specialized laboratory testing, can help clarify the diagnosis (**Table 47**, on page 79).

Electromyography (EMG), including both nerve conduction studies and needle electrode examination, can differentiate neuropathy from other neuromuscular disorders. In neuropathy, motor unit potentials are high amplitude and prolonged, whereas in myopathy, these potentials are low amplitude and brief. If neuropathy is present, EMG also can determine whether it is demyelinating or axonal. In demyelinating neuropathies, velocity of nerve conduction decreases, but in axonopathy, velocity remains unchanged. The presence of weakness, asymmetry, proximal findings, rapid course, or atypical features should prompt EMG testing. In patients with a slowly progressive distal symmetric sensory neuropathy with negative family history, however, EMG may not be required.

Nerve biopsy should only be considered in rare settings in which concern for a vasculitic, infectious, or infiltrative neuropathy exists. Autonomic tests, including

TABLE 46. Common Symptoms and Signs of Neuromuscular Disorders

Symptoms and Signs	Differential Diagnosis
Weakness	
Distal extremities	Diabetic, toxic and systemic polyneuropathy, hereditary neuropathy
Proximal extremities	Myopathy, polyradiculopathy, inflammatory demyelinating neuropathy, diabetic amyotrophy
Multifocal with pain (mononeuropathy multiplex)	Vasculitis, rheumatoid arthritis, diabetes
Focal asymmetric	ALS, inclusion body myositis, radiculopathy, multifocal motor neuropathy
Fluctuating	Myasthenia gravis
Muscles of eye movement	Myasthenia gravis, mitochondrial myopathy, thyroid disease
Bulbar (tongue, palate, lips)	ALS, myasthenia gravis, inclusion body myositis
Cranial nerves (especially seventh and third)	Diabetes, Lyme disease, sarcoidosis, HIV infection, Sjögren syndrome
Neck extensors	ALS, myasthenia gravis (especially with anti-MuSK antibody)
Fasciculation	ALS, radiculopathy, benign fasciculation syndrome
Sensory	
Stocking-glove gradient	Diabetic, toxic, systemic, or cryptogenic polyneuropathy; hereditary neuropathy
Dermatomal pattern	Radiculopathy, peripheral nerve lesion
Distal pain without hyporeflexia	Small fiber neuropathy (diabetes mellitus, alcoholism, Sjögren syndrome, sarcoidosis)
Marked proprioceptive loss in single limb	Dorsal root ganglionopathy (paraneoplastic, Sjögren syndrome, HIV)
Autonomic	
Orthostatic hypotension, resting tachycardia, excessive or impaired sweating, gastroparesis, constipation, erectile dysfunction	Diabetes, alcoholism, amyloidosis, autoimmune dysautonomia with antiganglionic acetylcholine receptor antibody, paraneoplastic antibodies

ALS = amyotrophic lateral sclerosis; MuSK = muscle-specific kinase.

quantitative sudomotor axon reflex and tilt table tests, can help confirm autonomic neuropathy but are rarely performed in practice.

KEY POINTS

HVC
- Electromyography (EMG) can differentiate neuropathy from other neuromuscular disorders, and if neuropathy is present, EMG can determine whether it is axonal or demyelinating; EMG may not be necessary in patients with a slowly progressive distal symmetric sensory neuropathy and a negative family history.

- The presence of weakness, asymmetry, proximal findings, a rapid course, or atypical features should prompt testing with electromyography in a patient with a suspected peripheral neuropathy.

Mononeuropathies

Mononeuropathies involve a single nerve and can cause both motor and sensory symptoms within the territory of the affected nerve. Sequential involvement of multiple nerves may be seen in mononeuropathy multiplex, a condition most often associated with pain and caused by vasculitis.

Plexopathies originate at the level of the brachial or lumbosacral plexus and involve multiple sensory and motor nerves simultaneously.

Carpal Tunnel Syndrome

Carpal tunnel syndrome results from focal compression of the median nerve at the wrist. Most often, paresthesia and pain are experienced in the first three digits but may radiate to the entire hand or proximally. With milder symptoms, diagnosis of carpal tunnel syndrome can be made clinically, and treatment is supportive, including neutral positioning, wrist splints, and pain control. The presence of weakness, thenar atrophy, refractory pain, or active denervation evident on EMG should prompt surgical decompression. See MKSAP 18 General Internal Medicine for further information about carpal tunnel syndrome.

KEY POINT

- In patients with carpal tunnel syndrome and mild symptoms, a clinical diagnosis and supportive care is appropriate; the presence of weakness, thenar atrophy, refractory pain, or active denervation evident on electromyography should prompt decompression surgery. HVC

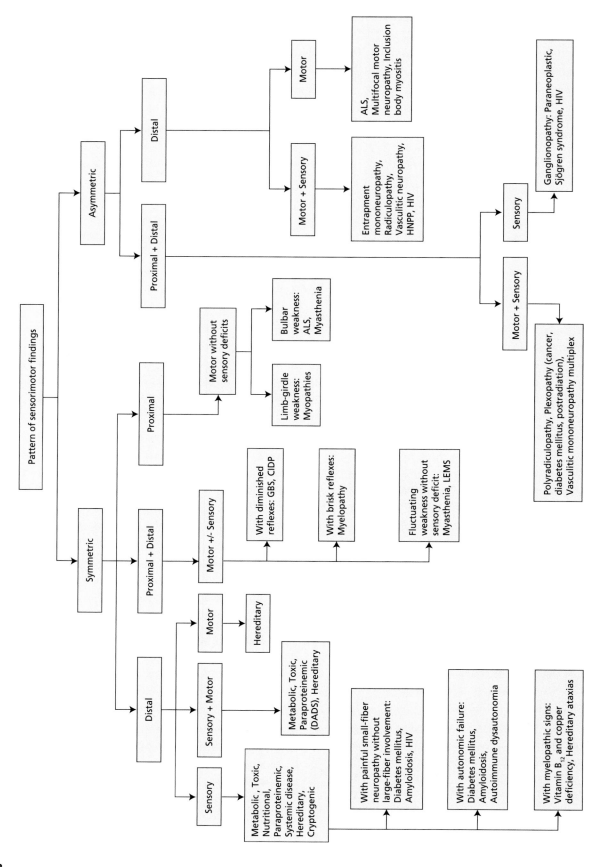

FIGURE 28. Algorithmic approach to peripheral neuropathies. ALS = amyotrophic lateral sclerosis; CIDP = chronic inflammatory demyelinating polyradiculoneuropathy; DADS = distal acquired demyelinating symmetric neuropathy; GBS = Guillain-Barré syndrome; HNPP = hereditary neuropathy with predisposition to pressure palsy; LEMS = Lambert-Eaton myasthenic syndrome.

TABLE 47. Laboratory Testing in Peripheral Neuropathy

Underlying Cause	Clinical Presentation	Laboratory Testing
Diabetes mellitus, impaired glucose tolerance	Distal symmetric polyneuropathy, mononeuropathy, lumbosacral radiculoneuropathy	Glucose tolerance test, hemoglobin A_{1c} measurement
Uremia, thyroid disease, anemia, liver disease	Distal symmetric polyneuropathy	Serum creatinine, TSH, and free thyroxine (T_4) levels; hematocrit, liver chemistry tests
Connective tissue disease, polyarteritis nodosa, vasculitis, Sjögren syndrome, cryoglobulinemia	Vasculitic mononeuropathy multiplex, Sjögren ganglionopathy	ESR and rheumatoid factor determination; antinuclear antibody, ANCA, anti-Ro/SSA antibody, anti-LA/SSB antibody, and cryoglobulin measurements
Syphilis	Posterior column disease resembling large-fiber neuropathy	RPR, CSF VDRL
MGUS, amyloidosis, multiple myeloma, lymphoproliferative disease, POEMS syndrome	Paraproteinemic neuropathy	SPEP, UPEP, IFE, serum free light chain assay
Vitamin B_{12}, folate, vitamin E, or copper deficiency	Myeloneuropathy with brisk reflexes	Serum copper, vitamin B_{12}, folate, vitamin E, methylmalonic acid/homocysteine levels
CIDP, GBS	Progressive symmetric proximal and distal motor and sensory polyradiculoneuropathy	CSF cell and protein, serum antiganglioside antibodies
Miller-Fisher variant of GBS	Ophthalmoplegia, ataxia, areflexia	Serum anti-GQ1B antibody
Multifocal motor neuropathy	Asymmetric pure motor weakness	Serum anti-GM1 antibody
Distal acquired demyelinating symmetric neuropathy	Distal sensory loss, tremor, sensory ataxia	SPEP, IFE, serum anti-MAG antibody
Amyloidosis	Autonomic and small-fiber neuropathy	Serum free light chains, abdominal fat pad biopsy (acquired), transthyretin gene testing (familial)
Infectious neuropathy	Variable, cranial nerve palsy, myelopathy with flaccid weakness in West Nile virus	Serum HIV antibody, serum Lyme antibody with Western blot confirmation, CSF West Nile virus antibody, skin biopsy in leprosy, IGRA, CSF acid-fast smear
Toxic neuropathy	Symmetric sensory or sensorimotor neuropathy, acute motor neuropathy (lead)	Serum lead, arsenic, mercury, and thallium measurements; 24-hour urine toxicology; history of exposure to ethanol, chemotherapy agents, colchicine, amiodarone, quinolones
Celiac disease	Sensory neuropathy and ataxia	IgA tissue transglutaminase antibodies and endomysial antibodies
Porphyria	Acute painful polyradiculopathy	Urine porphobilinogen and δ-aminolevulinic acid
Paraneoplastic disease	Subacute progressive sensory neuropathy, asymmetric ganglionopathy	Serum anti-Hu and anti-CRMP5 measurement; CSF oligoclonal bands

ANCA = anti-neutrophil cytoplasmic antibody; CIDP = chronic inflammatory demyelinating polyradiculoneuropathy; CRMP5 = collapsin response mediator protein 5; CSF = cerebrospinal fluid; ESR = erythrocyte sedimentation rate; GBS = Guillain-Barré syndrome, IFE = immune fixation electrophoresis; IGRA = interferon-γ release assay; MAG = myelin-associated glycoprotein; MGUS = monoclonal gammopathy of unknown significance; POEMS = polyneuropathy, organomegaly, endocrinopathy, monoclonal protein plasma cell disorder, and skin lesions ; RPR = rapid plasma reagin; SPEP = serum protein electrophoresis; SSA = Sjögren syndrome–related antigen A; SSB = Sjögren syndrome–related antigen B; TSH = thyroid-stimulating hormone; UPEP = urine protein electrophoresis; VDRL = Venereal Disease Research Laboratory test.

Bell Palsy

Bell palsy is idiopathic paralysis of the facial nerve (cranial nerve VII) that leads to unilateral paralysis of upper and lower facial muscles. In contrast, upper facial muscles are spared in central facial weakness (stroke) because of their bilateral innervation. Altered taste and hyperacusis also may occur in Bell palsy because of involvement of chorda tympani and stapedius muscles. Between 70% and 90% of patients with Bell palsy fully recover within a few weeks. In classic Bell palsy,

initial brain imaging and laboratory testing are not required. Treatment with a 10-day course of oral prednisone, started within 72 hours of onset, is recommended to expedite both the rate and speed of full recovery. The utility of adding antiviral treatment to prednisone is controversial, and guidelines differ in their recommendations. There may be a small benefit to adding antiviral treatment in patients with severe palsy. Use of an eye patch and artificial tears to prevent corneal dryness are recommended. Synkinesis (concomitant movement of perioral and periorbital muscles) may result from aberrant reinnervation after Bell palsy.

Secondary causes for facial nerve palsy include diabetes mellitus, Lyme disease, sarcoidosis, HIV, vasculitis, and malignancy. If a secondary cause is suspected on the basis of history (subacute onset over days, comorbidities, rash) or clinical examination (deficits unrelated to the facial nerve), additional testing is indicated and prednisone is typically avoided. Brain MRI with contrast also is recommended in patients with lingering or worsening weakness after 2 months.

KEY POINT

HVC
- In classic Bell palsy, initial brain imaging and laboratory testing is not required; treatment with a 10-day course of oral prednisone, started within 72 hours of onset, may expedite both the rate and speed of full recovery.

Brachial and Lumbosacral Plexopathies

Common causes of brachial and lumbosacral plexopathy include diabetes, malignancy, radiation, and trauma. Imaging is mandatory to rule out structural lesions and malignancy. Idiopathic brachial plexitis (also known as neuralgic amyotrophy) presents with subacute severe scapular pain followed by pronounced weakness and atrophy in shoulder-girdle and upper extremity muscles. It is likely immune mediated, and a triggering event, such as infection or surgery, usually precedes this presentation, although the infection or surgery is not in the region of the brachial plexus. EMG can confirm the diagnosis, and imaging can rule out alternative causes. Treatment is supportive. Gradual recovery (90% by 3 years) is common. Idiopathic lumbosacral radiculoplexus neuropathy is immune mediated and very similar in presentation to diabetic amyotrophy. (See Neuropathies of Diabetes Mellitus and Impaired Glucose Tolerance.)

Polyneuropathies

Polyneuropathies arise from various disorders causing injury to peripheral nerves (see Table 47). Polyneuropathies may affect either large nerve fibers (and lead to impaired proprioception, hyporeflexia, and weakness) or small nerve fibers (and cause pain, dysesthesia, and dysautonomia). Additionally, they may be primarily axonal or demyelinating. If axonal, the distal axonal segments are affected first, which leads to a length-dependent stocking-glove pattern of involvement. A sensory-predominant distal symmetric neuropathy is typically seen with metabolic, toxic, and systemic neuropathies. Demyelinating neuropathies, which result from injury to the myelin sheath of the peripheral nerve, can cause non–length-dependent weakness and sensory loss.

Neuropathies of Diabetes Mellitus and Impaired Glucose Tolerance

Diabetes mellitus causes various types of neuropathy (**Table 48**). The most common presentation is symmetric distal neuropathy involving small and large sensory fibers and, to a lesser extent, distal motor nerves. Clinical examination may reveal length-dependent loss of light touch and vibration sensation, loss of the ankle reflex, and—in advanced disease—distal weakness. Pain and paresthesia may predominate, especially when small fibers are involved. Patients with a pure small-fiber variant of symmetric distal neuropathy may have normal distal sensory and reflex findings on examination and normal results on EMG at presentation; this pattern also can be seen at various stages of diabetes and even in patients with impaired glucose tolerance. Between 11% and 25% of patients with glucose intolerance have evidence of small-fiber neuropathy on specialized testing, but only a minority (5%-10%) are symptomatic.

Autonomic diabetic neuropathy can cause orthostatic hypotension, erectile dysfunction, abnormal hidrosis, and gastroparesis. Dysautonomia also can mask symptoms of hypoglycemia and may predispose patients to silent myocardial infarction. Diabetic mononeuropathy can involve the cranial nerves (especially III, VI, and VII) and truncal nerve roots (with a dermatomal pattern of pain and paresthesia in the chest or abdomen) and predispose patients to entrapment neuropathies, such as carpal tunnel syndrome.

Diabetic amyotrophy, also known as proximal lumbosacral radiculoneuropathy, is associated with subacute painful involvement of the lumbosacral plexus followed by resolution of pain and onset of marked asymmetric weakness with atrophy and weight loss. The differential diagnosis of diabetic amyotrophy includes polyradiculopathy, retroperitoneal hematoma, neoplasm, carcinomatous meningitis, and inflammatory neuropathy. Spontaneous recovery over 1 to 3 years is typical but may be incomplete.

Tight glycemic control, exercise, and management of dyslipidemia, obesity, and metabolic syndrome can slow the progression and improve the symptoms of diabetic polyneuropathy. Management of diabetic amyotrophy consists of supportive measures, physical therapy, and pain control but does not involve immunosuppression. See MKSAP 18 Endocrinology and Metabolism for further information about diabetic neuropathy, including neuropathic pain treatment.

KEY POINTS

- The most common form of neuropathy secondary to diabetes is a symmetric distal neuropathy involving small and large sensory fibers and, to less extent, distal motor nerves; examination may reveal length-dependent loss of light touch and vibration sensation, loss of the ankle reflex, and—in advanced disease—distal weakness

- Tight glycemic control, exercise, and management of dyslipidemia, obesity, and metabolic syndrome can slow the progression and improve the symptoms of diabetic polyneuropathy.

TABLE 48.	Peripheral Nerve Dysfunction in Diabetes Mellitus		
Classification	**Sign and Symptoms**	**Diagnosis**	**Management**
Autonomic neuropathy	Orthostatic hypotension, early satiety, nausea and vomiting (gastroparesis), constipation (colonic dysmotility), erectile dysfunction, hyperhidrosis or hypohidrosis	Orthostatic blood pressure determination, QSART, tilt table	Fludrocortisone; midodrine; compression stocking; supportive management of bowel, bladder, and sexual symptoms; glycemic control
Diabetic lumbosacral radiculoneuropathy (diabetic amyotrophy)	Severe pain followed by weakness and muscle wasting in proximal lower extremities; weight loss, with or without proximal sensory loss	Clinical examination, EMG, lumbar spinal MRI, CT of abdomen and pelvis (to rule out retroperitoneal hematoma)	Pain control, physical therapy, supportive measures, not associated with level of glycemic control, not responsive to immunotherapy
Mononeuropathy	Sensory loss; paresthesia or pain in the distribution of a single nerve, followed by weakness (median or peroneal nerve); cranial nerve palsy (especially cranial nerves III, VI, or VII)	Clinical examination, EMG, brain MRI	Avoidance of compressive positions, bracing, pain control, decompressive surgery, observation in cranial palsies
Radiculopathy	Sensory loss, pain, and weakness in the distribution of nerve roots; thoracic radiculopathy causing patchy truncal numbness is common	Clinical examination, EMG, MRI of nerve roots (to rule out root compression)	Pain control, glycemic control, observation
Sensorimotor peripheral neuropathy	Asymptomatic (sometimes); distal length dependent; sensory loss and weakness; often painful; possible loss of ankle reflex	Clinical, EMG, oral glucose tolerance test, hemoglobin A_{1c}	Regular monitoring of feet, supportive measures, neuropathic pain medication (see Small-fiber neuropathy below)
Small-fiber neuropathy	Burning distal extremity pain without weakness, may be non-length-dependent, sparing of ankle reflex	Clinical, QSART, skin biopsy (intraepidermal nerve fiber density)	Pregabalin, duloxetine, tapentadol (FDA-approved), tricyclic antidepressants, venlafaxine, gabapentin, and topical capsaicin

EMG = electromyography; QSART = quantitative sudomotor axon reflex test.

Hereditary Neuropathies

Charcot-Marie-Tooth disease consists of more than 70 genetic disorders in which peripheral neuropathy is the only or main clinical manifestation. The most common inherited neuropathy, Charcot-Marie-Tooth disease type 1 is an autosomal dominant demyelinating neuropathy presenting with early onset, slowly progressive distal weakness, areflexia, and sensory loss without pain or paresthesia. Foot deformities, such as hammer toes, high arches, and distal leg atrophy (stork legs) are common (**Figure 29**). EMG typically reveals a uniform slowing of nerve conduction velocities, and genetic testing is confirmatory.

Inflammatory Polyradiculoneuropathies

Guillain-Barré Syndrome

Guillain-Barré syndrome (GBS) is an acute autoimmune demyelinating polyradiculoneuropathy that presents with rapidly progressive flaccid weakness. Onset is often preceded by a respiratory or gastrointestinal infection, triggering a T-cell–mediated autoimmune attack against peripheral nerve and root myelin. Weakness is ascending, starting in the lower extremities, spreading to the upper limbs and bulbar and respiratory muscles, and reaching its nadir in less than 4 weeks. The weakness may occur first in the proximal muscles. Paresthesias and early low back pain are common. Dysautonomia can be severe and predispose patients to labile blood pressure and arrhythmias. Progressive respiratory and bulbar weakness may lead to rapid respiratory failure. On examination, diffuse areflexia is a key finding; there is not marked sensory loss, even in the setting of paresthesias. GBS variants include demyelinating polyradiculoneuropathy involving only or sparing the legs and the Miller-Fisher variant, which presents with ataxia, cranial neuropathies, and antibodies to GQ1b ganglioside protein (a highly sensitive finding).

The differential diagnosis of GBS includes botulism (descending weakness), myasthenic crisis (without pain and paresthesia), acute myelopathies (hyperreflexia and upper motor neuron signs), West Nile virus (asymmetric paralysis), carcinomatous and sarcoid meningitis (slower course), Lyme disease, HIV seroconversion, porphyria, and tick paralysis.

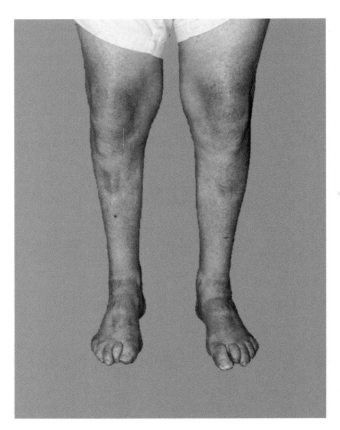

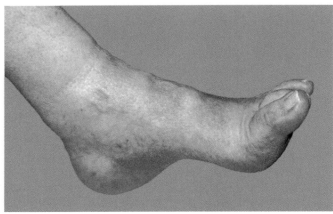

FIGURE 29. High arches, hammertoes, and distal leg atrophy in a patient with inherited neuropathy.

CONT.

CSF analysis shows a pattern of a highly elevated protein level with a normal or mildly elevated leukocyte count (albuminocytologic dissociation) in 90% of patients. EMG is the confirmatory test and shows a predominantly demyelinating pattern; sensitivity is initially low but 90% by week 5. Initiation of treatment should not await EMG confirmation; a negative early study should be repeated later if the diagnosis remains suspected. Additional studies, such as spinal MRI and serologic testing for Lyme disease, HIV, and myasthenia antibodies, may be considered in appropriate clinical settings.

Therapy includes supportive management and immunotherapy. All patients with GBS should be hospitalized for close respiratory and cardiovascular monitoring. Decisions about intubation should be guided by measurement of forced vital capacity and negative inspiratory force and be made before emergence of hypoxemia. Both plasmapheresis and intravenous immune globulin (IVIG) have equal efficacy in shortening the time to recovery and the duration of ventilation. Serial treatment with IVIG after plasma exchange is not superior to either treatment alone and should not be considered unless symptoms worsen after initial improvement or stabilization. Glucocorticoids are contraindicated in GBS and may worsen outcome. Prognosis is favorable, with 80% of patients resuming ambulation by 6 months after onset. Relapse occurs in 6% of patients with GBS and requires repeated treatment. **H**

KEY POINTS

- Guillain-Barré syndrome is an acute autoimmune demyelinating polyradiculoneuropathy that presents with rapidly progressive ascending flaccid weakness.
- All patients with Guillain-Barré syndrome should be hospitalized for close respiratory and cardiovascular monitoring; plasmapheresis and intravenous immune globulin have equal efficacy in shortening the time to recovery and the duration of ventilation.
- Glucocorticoids are contraindicated in Guillain-Barré syndrome and may worsen outcome.

Chronic Inflammatory Demyelinating Polyradiculoneuropathy

Chronic inflammatory demyelinating polyradiculoneuropathy (CIDP) is a potentially treatable autoimmune neuropathy. CIDP often presents with a progressive or relapsing symmetric proximal and distal weakness and sensory symptoms with diffuse areflexia. Its temporal course is often subacute with progression after 8 weeks of onset. Atypical forms include multifocal asymmetric and distal symmetric variants, but respiratory failure is rare. CIDP may be isolated or occur in the setting of several other systemic conditions, including diabetes mellitus, lymphoma, and HIV. CSF findings are similar to those of GBS, and a demyelinating pattern on EMG is the key to diagnosis. Nerve biopsy is often unnecessary but, in complex presentations, can differentiate CIDP from vasculitis or amyloidosis. First-line treatments include glucocorticoids, periodic IVIG, or plasma exchange, which all have similar efficacy. Treatment is typically continued for at least 6 months. Half of patients achieve remission, but the other half relapse and require resumption of immunotherapy. Second-line therapies, including azathioprine, mycophenolate mofetil, cyclosporine, or cyclophosphamide, are often used off-label to treat refractory disease.

Critical Illness Neuropathy

Prolonged intensive care treatment, particularly in association with sepsis and multiorgan failure, can lead to diffuse weakness, an inability to wean patients from ventilators, and prolonged posthospitalization weakness. Weakness may be secondary to critical illness myopathy, critical illness axonal polyneuropathy, or a combination of the two. Critical illness myopathy is more common, less severe, and potentially caused by channelopathy (a disease involving dysfunction of a cellular ion channel) triggered by sepsis and systemic disease. Critical illness neuropathy, on the other hand, is associated with microcirculatory axonal damage and a more protracted recovery. EMG can differentiate between the two, but often components of both are simultaneously present; in rare cases, nerve and muscle biopsy may be necessary. Differential diagnosis includes GBS, myasthenia gravis, vasculitis, and central weakness. No definitive treatment is available, but appropriate glycemic control, early mobilization and therapy, and minimizing glucocorticoid use improve prognosis. One third of patients with critical illness neuropathy die during the acute phase of the disease, with the remainder experiencing a full or partial slow recovery within months to years. 🔲

KEY POINTS

- Critical illness axonal polyneuropathy often coexists with critical illness myopathy and can lead to diffuse weakness, an inability to wean patients from ventilators, and prolonged posthospitalization weakness.

- No definitive treatment is available for critical illness neuropathy, but appropriate glycemic control, early mobilization and therapy, and minimizing glucocorticoid use improve prognosis.

Paraproteinemic Neuropathy

Paraproteinemic neuropathy frequently presents as a symmetric distal sensory neuropathy, but sensorimotor, multifocal motor, or cranial nerve variants also are possible. Therefore, all patients with peripheral neuropathy should be screened for paraproteinemia. Neuropathies associated with monoclonal proteins occur in monoclonal gammopathy of undetermined significance, multiple myeloma, Waldenström macroglobulinemia, amyloidosis, and other hematologic malignancies. (See MKSAP 18 Hematology and Oncology). Diagnosis depends on the detection of monoclonal proteins, and treatment is based on the underlying condition. A CIDP-like severe polyneuropathy may occur in paraproteinemic neuropathy in association with organomegaly, endocrinopathy, monoclonal plasma cell disorder, and skin changes (POEMS syndrome); this syndrome always is associated with λ paraproteinemia. Treatment is similar to that of multiple myeloma and may reverse neuropathic symptoms. Another neuropathic disorder associated with paraproteins is distal acquired demyelinating symmetric neuropathy. Patients with this condition generally are responsive to immunosuppressive therapy (glucocorticoids, IVIG, and rituximab), except for those with antibodies to myelin-associated glycoprotein; their disease is medication refractory.

Autonomic Neuropathy

Autonomic neuropathies manifest as diffuse or focal impairment of cholinergic or sympathetic autonomic systems. Whereas diabetes, amyloidosis, and HIV are common disorders underlying secondary autonomic neuropathy, primary autoimmune ganglionopathy is an important and potentially treatable cause of autonomic neuropathy that is often associated with antibodies against ganglionic nicotinic acetylcholine receptors. The presentation may range from acute pandysautonomia to chronic focal autonomic dysfunction. Antibody testing and skin biopsy help with diagnosis. Response to IVIG, plasmapheresis, or immunosuppression is common.

Amyloid neuropathy is caused by extracellular deposition of amyloid protein in peripheral nerves and other tissues. Amyloidosis starts with painful small-fiber neuropathy and progressively causes major autonomic impairment and weakness and multiorgan involvement. Primary amyloidosis is associated with monoclonal proteins, whereas familial amyloidosis is secondary to transthyretin gene mutation. See MKSAP 18 Hematology and Oncology.

Amyotrophic Lateral Sclerosis

Amyotrophic lateral sclerosis (ALS) is a neurodegenerative disease of motor neurons that causes progressive weakness, atrophy, and (eventually) death. This motor neuron disease often begins as isolated extremity or bulbar weakness (dysphagia, dysarthria) but relentlessly spreads to other regions. Upper (hyperreflexia, spasticity, and extensor plantar response) and lower (atrophy and fasciculation) motor neuron signs and the absence of sensory deficits are characteristic. Frontotemporal dementia occurs in 50% of affected patients, but oculomotor palsy, incontinence, and tremor are atypical. Diagnosis is based on clinical evidence of both upper and lower motor neuron signs on examination and EMG evidence of lower motor neuron signs in at least two (probable ALS) or more (definite ALS) regions. Alternative diagnoses also must be excluded by brain and cervical spinal imaging and laboratory testing; cervical cord compression (causing lower motor neuron signs at the level of compression and some upper signs below that level), vitamin B_{12} and copper deficiencies, Lyme disease, hyperparathyroidism, and thyrotoxicosis must be excluded. Multifocal motor neuropathy is a treatable ALS mimic characterized by severe weakness with minimal atrophy, absence of upper motor neuron signs, and EMG evidence of motor conduction block. Benign fasciculation syndrome causes widespread fasciculation without weakness or upper motor neuron signs and should not be confused with ALS.

Treatment of ALS is supportive and should involve multidisciplinary care. Riluzole, a glutamate release blocker, is an FDA-approved treatment for ALS and may increase survival by 3 months. Edaravone, an intravenous free radical scavenger, recently received FDA approval on the basis of evidence showing that it slowed functional decline in ALS within a 6-month period. Whether this agent can slow the course of ALS over a longer period or can reduce mortality remains under investigation. Noninvasive ventilation, nutritional support (including percutaneous endoscopic gastrostomy), and treatment of pseudobulbar affect by dextromethorphan-quinidine also have shown some benefit. Prognosis and goals of care should be discussed with the patient early in the disease course to avoid unnecessary diagnostic and therapeutic measures.

KEY POINTS

- Amyotrophic lateral sclerosis (ALS) is a neurodegenerative disease of motor neurons that causes progressive weakness, atrophy, and (eventually) death; 50% of patients with ALS will develop frontotemporal dementia.

- Although treatment of amyotrophic lateral sclerosis (ALS) remains largely supportive, the glutamate release blocker riluzole may increase survival by 3 months, and the intravenous free radical scavenger edaravone has been shown to slow functional decline within a 6-month period; both drugs have received FDA approval for use in ALS.

Neuromuscular Junction Disorders
Myasthenia Gravis

Myasthenia gravis (MG) is an autoimmune disease of the postsynaptic neuromuscular junction associated with antibodies to the postsynaptic acetylcholine receptors. Onset most commonly occurs in the third decade of life in women and after age 50 years in men. Ptosis and diplopia are the first manifestations in two thirds of patients, although only half of these patients develop generalized myasthenia, typically within 2 years. Early bulbar and cervical involvement is seen in 10% of patients. Fluctuating painless weakness without sensory loss is typical. Weakness may be missed on clinical examination unless fatigability is assessed by sustained or repeated activation of muscles. The presence of respiratory symptoms should prompt close monitoring of respiratory parameters because of the risk of rapid respiratory failure (myasthenic crisis). This crisis can occur as part of the natural history of bulbar or generalized myasthenia or be triggered by external factors,

including infection, surgery, or certain medications (especially aminoglycosides, quinolones, magnesium, beta blockers, and hydroxychloroquine).

Diagnosis of MG is based on clinical, serologic, and EMG findings. Disease-specific antibodies are found in 90% of patients; of these, 85% have typical MG with acetylcholine receptor antibodies, but 5% have anti–muscle-specific kinase (MuSK) antibodies. MuSK-positive myasthenia is more likely to cause focal or severe bulbar, cervical, or respiratory weakness. The characteristic EMG finding of MG is a decremental response to repetitive stimulation. All patients with MG should undergo chest CT to screen for thymoma, a tumor associated with the disease.

Symptomatic treatment of ocular and mild generalized myasthenia usually starts with the cholinesterase inhibitor pyridostigmine. In those with more advanced disease, immunosuppressive therapy is required. Oral glucocorticoids often are used as first-line treatment but can cause transient exacerbation at high doses and should be titrated upward slowly in patients with mild to moderate weakness. In the presence of prominent bulbar or generalized weakness and in myasthenic crisis, treatment with IVIG or plasmapheresis should precede initiation of glucocorticoids. The immunosuppressant agents azathioprine, mycophenolate mofetil, and cyclosporine are effective long-term maintenance therapies. However, these drugs have a delayed onset of action, and bridging therapy with concomitant glucocorticoids, IVIG, or plasmapheresis is usually required.

Thymectomy should be performed in all patients with thymoma. Benefits of thymectomy in patients without thymoma are not firmly established, but a recent randomized controlled trial confirmed that thymectomy improves clinical outcome and reduces immunosuppression requirements in patients with generalized MG who are younger than 65 years and within 3 years of diagnosis.

MuSK-positive myasthenia responds well to plasmapheresis and glucocorticoids but requires aggressive maintenance immunosuppression. Prolonged remission has been reported with rituximab (off-label use); thymectomy and pyridostigmine are not helpful.

KEY POINTS

- Onset of myasthenia gravis (MG) most commonly occurs in the third decade of life in women and after age 50 years in men, with ptosis, diplopia, and fluctuating painless weakness without sensory loss being typical symptoms; all patients with MG should undergo chest CT to screen for thymoma, a tumor associated with the disease.

- Symptomatic treatment of ocular and mild generalized myasthenia gravis usually starts with the cholinesterase inhibitor pyridostigmine; in those with more advanced disease, immunosuppressive therapy is required, as is thymectomy for those with thymoma.

Lambert-Eaton Myasthenic Syndrome

Lambert-Eaton myasthenic syndrome is an autoimmune disorder of the presynaptic neuromuscular junction associated with antibodies against the voltage-gated calcium channel. This disorder presents similarly to MG, except that weakness improves with exercise, and hyporeflexia and dysautonomia are present. Diagnosis is confirmed by detection of serum anti–voltage-gated calcium channel antibodies (90%) and the EMG finding of augmented motor response to rapid repetitive stimulation. Malignancy, especially small cell lung cancer, is found in half of patients.

Treatment consists of treating any underlying malignancy or, in nonparaneoplastic disease, immunosuppression, IVIG, or plasmapheresis. H

Myopathies
Overview

Classification of myopathies is based on clinical and pathologic characteristics and acquired versus inherited causes (**Table 49**). Most myopathies involve symmetric weakness of the proximal limb muscles. A normal sensory and reflex

TABLE 49. Classification of Myopathies		
Class	**Examples**	**Features**
Inherited myopathies		
Muscular dystrophies	Duchenne	Early onset, fulminant
	Becker, Emery-Dreifuss	Early onset, survival to adulthood, cardiac disease
	Limb-girdle, facioscapulohumeral, oculopharyngeal	Variable onset, slow course
Myotonic dystrophy	Type 1	Myotonia, distal weakness, ptosis with lower facial weakness, variable cognitive impairment, cataract, arrhythmia with cardiomyopathy, diabetes mellitus, thyroid disease
	Type 2	Myotonia, proximal weakness, milder course, systemic features similar to those of type 1
Congenital myopathies	Nemaline myopathy, centronuclear myopathy, central core myopathy, distal myopathies	Childhood onset, focal weakness in distal forms, predisposition to exercise-induced cramping and malignant hyperthermia in central core myopathy
Metabolic myopathies	Acid maltase deficiency (Pompe disease), CPT II deficiency, McArdle disease (myophosphorylase deficiency), other lipid and glycogen storage disorders	Exercise intolerance, myoglobinuria, myalgia, progressive proximal and respiratory weakness in acid maltase deficiency
Mitochondrial myopathies	MERRF, MELAS, MNGIE, Kearns-Sayre syndrome	Childhood or early adulthood onset, fluctuating course, wide spectrum with variable systemic comorbidity, ophthalmoplegia, bulbar symptoms, elevated serum lactic acid level
Acquired myopathies		
Inflammatory	Dermatomyositis, polymyositis, immune-mediated necrotizing myopathy	Highly elevated creatine kinase level, subacute course, association with malignancy, dermatologic signs in dermatomyositis
	Inclusion body myositis	Onset usually after age 50 years, asymmetric progressive weakness with atrophy, distal arm and quadriceps involvement
Endocrine-related	Hypothyroidism, hyperthyroidism, hyperparathyroidism, Addison disease, Cushing syndrome, acromegaly, vitamin D deficiency, hypokalemia	
Systemic disease	Systemic lupus erythematosus, mixed connective tissue disease, systemic sclerosis, critical illness, paraneoplastic	
Toxic and drug-related	Ethanol, statins, glucocorticoids, anti-HIV and antimalarial agents, interferons, amphotericin B, amiodarone, immunophilins	Statin myopathy as possible cause of mildly to highly elevated creatine kinase level

CPT II deficiency = carnitine palmitoyltransferase II deficiency; MELAS = mitochondrial encephalopathy, lactic acidosis, and stroke-like episodes syndrome; MERRF = myoclonic epilepsy with ragged red fibers; MNGIE = mitochondrial neurogastrointestinal encephalopathy.

examination can differentiate myopathy from neuropathy. Additional features that can indicate a specific diagnosis include the clinical course; the presence of pain and stiffness; atypical distribution in ocular, bulbar, or distal limb muscles; and episodic symptoms (**Table 50**).

Diagnosis is based on systematic clinical assessment, muscle-related serum markers (creatine kinase [CK], aldolase), EMG findings, muscle biopsy, and, in certain cases, genetic testing. The serum CK level is elevated in many forms of myopathy and can be followed to monitor disease activity and response to treatment in inflammatory myopathies. Mild elevation of the serum CK level (<5 times normal) is not specific to myopathies and also can be seen in ALS, CIDP, muscle trauma, and persistent elevation of the serum CK level without weakness (benign hyperCKemia). EMG can confirm the presence of changes associated with myopathy (low amplitude, short duration, polyphasic shape of motor unit potentials), determine distribution of involved muscles, and rule out neuropathy or a neuromuscular junction disorder. The serum CK level should be checked before EMG to prevent procedure-related false positive results. Muscle biopsy is the most helpful test to confirm the diagnosis of myopathy, but in some hereditary myopathies, genetic testing can provide the confirmation without need for biopsy.

KEY POINT

- Diagnosis of a myopathy is based on systematic clinical assessment, muscle-related serum markers, electromyographic findings, muscle biopsy, and (sometimes) genetic testing.

TABLE 50. Clinical Features of Myopathies	
Clinical Features	**Differential Diagnosis**
Pain	Metabolic, toxic, infectious, inflammatory, and mitochondrial myopathies
Stiffness	Myotonic dystrophy, myotonic channelopathies, hyperkalemic periodic paralysis, hypothyroidism; differential diagnosis: stiff person syndrome
Rapid course	Inflammatory, toxic, autoimmune, and endocrine myopathies
Very slow course, plus or minus focal atrophy	Muscular dystrophies, congenital myopathies, metabolic myopathies
Fluctuating weakness	Mitochondrial myopathy, myasthenia gravis
Myoglobinuria	Toxic and infectious myopathy, trauma, metabolic myopathies (CPT II deficiency, McArdle disease, central core myopathy)
Respiratory muscle involvement	Muscular dystrophies, inflammatory, mitochondrial, and metabolic myopathies (acid maltase deficiency, debrancher deficiency)

CPT II deficiency = carnitine palmitoyltransferase II deficiency.

Inflammatory Myopathy

Polymyositis, dermatomyositis, immune-mediated necrotizing myopathy, and inclusion body myositis are idiopathic inflammatory myopathies. Polymyositis and dermatomyositis present with acute or subacute proximal muscle weakness. Diagnosis is based on an elevated serum CK level, EMG findings, and muscle biopsy findings. Immune-mediated necrotizing myopathy typically presents with progressive proximal weakness and an elevated serum CK level; diagnosis is based on muscle biopsy findings of necrotic fibers with limited inflammation. Onset can be triggered by statins, but weakness continues to progress after removal of the drug. In this setting, the presence of the disease-specific serum antibody to hydroxymethylglutaryl coenzyme A reductase can support the diagnosis. Treatment with immunosuppression reverses the myopathy.

Inclusion body myositis has a slowly progressive course and causes early weakness and atrophy of distal upper extremity flexors, quadriceps, and bulbar muscles. Muscle biopsy reveals inflammation and characteristic inclusion bodies. See MKSAP 18 Rheumatology for further information on inflammatory myopathy.

Endocrine-Related Myopathy

Hypothyroid myopathy can cause diffuse myalgia, proximal weakness, and myoedema (muscle mounding after percussion). Hyperthyroidism also can cause myopathy in association with fasciculation, ophthalmoplegia and hyperreflexia.

Glucocorticoid-Induced Myopathy

Exposure to chronic high-dose exogenous glucocorticoids can cause myopathy of unclear mechanism. This disorder is associated with proximal weakness and myalgia but normal CK levels and (mostly) normal EMG findings. Dexamethasone is more likely than prednisone or hydrocortisone to cause this type of myopathy. In patients treated with glucocorticoids for inflammatory myopathies, persistence of weakness after normalization of the CK level may indicate glucocorticoid-induced myopathy, and a trial of glucocorticoid tapering may be warranted.

KEY POINT

- Glucocorticoid-induced myopathy is associated with proximal weakness and myalgia but normal creatine kinase levels and (mostly) normal electromyographic findings; dexamethasone is more likely than prednisone or hydrocortisone to cause this type of myopathy.

Toxic Myopathy

Toxic myopathy can be triggered by statins and other drugs (see Table 49). Statins can cause acute toxic myopathy associated with rhabdomyolysis. The lipophilic statins metabolized by the cytochrome P450 3A4 isozyme system (simvastatin, atorvastatin, and lovastatin) have a higher propensity to cause myopathy than the hydrophilic agents pravastatin and rosuvastatin. The risk of myopathy increases with higher dosages, the addition of fenofibrate or gemfibrozil, and the addition of cytochrome P450 3A4 isozyme inhibitors. Serum CK levels can be mildly or highly elevated in toxic myopathy.

Inherited Myopathies

Inherited myopathies are listed in Table 49. Many of these disorders develop early in life, but some present in adulthood. Myotonic dystrophies are systemic diseases associated with myotonia, an impairment of muscle relaxation causing stiffness and a delayed hand-grip release. Myotonic dystrophy type 1 causes distal weakness and is associated with cataracts, frontal balding, cardiac and endocrine disease, and mild cognitive impairment. Progression of weakness is slow, but diagnosis should prompt close monitoring for cardiac and pulmonary disease that can cause premature mortality.

Mitochondrial myopathy presents with significant variability and can cause fatigue, myalgia, ophthalmoplegia, and various extramuscular manifestations. Mitochondrial myopathies should be suspected in the presence of a fluctuating course, multiorgan involvement, and maternal transmission.

Adult-onset metabolic myopathies may present with isolated exercise-induced weakness, cramps, and myoglobinuria and include many deficiencies of key metabolic pathways, such as glycogen storage and fatty acid oxidation; the most common types are carnitine palmitoyltransferase II deficiency and McArdle disease.

Acid maltase deficiency (Pompe disease) has an adult-onset form associated with proximal and respiratory muscle weakness. Diagnosis is based on assessment of α-glucosidase activity and genetic testing. Alglucosidase alfa is FDA approved to prevent progression of weakness.

Neuro-oncology

Approach to Intracranial Tumors

Both benign and malignant intracranial tumors can have devastating neurologic consequences because of the obvious space constraints within the skull and potential surgical inaccessibility (if in the thalamus or brainstem, for example). Presenting symptoms of intracranial tumors appear in **Table 51**. Intracranial tumors most often present with a slow, progressive course of neurologic symptoms. Acute symptoms typically occur when a tumor causes seizure or hemorrhage.

Headache is a common symptom, although the classic early morning headache is uncommon. Elevated intracranial pressure (ICP) can cause the headache to increase with coughing, sneezing, straining, or the Valsalva maneuver. Elevated ICP also is associated with nausea, vomiting, blurry vision, papilledema, and an inability to abduct the

TABLE 51. Presenting Symptoms/Findings of Central Nervous System Tumors

Tumor Location	Symptoms/Findings
Brainstem	Cranial nerve findings, elevated intracranial pressure[a]
Cerebellum	Ataxia, falls, imbalance, elevated intracranial pressure[a]
Frontal lobe	Weakness, personality change, cognitive symptoms, or psychiatric symptoms
Occipital lobe	Homonymous hemianopia
Parietal lobe	Numbness, paresthesia
Temporal lobe	Amnesia
Dominant hemisphere	Aphasia

[a]Symptoms of elevated intracranial pressure include nausea, vomiting, blurry vision, papilledema, and inability to abduct the eyes (bilateral abducens nerve [cranial nerve VI] palsy).

eyes (bilateral abducens nerve [cranial nerve VI] palsy). Elevated ICP also can lead to life-threatening herniation, syncope, or cerebellar "fits" (episodic extension, flexion and stiffening of limbs; loss of consciousness; slowed or irregular respiration; and pupil dilation), which may be confused with seizures.

Head CT without contrast may be useful emergently to assess for hemorrhage or herniation but is not very sensitive for detecting the presence of a mass lesion, especially in the posterior fossa. Brain MRI is the preferred diagnostic modality; contrast administration improves diagnostic sensitivity. Management is determined by tumor location and pathology.

KEY POINT

- Head CT without contrast may be useful emergently to assess for hemorrhage or herniation, but brain MRI is the preferred diagnostic modality for the evaluation of intracranial tumors.

Metastatic Brain Tumors

Brain metastases are the most common intracranial tumors. The most likely sources are lung, breast, and kidney cancers and melanoma. Metastases can be solitary but are more often multiple. These metastases typically appear as ring-enhancing lesions on postcontrast MRIs, usually at the gray-white cortical junction. Survival is generally measured in weeks to months. Most brain metastases are treated with whole-brain or more targeted radiation (stereotactic radiosurgery). Resection may increase survival in younger patients with good baseline function and a single or limited number of metastases; it may also be considered when the underlying diagnosis is uncertain.

Carcinomatous meningitis is a rare diagnosis that requires a high index of suspicion to identify; presenting symptoms are variable and include headache, neurologic deficits, and altered mental status. MRI typically shows nodular meningeal enhancement. Patients with leukemia or lymphoma whose initial symptoms are cranial nerve deficits or radiculopathy may have evidence of nerve root enhancement on postcontrast MRI of the brain and/or spine. Cerebrospinal fluid (CSF) analysis with cytology and often flow cytometry is required to make the diagnosis; because of limited sensitivity of CSF cytology, repeat lumbar puncture is sometimes needed to establish the diagnosis.

KEY POINTS

- Brain metastases are the most common intracranial tumors that typically appear as ring-enhancing lesions on postcontrast MRIs at the gray-white cortical junction.

- Most brain metastases are treated with whole-brain or more targeted radiation (stereotactic radiosurgery), but resection of a single or limited number of intracranial metastases may increase survival in younger patients with good baseline function.

Primary Central Nervous System Tumors

Meningiomas

Meningioma is the most common primary type of central nervous system (CNS) tumor. Often found incidentally, meningiomas are benign dural-based tumors that typically show homogenous enhancement on postcontrast MRI. They have a smooth, rounded shape and often a "tail" that tracks along the dura outside the brain parenchyma (**Figure 30**). On noncontrast images, meningiomas may be hypointense or isointense

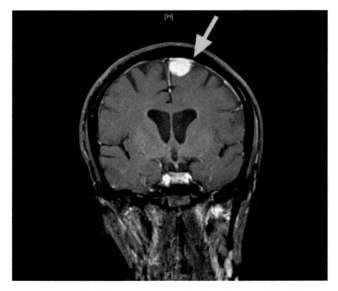

FIGURE 30. Coronal postcontrast T1-weighted MRI showing a left parafalcine meningioma. The tumor enhances homogeneously with contrast, which makes it look like a "lightbulb." Note the "dural tail" (*arrow*).

and thus not readily seen. Because of their characteristic MRI appearance, many meningiomas are followed clinically, without resection or biopsy, unless they are accompanied by significant clinical deficits, drug-resistant seizures, severe headaches, or peritumoral edema.

KEY POINT

- Meningioma is the most common primary type of central nervous system tumor and has a characteristic MRI appearance; the tumor is resected only if accompanied by significant clinical deficits, drug-resistant seizures, severe headaches, or peritumoral edema.

Glioblastoma Multiforme

Glioblastoma multiforme (**Figure 31**) is the most common and most aggressive glioma subtype in adults. Previous exposure to medical therapeutic radiation is the only consistent risk factor for developing gliomas. There is no evidence that environmental electromagnetic fields, cell phones, or smoking increase tumor risk. Gliomas rarely metastasize, and routine evaluation of patients with glioblastoma multiforme with lumbar puncture or MRI of the spinal cord is not recommended unless dictated by focal findings.

An MRI typically shows a large, space-occupying lesion with central necrosis, mass effect, and surrounding edema. Lower-grade gliomas may not enhance. Treatment is usually resection, if possible, followed by radiation and chemotherapy. Temozolomide, nitrosoureas, and bevacizumab can be used. Prognosis is dependent on pathologic type; 5-year survival rates for glioblastoma multiforme are less than 10%, and survival is often measured in months. Prognosis is better in patients who are younger than 45 years, have an excellent functional status, have minimal residual tumor after resection, and receive chemotherapy and radiation after surgery.

KEY POINTS

- Previous exposure to medical therapeutic radiation is the only consistent risk factor for developing gliomas, including glioblastoma multiforme.

- Prognosis in glioblastoma multiforme is better in patients who are younger than 45 years, have an excellent functional status, have minimal residual tumor after resection, and receive chemotherapy and radiation after surgery.

Primary Central Nervous System Lymphoma

Primary central nervous system lymphoma (PCNSL) initially occurs without systemic or lymph node involvement. Its typical pathologic appearance is diffuse large B-cell lymphoma. Immunodeficiency is the most consistent risk factor, but PCNSL incidence is increasing in older, immunocompetent patients. On MRI, PCNSL appears as a single, well-demarcated, deep white matter (periventricular) lesion without mass effect or edema. The radiologic appearance of PCNSL can be confused with inflammatory or demyelinating lesions.

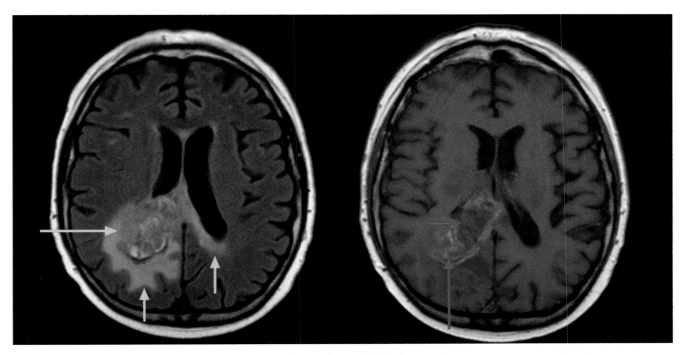

FIGURE 31. MRI showing a right parieto-occipital glioblastoma multiforme. *Left*, T2-weighted fluid-attenuated inversion recovery sequence shows a heterogenous intensity mass lesion (*longer yellow arrow*) with surrounding hyperintense edema that extends into both hemispheres (*shorter yellow arrows*). *Right*, T1-weighted sequence shows a hypointense core suggestive of central necrosis (*shorter red arrow*) with heterogenous enhancement (*longer red arrow*).

CONT.

PCNSL evaluation should include HIV testing, lumbar puncture (if not contraindicated because of elevated ICP), and ophthalmologic evaluation with vitreous fluid sampling. Lymphomatous cells in vitreous or CSF samples (from cytology and flow cytometry) can add to diagnostic sensitivity and may obviate the need for biopsy. Systemic staging should include bone marrow biopsy, testicular ultrasonography, and whole-body PET or CT. Empiric glucocorticoids should be avoided before biopsy because they can temporarily suppress lymphoma and prevent or delay a tissue diagnosis.

Surgery and typical chemotherapeutic regimens for systemic lymphoma are usually ineffective in PCNSL. High-dose intravenous (IV) methotrexate combined with rituximab is the mainstay of treatment and at times is followed by subsequent radiation. Intrathecal chemotherapy has not been prospectively studied. Despite being chemo- and radiosensitive, PCNSL typically has multiple recurrences and a generally poor prognosis. **H**

KEY POINTS

- Immunodeficiency is the most consistent risk factor for primary central nervous system lymphoma, but its incidence is increasing in older, immunocompetent patients.
- Empiric glucocorticoids should be avoided before biopsy because they can temporarily suppress lymphoma and prevent or delay a tissue diagnosis.

Medical Management of Complications of Central Nervous System Tumors

Seizures

Seizures are more common in low-grade than high-grade tumors. Tumors near the cortex, especially the temporal lobe or primary motor cortex, are especially associated with seizures. White matter and posterior fossa tumors, on the other hand, typically do not cause seizures. Gangliogliomas and dysembryoplastic neuroepithelial tumors provoke medication-resistant seizures in more than 90% of patients, and these tumors should be resected, if possible. Seizures may not be directly caused by the CNS tumor but rather by associated conditions or treatment, such as electrolyte disturbances, infection, chemotherapy, or paraneoplastic encephalitis.

In patients with CNS tumors not associated with seizures, prophylactic antiepileptic drugs (AEDs) are not recommended, although they may be used for 1 week immediately postresection. In patients with seizures, older AEDs (phenobarbital, phenytoin, valproic acid, carbamazepine) should be avoided because of drug interactions and adverse effects. Levetiracetam and lacosamide are the preferred AEDs because of their lack of drug interactions, IV availability, better tolerability, and rapid titration to a therapeutic dose. Unprovoked seizures occurring after resection typically require lifelong AED treatment. **H**

KEY POINTS

- Gangliogliomas and dysembryoplastic neuroepithelial tumors provoke medication-resistant seizures in more than 90% of patients; therefore, patients with these tumors should be referred for resection, if possible.

- In patients with central nervous system tumors not associated with seizures, prophylactic antiepileptic drugs are not recommended, although they may be used for 1 week immediately postresection.

Edema and Herniation

CONT.

Brain edema can lead to focal neurologic deficits, elevated ICP, or herniation. Brain herniation inevitably leads to death if unrecognized. It manifests as an abrupt decline in mental status, unreactive dilated pupils, and motor weakness with flexor or extensor posturing. Emergent treatment includes elevation of the head of the bed to 30 degrees, hyperventilation (usually with mechanical ventilation) to an arterial P_{CO_2} greater than 26 mm Hg (3.5 kPa), infusion of either hypertonic saline or mannitol, and administration of glucocorticoids. These treatments can be life-saving and often are used as a bridge to emergent surgery. Among the glucocorticoids, dexamethasone is preferred because of its lack of mineralocorticoid effects. Antiangiogenic agents, such as bevacizumab, can be used as glucocorticoid-sparing agents but take weeks or months to have an effect. Both glucocorticoids and antiangiogenic agents may seal the blood-brain barrier and thus "hide" the previously contrast-enhancing residual tumor. 🅷

KEY POINTS

- In patients with central nervous system tumors, brain herniation inevitably leads to death if unrecognized.

- Emergent treatment of brain herniation includes elevation of the head of the bed, hyperventilation, infusion of either hypertonic saline or mannitol, and administration of glucocorticoids.

Venous Thromboembolism

Certain characteristics are associated with increased risk of venous thromboembolism in patients with CNS tumors (**Table 52**). Despite the risk of intracranial hemorrhage, therapeutic anticoagulation is generally recommended in confirmed thromboembolic disease. Anticoagulation has historically been avoided in melanoma, choriocarcinoma, papillary thyroid carcinoma, and renal carcinoma because of an assumed increased risk of hemorrhage. However, recent studies have not shown that anticoagulation increases hemorrhage risk in patients with these cancers. Besides the usual contraindications, anticoagulation should be avoided in patients with previous intracranial hemorrhage and a platelet count less than 50,000/µL (50×10^9/L). The presence of a CNS tumor is a contraindication for thrombolytic therapy in pulmonary embolism, although exceptions may be made for low-risk tumors, such as meningiomas. Although evidence does

TABLE 52. Risk Factors for Venous Thromboembolism in Patients with Central Nervous System Tumors
Age >75 years
Prolonged immobility or leg weakness
Indwelling vascular catheter
Prior venous thromboembolism
Glioblastoma multiforme
Glioma >5 cm
Chemotherapy, particularly hormonal or antiangiogenic agents
Recurrent tumor
Incomplete resection
Immediate postresection period

not support routine use of preanticoagulation neuroimaging to assess for hemorrhage, noncontrast head CT is the most cost-effective test in this situation.

Low-molecular-weight heparin is generally preferred over unfractionated heparin. Exceptions include kidney impairment and a higher hemorrhage risk when rapid reversal may be required. Inferior vena cava filters have considerably high rates of complications and should be reserved for patients with an absolute contraindication to anticoagulation. Warfarin or low-molecular-weight heparin may be considered for long-term therapy, although medication interactions between warfarin and chemotherapy or AEDs are a concern. Evidence is insufficient to recommend the non–vitamin K antagonist oral anticoagulants for patients with CNS tumors.

Prophylactic anticoagulation in combination with mechanical devices is recommended in hospitalized patients with CNS tumors as soon as possible after resection. Chronic outpatient prophylactic anticoagulation is not recommended. 🅷

KEY POINTS

- Despite the risk of intracranial hemorrhage, therapeutic anticoagulation is generally recommended in confirmed venous thromboembolic disease.

- Prophylactic anticoagulation in combination with mechanical devices is recommended in hospitalized patients with central nervous system tumors as soon as possible after resection.

Paraneoplastic Neurologic Syndromes

Antibody-mediated neurologic syndromes may occur as primary autoimmune or paraneoplastic disorders. Various syndromes have been described with different neurologic manifestations and findings on serum and CSF studies (**Table 53**). Suggestive symptoms include new-onset status epilepticus in a patient without epilepsy, acute psychosis in a healthy patient, acute movement disorder (ataxia, chorea,

TABLE 53. Common Autoimmune and Paraneoplastic Neurologic Disorders

Clinical Presentation	Associated Cancers	Autoantibody Targets
Psychosis, chorea, dysautonomia[a]	Ovarian teratoma	NMDA receptor[b]
Executive dysfunction, personality change, brainstem/limbic encephalitis, myoclonus, neuropathy, hyponatremia[a]	SCLC	VGKC receptor complex[b] (includes LGI1, CASPR2, contactin-2)
Brainstem encephalitis, autonomic or sensory neuropathy[a]	SCLC	ANNA-1 (Hu)
Ataxia, brainstem encephalitis	Breast cancer, SCLC, gynecologic cancer	ANNA-2 (Ri)
Ataxia	Gynecologic cancer, breast cancer	PCA-1 (Yo)
Brainstem encephalitis[a]	Testicular cancer	Ma1, Ma2
Dementia, personality change, chorea, ataxia, neuropathy	SCLC, thymoma	CRMP5
Stiff-person syndrome, type 1 diabetes mellitus, ataxia, brainstem encephalitis, ophthalmoplegia, parkinsonism	Thymoma, breast cancer	GAD[b]

ANNA = antineuronal nuclear antigen; CASPR = contactin associated protein-like; CRMP = collapsin response mediator protein; GAD = glutamic acid decarboxylase; LGI = leucine-rich, glioma inactivated; NMDA = N-methyl-D-aspartate; PCA = Purkinje-cell antibody; SCLC = small cell lung cancer; VGKC = voltage-gated potassium channel.

[a]May present with limbic encephalitis (acute or subacute mood and behavioral changes, short-term memory problems, cognitive dysfunction), in addition to the presentations listed.

[b]Not necessarily associated with paraneoplastic syndromes; may be primary autoimmune, without cancer.

CONT.

myoclonus, tremor), acute progressive peripheral neuropathy, and systemic signs of malignancy (severe anorexia, weight loss, lymphadenopathy).

Evaluation should include brain MRI with contrast, antibody testing of the blood and CSF, and imaging (full-body CT, body and brain PET, and ultrasonography, as appropriate) for tumor detection. Treating the symptoms directly is ineffective without appropriate tumor resection and immunotherapy. Even when the tumor is removed, immunotherapy may be needed. Acute management with IV immune globulin or IV methylprednisolone is often helpful. Chronic treatment with azathioprine, mycophenolate, cyclophosphamide, or rituximab may be considered. **H**

KEY POINT

- Treatment of paraneoplastic neurologic syndromes usually requires appropriate tumor resection and immunotherapy.

Bibliography

Headache and Facial Pain

Becker WJ. Acute migraine treatment in adults. Headache. 2015;55:778-93. [PMID: 25877672] doi:10.1111/head.12550

Chiang CC, Schwedt TJ, Wang SJ, Dodick DW. Treatment of medication-overuse headache: A systematic review. Cephalalgia. 2016;36:371-86. [PMID: 26122645] doi:10.1177/0333102415593088

Ducros A, Wolff V. The typical thunderclap headache of reversible cerebral vasoconstriction syndrome and its various triggers. Headache. 2016;56:657-73. [PMID: 27015869] doi:10.1111/head.12797

Maarbjerg S, Gozalov A, Olesen J, Bendtsen L. Trigeminal neuralgia–a prospective systematic study of clinical characteristics in 158 patients. Headache. 2014;54:1574-82. [PMID: 25231219] doi:10.1111/head.12441

Markey KA, Mollan SP, Jensen RH, Sinclair AJ. Understanding idiopathic intracranial hypertension: mechanisms, management, and future directions. Lancet Neurol. 2016;15:78-91. [PMID: 26700907] doi:10.1016/S1474-4422(15)00298-7

Marmura MJ, Silberstein SD, Schwedt TJ. The acute treatment of migraine in adults: the American Headache Society evidence assessment of migraine pharmacotherapies. Headache. 2015;55:3-20. [PMID: 25600718] doi:10.1111/head.12499

Mokri B. Spontaneous CSF leaks: low CSF volume syndromes. Neurol Clin. 2014;32:397-422. [PMID: 24703536] doi:10.1016/j.ncl.2013.11.002

Nye BL, Ward TN. Clinic and emergency room evaluation and testing of headache. Headache. 2015;55:1301-8. [PMID: 26422648] doi:10.1111/head.12648

Orr SL, Friedman BW, Christie S, Minen MT, Bamford C, Kelley NE, et al. Management of adults with acute migraine in the emergency department: The American Headache Society evidence assessment of parenteral pharmacotherapies. Headache. 2016;56:911-40. [PMID: 27300483] doi:10.1111/head.12835

Pareja JA, Álvarez M. The usual treatment of trigeminal autonomic cephalalgias. Headache. 2013;53:1401-14. [PMID: 24090529] doi:10.1111/head.12193

Silberstein SD, Holland S, Freitag F, Dodick DW, Argoff C, Ashman E; Quality Standards Subcommittee of the American Academy of Neurology and the American Headache Society. Evidence-based guideline update: pharmacologic treatment for episodic migraine prevention in adults: report of the Quality Standards Subcommittee of the American Academy of Neurology and the American Headache Society. Neurology. 2012;78:1337-45. [PMID: 22529202] doi:10.1212/WNL.0b013e3182535d20

Head Injury

Giza CC, Kutcher JS, Ashwal S, Barth J, Getchius TS, Gioia GA, et al. Summary of evidence-based guideline update: evaluation and management of concussion in sports: report of the Guideline Development Subcommittee of the American Academy of Neurology. Neurology. 2013;80:2250-7. [PMID: 23508730] doi:10.1212/WNL.0b013e31828d57dd

Harmon KG, Drezner JA, Gammons M, Guskiewicz KM, Halstead M, Herring SA, et al. American Medical Society for Sports Medicine position statement: concussion in sport. Br J Sports Med. 2013;47:15-26. [PMID: 23243113] doi:10.1136/bjsports-2012-091941

Holtkamp MD, Grimes J, Ling G. Concussion in the military: an evidence-base review of mTBI in US military personnel focused on posttraumatic headache. Curr Pain Headache Rep. 2016;20:37. [PMID: 27084376] doi:10.1007/s11916-016-0572-x

Jaramillo CA, Eapen BC, McGeary CA, McGeary DD, Robinson J, Amuan M, et al. A cohort study examining headaches among veterans of Iraq and Afghanistan wars: Associations with traumatic brain injury, PTSD, and depression. Headache. 2016;56:528-39. [PMID: 26688427] doi:10.1111/head.12726

Lucas S, Hoffman JM, Bell KR, Dikmen S. A prospective study of prevalence and characterization of headache following mild traumatic brain injury. Cephalalgia 2014 Feb;34(2):93-102. Epub 2013 Aug 6. [PMID: 23921798] doi:10.1177/0333102413499645

Seizures and Epilepsy

Fisher RS, Acevedo C, Arzimanoglou A, Bogacz A, Cross JH, Elger CE, et al. ILAE official report: a practical clinical definition of epilepsy. Epilepsia. 2014;55:475-82. [PMID: 24730690] doi:10.1111/epi.12550

Glauser T, Shinnar S, Gloss D, Alldredge B, Arya R, Bainbridge J, et al. Evidence-based guideline: treatment of convulsive status epilepticus in children and adults: Report of the Guideline Committee of the American Epilepsy Society. Epilepsy Curr. 2016;16:48-61. [PMID: 26900382] doi:10.5698/1535-7597-16.1.48

Herman ST, Abend NS, Bleck TP, Chapman KE, Drislane FW, Emerson RG, et al; Critical Care Continuous EEG Task Force of the American Clinical Neurophysiology Society. Consensus statement on continuous EEG in critically ill adults and children, part I: indications. J Clin Neurophysiol. 2015;32:87-95. [PMID: 25626778] doi:10.1097/WNP.0000000000000166

Jobst BC, Cascino GD. Resective epilepsy surgery for drug-resistant focal epilepsy: a review. JAMA. 2015;313:285-93. [PMID: 25602999] doi:10.1001/jama.2014.17426

Krumholz A, Wiebe S, Gronseth GS, Gloss DS, Sanchez AM, Kabir AA, et al. Evidence-based guideline: Management of an unprovoked first seizure in adults: Report of the Guideline Development Subcommittee of the American Academy of Neurology and the American Epilepsy Society. Neurology. 2015;84:1705-13. [PMID: 25901057] doi:10.1212/WNL.0000000000001487

Vélez-Ruiz NJ, Pennell PB. Issues for women with epilepsy. Neurol Clin. 2016;34:411-25, ix. [PMID: 27086987] doi:10.1016/j.ncl.2015.11.009

Vossler DG, Anderson GD, Bainbridge J. AES position statement on generic substitution of antiepileptic drugs. Epilepsy Curr. 2016;16:209-11. [PMID: 27330454] doi:10.5698/1535-7511-16.3.209

Stroke

Demaerschalk BM, Kleindorfer DO, Adeoye OM, Demchuk AM, Fugate JE, Grotta JC, et al; American Heart Association Stroke Council and Council on Epidemiology and Prevention. Scientific rationale for the inclusion and exclusion criteria for intravenous alteplase in acute ischemic stroke: a statement for healthcare professionals from the American Heart Association/American Stroke Association. Stroke. 2016;47:581-641. [PMID: 26696642] doi:10.1161/STR.0000000000000086

Hemphill JC 3rd, Greenberg SM, Anderson CS, Becker K, Bendok BR, Cushman M, et al; American Heart Association Stroke Council. Guidelines for the management of spontaneous intracerebral hemorrhage: a guideline for healthcare professionals from the American Heart Association/American Stroke Association. Stroke. 2015;46:2032-60. [PMID: 26022637] doi:10.1161/STR.0000000000000069

Kernan WN, Ovbiagele B, Black HR, Bravata DM, Chimowitz MI, Ezekowitz MD, et al; American Heart Association Stroke Council, Council on Cardiovascular and Stroke Nursing, Council on Clinical Cardiology, and Council on Peripheral Vascular Disease. Guidelines for the prevention of stroke in patients with stroke and transient ischemic attack: a guideline for healthcare professionals from the American Heart Association/American Stroke Association. Stroke. 2014;45:2160-236. [PMID: 24788967] doi:10.1161/STR.0000000000000024

Meschia JF, Bushnell C, Boden-Albala B, Braun LT, Bravata DM, Chaturvedi S, et al; American Heart Association Stroke Council. Guidelines for the primary prevention of stroke: a statement for healthcare professionals from the American Heart Association/American Stroke Association. Stroke. 2014;45:3754-832. [PMID: 25355838] doi:10.1161/STR.0000000000000046

Powers WJ, Rabinstein AA, Ackerson T, Adeoye OM, Bambakidis NC, Becker K, et al; American Heart Association Stroke Council. 2018 Guidelines for the early management of patients with acute ischemic stroke: a guideline for healthcare professionals from the American Heart Association/American Stroke Association. Stroke. 2018 Jan 24. [Epub ahead of print] [PMID: 29367334] doi:10.1161/STR.0000000000000158

Thompson BG, Brown RD Jr, Amin-Hanjani S, Broderick JP, Cockroft KM, Connolly ES Jr, et al; American Heart Association Stroke Council, Council on Cardiovascular and Stroke Nursing, and Council on Epidemiology and Prevention. Guidelines for the management of patients with unruptured intracranial aneurysms: a guideline for healthcare professionals from the American Heart Association/American Stroke Association. Stroke. 2015;46:2368-400. [PMID: 26089327] doi:10.1161/STR.0000000000000070

Yaghi S, Willey JZ, Khatri P. Minor ischemic stroke: triaging, disposition, and outcome. Neurol Clin Pract. 2016;6:157-163. [PMID: 27104067] doi:10.1212/CPJ.0000000000000234

Whelton PK, Carey RM, Aronow WS, Casey DE Jr, Collins KJ, Dennison Himmelfarb C, et al. 2017 ACC/AHA/AAPA/ABC/ACPM/AGS/APhA/ASH/ASPC/NMA/PCNA Guideline for the prevention, detection, evaluation, and management of high blood pressure in adults: a report of the American College of Cardiology/American Heart Association Task Force on Clinical Practice Guidelines. J Am Coll Cardiol. 2017 Nov 7. pii; S735-1097(17)41519-1. [PMID: 29146535] doi:10.1016/j.jacc.2017.11.006

Cognitive Impairment

Corbett A, Smith J, Creese B, Ballard C. Treatment of behavioral and psychological symptoms of Alzheimer's disease. Curr Treat Options Neurol. 2012;14:113-25. [PMID: 22328204] doi:10.1007/s11940-012-0166-9

Geschwind MD, Shu H, Haman A, Sejvar JJ, Miller BL. Rapidly progressive dementia. Ann Neurol. 2008;64:97-108. [PMID: 18668637] doi:10.1002/ana.21430

Inouye SK, van Dyck CH, Alessi CA, Balkin S, Siegal AP, Horwitz RI. Clarifying confusion: the confusion assessment method. A new method for detection of delirium. Ann Intern Med. 1990;113:941-8. [PMID: 2240918]

Lin JS, O'Connor E, Rossom RC, Perdue LA, Eckstrom E. Screening for cognitive impairment in older adults: A systematic review for the U.S. Preventive Services Task Force. Ann Intern Med. 2013;159:601-12. [PMID: 24145578]doi:10.7326/0003-4819-159-9-201311050-00730

Morley JE, Morris JC, Berg-Weger M, Borson S, Carpenter BD, Del Campo N, et al. Brain health: the importance of recognizing cognitive impairment: an IAGG consensus conference. J Am Med Dir Assoc. 2015;16:731-9. [PMID: 26315321] doi:10.1016/j.jamda.2015.06.017

Ott BR, Daiello LA, Dahabreh IJ, Springate BA, Bixby K, Murali M, et al. Do statins impair cognition? A systematic review and meta-analysis of randomized controlled trials. J Gen Intern Med. 2015;30:348-58. [PMID: 25575908] doi:10.1007/s11606-014-3115-3

Rascovsky K, Hodges JR, Knopman D, Mendez MF, Kramer JH, Neuhaus J, et al. Sensitivity of revised diagnostic criteria for the behavioural variant of frontotemporal dementia. Brain. 2011;134:2456-77. [PMID: 21810890] doi:10.1093/brain/awr179

Ritter A, Pillai JA. Treatment of vascular cognitive impairment. Curr Treat Options Neurol. 2015;17:367. [PMID: 26094078] doi:10.1007/s11940-015-0367-0

Ströhle A, Schmidt DK, Schultz F, Fricke N, Staden T, Hellweg R, et al. Drug and exercise treatment of Alzheimer Disease and mild cognitive impairment: a systematic review and meta-analysis of effects on cognition in randomized controlled trials. Am J Geriatr Psychiatry. 2015;23:1234-49. [PMID: 26601726] doi:10.1016/j.jagp.2015.07.007

Movement Disorders

Albanese A, Bhatia K, Bressman SB, Delong MR, Fahn S, Fung VS, et al. Phenomenology and classification of dystonia: a consensus update. Mov Disord. 2013;28:863-73. [PMID: 23649720] doi:10.1002/mds.25475

Ali K, Morris HR. Parkinson's disease: chameleons and mimics. Pract Neurol. 2015;15:14-25. [PMID: 25253895] doi:10.1136/practneurol-2014-000849

Fasano A, Deuschl G. Therapeutic advances in tremor. Mov Disord. 2015;30:1557-65. [PMID: 26293405] doi:10.1002/mds.26383

Hermann A, Walker RH. Diagnosis and treatment of chorea syndromes. Curr Neurol Neurosci Rep. 2015;15:514. [PMID: 25620691] doi:10.1007/s11910-014-0514-0

Mills K, Mari Z. An update and review of the treatment of myoclonus. Curr Neurol Neurosci Rep. 2015;15:512. [PMID: 25398378] doi:10.1007/s11910-014-0512-2

Okun MS. Deep-brain stimulation for Parkinson's disease. N Engl J Med. 2012;367:1529-38. [PMID: 23075179] doi:10.1056/NEJMct1208070

Postuma RB, Berg D, Stern M, Poewe W, Olanow CW, Oertel W, et al. MDS clinical diagnostic criteria for Parkinson's disease. Mov Disord. 2015;30:1591-601. [PMID: 26474316] doi:10.1002/mds.26424

Todorova A, Jenner P, Ray Chaudhuri K. Non-motor Parkinson's: integral to motor Parkinson's, yet often neglected. Pract Neurol. 2014;14:310-22. [PMID: 24699931] doi:10.1136/practneurol-2013-000741

Trenkwalder C, Winkelmann J, Inoue Y, Paulus W. Restless legs syndrome—current therapies and management of augmentation. Nat Rev Neurol. 2015;11:434-45. [PMID: 26215616] doi:10.1038/nrneurol.2015.122

Saifee TA, Edwards MJ. Tardive movement disorders: a practical approach. Pract Neurol. 2011;11:341-8. [PMID: 22100943] doi:10.1136/practneurol-2011-000077

Multiple Sclerosis

Burton JM, O'Connor PW, Hohol M, Beyene J. Oral versus intravenous steroids for treatment of relapses in multiple sclerosis. Cochrane Database Syst Rev.

2012;12:CD006921. [PMID: 23235634] doi:10.1002/14651858.CD006921.pub3

Haselkorn JK, Hughes C, Rae-Grant A, Henson LJ, Bever CT, Lo AC, et al. Summary of comprehensive systematic review: rehabilitation in multiple sclerosis: report of the Guideline Development, Dissemination, and Implementation Subcommittee of the American Academy of Neurology. Neurology. 2015;85:1896-903. [PMID: 26598432] doi:10.1212/WNL.0000000000002146

Lublin FD, Reingold SC, Cohen JA, Cutter GR, Sørensen PS, Thompson AJ, et al. Defining the clinical course of multiple sclerosis: the 2013 revisions. Neurology. 2014;83:278-86. [PMID: 24871874] doi:10.1212/WNL.0000000000000560

Minden SL, Feinstein A, Kalb RC, Miller D, Mohr DC, Patten SB, et al; Guideline Development Subcommittee of the American Academy of Neurology. Evidence-based guideline: assessment and management of psychiatric disorders in individuals with MS: report of the Guideline Development Subcommittee of the American Academy of Neurology. Neurology. 2014;82:174-81. [PMID: 24376275] doi:10.1212/WNL.0000000000000013

Soilu-Hänninen M, Aivo J, Lindström BM, Elovaara I, Sumelahti ML, Färkkilä M, et al. A randomised, double blind, placebo controlled trial with vitamin D_3 as an add on treatment to interferon ß-1b in patients with multiple sclerosis. J Neurol Neurosurg Psychiatry. 2012;83:565-71. [PMID: 22362918] doi:10.1136/jnnp-2011-301876

Thompson AJ, Banwell BL, Barkhof F, Carroll WM, Coetzee T, Comi G, et al. Diagnosis of multiple sclerosis: 2017 revisions of the McDonald criteria. Lancet Neurol. 2018 Feb;17(2):162-173. [Epub 2017 Dec 21] [PMID: 29275977] doi:10.1016/S1474-4422(17)30470-2

Traboulsee A, Simon JH, Stone L, Fisher E, Jones DE, Malhotra A, et al. Revised recommendations of the consortium of MS centers task force for a standardized MRI protocol and clinical guidelines for the diagnosis and follow-up of multiple sclerosis. AJNR Am J Neuroradiol. 2016;37:394-401. [PMID: 26564433] doi:10.3174/ajnr.A4539

Tramacere I, Del Giovane C, Salanti G, D'Amico R, Filippini G. Immunomodulators and immunosuppressants for relapsing-remitting multiple sclerosis: a network meta-analysis. Cochrane Database Syst Rev. 2015:CD011381. [PMID: 26384035] doi:10.1002/14651858.CD011381.pub2

Yadav V, Bever C Jr, Bowen J, Bowling A, Weinstock-Guttman B, Cameron M, et al. Summary of evidence-based guideline: complementary and alternative medicine in multiple sclerosis: report of the guideline development subcommittee of the American Academy of Neurology. Neurology. 2014;82:1083-92. [PMID: 24663230] doi:10.1212/WNL.0000000000000250

Disorders of the Spinal Cord

Al-Qurainy R, Collis E. Metastatic spinal cord compression: diagnosis and management. BMJ. 2016 May 19;353:i2539. [PMID: 27199232] doi:10.1136/bmj.i2539

Briani C, Dalla Torre C, Citton V, et al. Cobalamin deficiency: clinical picture and radiological findings. Nutrients. 2013 Nov 15;5(11):4521-39. [PMID: 24248213] doi:10.3390/nu5114521

Evaniew N, Belley-Côté EP, Fallah N, Noonan VK, Rivers CS, Dvorak MF. Methylprednisolone for the treatment of patients with acute spinal cord injuries: a systematic review and meta-analysis. J Neurotrauma. 2016 Mar 1;33(5):468-81. [PMID: 26529320] doi:10.1089/neu.2015.4192

Hurlbert RJ, Hadley MN, Walters BC, et al. Pharmacological therapy for acute spinal cord injury. Neurosurgery. 2013 Mar;72 Suppl 2:93-105. [PMID: 23417182] doi:10.1227/NEU.0b013e31827765c6

Narvid J, Hetts SW, Larsen D, et al. Spinal dural arteriovenous fistulae: clinical features and long-term results. Neurosurgery. 2008 Jan;62(1):159-66. [PMID: 18300903] doi:10.1227/01.NEU.0000311073.71733.C4

Scott TF, Frohman EM, De Seze J, Gronseth GS, Weinshenker BG; Therapeutics and Technology Assessment Subcommittee of the American Academy of Neurology. Evidence-based guideline: clinical evaluation and treatment of transverse myelitis: report of the Therapeutics and Technology Assessment Subcommittee of the American Academy of Neurology. Neurology. 2011 Dec 13;77(24):2128-34. Epub 2011 Dec 7. [PMID: 22156988] doi:10.1212/WNL.0b013e31823dc535

Neuromuscular Disorders

Barohn RJ, Amato AA. Pattern-recognition approach to neuropathy and neuronopathy. Neurol Clin. 2013;31:343-61. [PMID: 23642713] doi:10.1016/j.ncl.2013.02.001

Fuller G, Morgan C. Bell's palsy syndrome: mimics and chameleons. Pract Neurol. 2016. [PMID: 27034243] doi:10.1136/practneurol-2016-001383

Kress JP, Hall JB. ICU-acquired weakness and recovery from critical illness. N Engl J Med. 2014;370:1626-35. [PMID: 24758618] doi:10.1056/NEJMra1209390

Latov N. Diagnosis and treatment of chronic acquired demyelinating polyneuropathies. Nat Rev Neurol. 2014;10:435-46. [PMID: 24980070] doi:10.1038/nrneurol.2014.117

Levine TD, Saperstein DS. Laboratory evaluation of peripheral neuropathy. Neurol Clin. 2013;31:363-76. [PMID: 23642714] doi:10.1016/j.ncl.2013.01.004

Mammen AL. Statin-associated autoimmune myopathy. N Engl J Med. 2016;374:664-9. [PMID: 26886523] doi:10.1056/NEJMra1515161

Peltier A, Goutman SA, Callaghan BC. Painful diabetic neuropathy. BMJ. 2014;348:g1799. [PMID: 24803311] doi:10.1136/bmj.g1799

Silvestri NJ, Wolfe GI. Myasthenia gravis. Semin Neurol. 2012;32:215-26. [PMID: 23117946] doi:10.1055/s-0032-1329200

van den Berg B, Walgaard C, Drenthen J, Fokke C, Jacobs BC, van Doorn PA. Guillain-Barré syndrome: pathogenesis, diagnosis, treatment and prognosis. Nat Rev Neurol. 2014;10:469-82. [PMID: 25023340] doi:10.1038/nrneurol.2014.121

Neuro-oncology

Englot DJ, Magill ST, Han SJ, Chang EF, Berger MS, McDermott MW. Seizures in supratentorial meningioma: a systematic review and meta-analysis. J Neurosurg. 2016 Jun;124(6):1552-61. Epub 2015 Dec 4. [PMID: 26636386] doi:10.3171/2015.4.JNS142742

Hoang-Xuan K, Bessell E, Bromberg J, Hottinger AF, Preusser M, Rudà R, et al; European Association for Neuro-Oncology Task Force on Primary CNS Lymphoma. Diagnosis and treatment of primary CNS lymphoma in immunocompetent patients: guidelines from the European Association for Neuro-Oncology. Lancet Oncol. 2015 Jul;16(7):e322-32. [PMID: 26149884] doi:10.1016/S1470-2045(15)00076-5

Jo JT, Schiff D, Perry JR. Thrombosis in brain tumors. Semin Thromb Hemost. 2014 Apr;40(3):325-31. [PMID: 24599439] doi:10.1055/s-0034-1370791

Leung D, Han X, Mikkelsen T, Nabors LB. Role of MRI in primary brain tumor evaluation. J Natl Compr Canc Netw. 2014 Nov;12(11):1561-8. [PMID: 25361803]

McKeon A. Autoimmune encephalopathies and dementias. Continuum (Minneap Minn). 2016 Apr;22(2 Dementia):538-58. [PMID: 27042907] doi:10.1212/CON.0000000000000299

Nabors LB, Portnow J, Ammirati M, Baehring J, Brem H, et al. Central nervous system cancers, version 1.2015. J Natl Compr Canc Netw. 2015 Oct;13(10):1191-202. [PMID: 26483059]

Owonikoko TK, Arbiser J, Zelnak A, Shu HK, Shim H, et al. Current approaches to the treatment of metastatic brain tumours. Nat Rev Clin Oncol. 2014 Apr;11(4):203-22. Epub 2014 Feb 25. [PMID: 24569448] doi: 10.1038/nrclinonc.2014.25

Sayegh ET, Fakurnejad S, Oh T, Bloch O, Parsa AT. Anticonvulsant prophylaxis for brain tumor surgery: determining the current best available evidence. J Neurosurg. 2014 Nov;121(5):1139-47. Epub 2014 Aug 29. [PMID: 25170671] doi: 10.3171/2014.7.JNS132829

Schiff D, Lee EQ, Nayak L, Norden AD, Reardon DA, Wen PY. Medical management of brain tumors and the sequelae of treatment. Neuro Oncol. 2015 Apr;17(4):488-504. Epub 2014 Oct 30. [PMID: 25358508] doi: 10.1093/neuonc/nou304

Weller M, van den Bent M, Hopkins K, Tonn JC, Stupp R, Falini A, et al; European Association for Neuro-Oncology (EANO) Task Force on Malignant Glioma. EANO guideline for the diagnosis and treatment of anaplastic gliomas and glioblastoma [erratum in: Lancet Oncol. 2014 Dec;15(13):e587]. Lancet Oncol. 2014 Aug;15(9):e395-403. [PMID: 25079102] doi: 10.1016/S1470-2045(14)70011-7

Neurology Self-Assessment Test

This self-assessment test contains one-best-answer multiple-choice questions. Please read these directions carefully before answering the questions. Answers, critiques, and bibliographies immediately follow these multiple-choice questions. The American College of Physicians (ACP) is accredited by the Accreditation Council for Continuing Medical Education (ACCME) to provide continuing medical education for physicians.

The American College of Physicians designates MKSAP 18 Neurology for a maximum of 22 *AMA PRA Category 1 Credits*™. Physicians should claim only the credit commensurate with the extent of their participation in the activity.

Successful completion of the CME activity, which includes participation in the evaluation component, enables the participant to earn up to 22 medical knowledge MOC points in the American Board of Internal Medicine's Maintenance of Certification (MOC) program. It is the CME activity provider's responsibility to submit participant completion information to ACCME for the purpose of granting MOC credit.

Earn Instantaneous CME Credits or MOC Points Online

Print subscribers can enter their answers online to earn instantaneous CME credits or MOC points. You can submit your answers using online answer sheets that are provided at mksap.acponline.org, where a record of your MKSAP 18 credits will be available. To earn CME credits or to apply for MOC points, you need to answer all of the questions in a test and earn a score of at least 50% correct (number of correct answers divided by the total number of questions). Please note that if you are applying for MOC points, you must also enter your birth date and ABIM candidate number.

Take either of the following approaches:

- Use the printed answer sheet at the back of this book to record your answers. Go to mksap.acponline.org, access the appropriate online answer sheet, transcribe your answers, and submit your test for instantaneous CME credits or MOC points. There is no additional fee for this service.

- Go to mksap.acponline.org, access the appropriate online answer sheet, directly enter your answers, and submit your test for instantaneous CME credits or MOC points. There is no additional fee for this service.

Earn CME Credits or MOC Points by Mail or Fax

Pay a $20 processing fee per answer sheet and submit the printed answer sheet at the back of this book by mail or fax, as instructed on the answer sheet. Make sure you calculate your score and enter your birth date and ABIM candidate number, and fax the answer sheet to 215-351-2799 or mail the answer sheet to Member and Customer Service, American College of Physicians, 190 N. Independence Mall West, Philadelphia, PA 19106-1572, using the courtesy envelope provided in your MKSAP 18 slipcase. You will need your 10-digit order number and 8-digit ACP ID number, which are printed on your packing slip. Please allow 4 to 6 weeks for your score report to be emailed back to you. Be sure to include your email address for a response.

If you do not have a 10-digit order number and 8-digit ACP ID number, or if you need help creating a username and password to access the MKSAP 18 online answer sheets, go to mksap.acponline.org or email custserv@acponline.org.

CME credits and MOC points are available from the publication date of July 31, 2018, until July 31, 2021. You may submit your answer sheet or enter your answers online at any time during this period.

*Each of the numbered items is followed by lettered answers. Select the **ONE** lettered answer that is **BEST** in each case.*

Item 1

A 19-year-old man is evaluated for a 2-week history of shaking episodes sometimes associated with falling that are followed by a period of unresponsiveness. He reports having a 30-minute episode just before getting in the car to go to this appointment. Episodes have been occurring daily, sometimes as often as four times per day, and last 20 to 45 minutes. According to the patient's mother, the episodes involve limb shaking with the eyes closed, intermittent cessation of breathing, and a reddening of the face. The patient remains standing for a few seconds after the shaking starts but on occasion becomes limp and falls. He does not respond when his name is called or his arms or legs are lightly touched. The shaking, which gradually increases and decreases in intensity, typically involves both arms and sometimes the legs. He is exhausted but oriented and responsive afterward and has rapid breathing.

All physical examination findings are normal.

Which of the following is the most likely diagnosis?

(A) Convulsive status epilepticus
(B) Generalized tonic clonic seizure
(C) Myoclonic seizure
(D) Psychogenic nonepileptic spell/event

Item 2

A 75-year-old man is hospitalized for treatment of extreme agitation and delirium after developing a urinary tract infection (UTI). He has a 1-year history of dementia with Lewy bodies. According to his wife, the patient has nighttime visual hallucinations 4 or 5 times per week but is rarely bothered by them. Home medications are simvastatin and aspirin.

On physical examination, blood pressure is 150/92 mm Hg and pulse rate is 98/min; other vital signs are normal. The patient is agitated and disoriented and appears to be having visual hallucinations. Although his agitation steadily increases, he does not become aggressive. His UTI is being treated appropriately. No other clear sources of the delirium are present.

Environmental interventions are instituted to help abate his symptoms.

Which of the following medications is most likely to be effective in treating his acute agitation?

(A) Alprazolam
(B) Diphenhydramine
(C) Donepezil
(D) Haloperidol

Item 3

A 59-year-old woman comes to the office for a follow-up evaluation of Parkinson disease, which was diagnosed 8 years ago and has been treated with carbidopa-levodopa, amantadine, and rasagiline. Primary symptoms are tremor, slowness, shuffling of the feet, and intermittent freezing of gait, which has caused her to fall several times; the tremor and slowness substantially improve after administration of carbidopa-levodopa, but she exhibits prominent involuntary, nonpatterned, dance-like movements for approximately 2 hours after a dose. She has tried increasing the carbidopa-levodopa dosage but could not tolerate the resultant nausea and orthostatic hypotension.

On initial physical examination, which takes place before she takes her scheduled dose of carbidopa-levodopa, a prominent tremor is noted. The patient's spontaneous and repetitive movements are very slow, and she has difficulty taking more than a few steps before needing assistance to maintain balance. A repeat examination performed 1 hour after she takes the medication reveals suppression of the tremor, remarkable improvement of speed and gait, and the presence of diffuse high-amplitude flowing involuntary movements in all extremities.

An MRI of the brain is unremarkable.

Which of the following is the most appropriate next step in her treatment?

(A) Apomorphine
(B) Deep brain stimulation
(C) Droxidopa
(D) Rotigotine patch

Item 4

A 22-year-old man is evaluated in the hospital after sustaining a traumatic brain injury in a motorcycle accident 4 hours earlier. The patient lost consciousness briefly at the scene but was wearing a helmet. He is now awake and reports a severe headache, nausea, vertigo, left-ear tinnitus and deafness, and rhinorrhea when he sits upright.

On physical examination, temperature is 38.1 °C (100.6 °F), blood pressure is 110/60 mm Hg, pulse rate is 104/min, and respiration rate is 20/min. Oxygen saturation is 95% with the patient breathing ambient air. Right hemotympanum and deafness are noted. Bruising is shown.

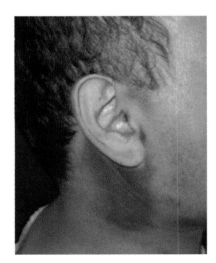

CONT. Results of laboratory studies show a normal complete blood count, comprehensive metabolic profile, and urinalysis; a urine drug screen is positive for opiates.

A noncontrast head CT scan shows a small right temporal bone fracture but no intracranial hemorrhage. Chest radiographs and a cervical spine CT scan are normal.

Which of the following is the most appropriate initial treatment?

(A) Acetaminophen

(B) Ceftriaxone

(C) Dexamethasone

(D) Naloxone

(E) Norepinephrine

Item 5

A 48-year-old man is hospitalized with new-onset right hemiparesis and difficulty speaking. He was well when last seen 20 hours earlier.

On physical examination, blood pressure is 138/76 mm Hg, pulse rate is 72 and regular, and respiration rate is 12/min. The patient has aphasia. A right visual field deficit and right facial, arm, and leg weakness are noted. Decreased pinprick sensation is present on the right. Reflexes also are decreased on the right; a right plantar extensor response is noted.

An electrocardiogram shows sinus rhythm. A CT scan of the head shows a hypodensity in the left frontal and parietal lobes, and a CT angiogram of the head and neck shows patent internal carotid arteries and 80% stenosis of the left middle cerebral artery.

Results of laboratory studies include a serum LDL cholesterol level of 108 mg/dL (2.80 mmol/L) and a hemoglobin A_{1c} value of 6.8%.

The patient is given aspirin.

Which of the following is the most appropriate next step in treatment?

(A) Atorvastatin

(B) Intracranial stenting

(C) Methylphenidate

(D) Warfarin

Item 6

A 51-year-old woman is evaluated for a 1-year history of daily afternoon fatigue that necessitates frequent naps and impairs her concentration at the office, where she works as a lawyer. Lifestyle adjustments, such as improving sleep hygiene, getting regular exercise, yoga, and vitamin supplementation have not resolved this symptom. She has a 5-year history of multiple sclerosis. Medications are glatiramer acetate and a vitamin D supplement.

On physical examination, vital signs are normal. Depression screening is negative. The remainder of the physical examination is noncontributory.

Results of laboratory studies, including hemoglobin and serum thyroid-stimulating hormone levels, are unremarkable.

Which of the following is the most appropriate management?

(A) Baclofen

(B) Memantine

(C) Modafinil

(D) Substitution of an interferon beta for the glatiramer acetate

(E) Tetrahydrocannabinol-cannabidiol combination

Item 7

A 22-year-old man is evaluated in the emergency department 40 minutes after having a first-time generalized tonic-clonic seizure. According to his mother, the patient exhibited shaking for 5 minutes. He has never had a seizure previously or any episode of jerking, staring, confusion, or memory loss. He has had no recent illness and has no history of neurologic problems. Birth and development were normal. There is no family history of seizures or epilepsy. He takes no medication and does not use illicit drugs.

On physical examination, vital signs are normal. Neurologic examination findings are unremarkable.

Results of laboratory studies show a normal complete blood count and comprehensive metabolic panel and a negative urine drug screen.

Which of the following is the most appropriate initial step in management?

(A) Head CT

(B) Intravenous levetiracetam

(C) Intravenous lorazepam

(D) Lumbar puncture

Item 8

A 53-year-old woman is brought to the office by her husband for follow-up evaluation of behavioral-variant frontotemporal dementia, which was diagnosed 9 months ago. Her clinical symptoms of occasional aphasia, minor memory impairment, behavioral disinhibition, and obsessive-compulsive behaviors have worsened since diagnosis and have become disruptive. She is currently estranged from her son and his family after bringing a large bag filled with plastic bottles collected from his neighbors' trash cans to her granddaughter's birthday party 2 weeks ago. Her husband asks about possible medications to control her symptoms.

Which of the following is the most appropriate medication to recommend?

(A) Citalopram

(B) Donepezil

(C) Memantine

(D) Methylphenidate

(E) Olanzapine

Item 9

A 72-year-old woman is evaluated in the emergency department 5 hours after developing difficulty speaking and facial weakness on the right. She takes no medication.

CONT.

On physical examination, vital signs are normal. The patient is awake and attentive. Spontaneous speech is slow. Right-sided facial weakness and dysarthria are noted.

Hemoglobin level, platelet count, and coagulation profile are within normal limits.

An electrocardiogram is normal. A CT scan of the head shows an acute left frontal ischemic stroke. A carotid duplex ultrasound reveals less than 40% stenosis in both internal carotid arteries; a transcranial Doppler ultrasound is normal. A transthoracic echocardiogram shows an ejection fraction of 50% but is otherwise unremarkable.

Aspirin and rosuvastatin are initiated, and the patient is admitted to the telemetry unit for 3 days, during which time she remains in sinus rhythm.

Which of the following is the most appropriate next step in management?

(A) Addition of clopidogrel
(B) Outpatient cardiac telemetry
(C) Substitution of apixaban for aspirin
(D) Transesophageal echocardiography

Item 10

A 47-year-old woman is evaluated in the emergency department for abrupt-onset severe headaches lasting 6 to 8 hours that have occurred three times in the past 4 days. The pain developed spontaneously, reached maximum intensity within 10 seconds, and is holocranial and throbbing. She reports associated nausea and photophobia but no changes in mentation, vision, sensation, or motor function. The first two episodes occurred while showering and the third while at the dinner table 2 hours ago. The patient has anxiety but no personal or family history of headache. She started taking sertraline 1 month ago for anxiety but discontinued it after headache onset.

On physical examination, temperature is 37.8 °C (100.0 °F), blood pressure is 130/80 mm Hg, and pulse rate is 72/min. All other physical examination findings, including those from a neurologic examination, are normal.

A head CT scan and results of lumbar puncture also are normal.

Which of the following is the most appropriate management?

(A) Digital subtraction angiography
(B) Magnetic resonance angiography of the brain
(C) Methylprednisolone sodium succinate
(D) Sumatriptan
(E) Valproic acid

Item 11

A 39-year-old woman is evaluated in the emergency department for a 3-day history of worsening imbalance, falling, and vertigo. Multiple sclerosis was diagnosed 5 years ago and has been treated with interferon beta-1a since that time. She also takes gabapentin for neuropathic pain.

On physical examination, temperature is 37.3 °C (99.1 °F); all other vital signs are normal. Internuclear ophthalmoplegia is noted on the left. The patient exhibits imbalance in her primary gait and is unable to perform tandem gait or to maintain balance during Romberg testing when she opens her eyes.

Which of the following is the most appropriate immediate treatment?

(A) High-dose oral prednisone
(B) Low-dose oral prednisone
(C) Plasmapheresis
(D) Vitamin D administration

Item 12

A 41-year-old woman is evaluated for a 2-year history of tremor in the dominant right hand. She says that the tremor has begun interfering with her work as a hairdresser, especially when she uses scissors. She also reports tightness in the forearm. The patient is able to eat, write, and type without difficulty and has had no trauma, imbalance, slowness of movement, or change in gait speed. Alcohol has no effect on the tremor. There is no family history of tremor.

On physical examination, vital signs are normal. A right upper extremity tremor is noted, as are rhythmic flexion of the wrist, involuntary flexion of the fingers, and pronation of the forearm. The tremor is present both at rest and during action and resolves by changing the position of an outstretched arm. No dysmetria, dysdiadochokinesia, bradykinesia, rigidity, shuffling gait, or reduced arm swing is noted. Her handwriting is neither tremulous nor micrographic.

An MRI of the brain is unremarkable.

Which of the following is the most likely diagnosis?

(A) Cerebellar tremor
(B) Dystonic tremor
(C) Essential tremor
(D) Parkinson disease
(E) Rubral tremor

Item 13

A 21-year-old man is evaluated in the emergency department for persistent convulsive status epilepticus that began 30 minutes before his arrival. An airway has been secured, and he has received intravenous glucose, thiamine, and two doses of intravenous lorazepam. After receiving the second dose of lorazepam, he continues shaking for another 5 minutes. Medications are levetiracetam and acetaminophen; the patient is allergic to phenytoin.

On physical examination, temperature is normal, blood pressure is 155/89 mm Hg, pulse rate is 108/min, respiration rate is 16/min, and oxygen saturation with the patient breathing 6 L of oxygen via a nasal cannula is 97%. The pupils are reactive but he remains comatose.

Results of a urine drug screen are negative.

CONT.

Which of the following is the most appropriate next step in management?

(A) Brain MRI

(B) Electroencephalography

(C) Fosphenytoin

(D) Lacosamide

(E) Valproic acid

Item 14

A 78-year-old man is evaluated for recent difficulty with memory. The patient has hypertension treated with hydrochlorothiazide. He reports decreased appetite, problems falling asleep, and withdrawal from social activities since his wife's death 13 months ago, at which time he had to assume several new responsibilities, including managing the finances and cooking. He is concerned because he received a missed payment notice on last month's utility bill and is worried that he is developing dementia; his 85-year-old brother has Alzheimer disease that was diagnosed 2 years ago. On a screening evaluation 6 months ago, the patient scored 28/30 (normal, ≥24) on a Mini–Mental State Examination, and his Geriatric Depression Scale Short Form score was 9 (normal, <6); he has lost 2.3 kg (5.1 lb) since that time.

Physical examination findings, including vital signs and results of neurologic examination, are unremarkable.

Results of laboratory studies, including a complete blood count and measurement of thyroid-stimulating hormone and vitamin B_{12} levels, are normal.

Which of the following is the most appropriate next step in management?

(A) Begin an acetylcholinesterase inhibitor

(B) Begin treatment for depression

(C) Obtain a brain MRI without contrast

(D) Obtain neuropsychological testing

Item 15

A 51-year-old woman is evaluated in the emergency department for a 1-month history of new-onset abnormal movements, paranoia, hallucinations, and progressive confusion. She was healthy before onset of symptoms and takes no medication.

On physical examination, vital signs are normal. The patient is alert but oriented to person and place only, recalls none of three objects after 5 minutes, requires constant redirection to follow commands and sustain attention, is having ongoing visual and auditory hallucinations, and exhibits intermittent slow, writhing (choreiform) movements of the arms. Muscle strength is normal, as are sensation and deep tendon reflexes.

Results of standard laboratory studies, including a complete blood count and comprehensive metabolic panel, are unremarkable. Results of brain MRI and lumbar puncture are normal. Subsequent testing for serum anti–N-methyl-D-aspartate receptor antibody is positive.

Which of the following is the most likely diagnosis?

(A) Breast adenocarcinoma

(B) Non–small cell lung cancer

(C) Ovarian teratoma

(D) Small cell lung cancer

Item 16

A 24-year-old woman has a 4-year history of monthly headaches. The pain is bitemporal, throbbing, and worsened by bending or ascending stairs. Approximately half of the headaches have been severe with associated nausea. She has no precursor symptoms, no photophobia or phonophobia, and no visual or neurologic symptoms. Over the past year, the headaches have not changed in character but have gradually become more frequent, increasing from 4 to 10 days per month. Episodes last as long as 8 hours and typically respond to ibuprofen within 1 hour. She takes no other medication.

All physical examination findings, including vital signs and those from a neurologic examination, are unremarkable.

Which of the following is the most appropriate treatment?

(A) Citalopram

(B) Gabapentin

(C) Metoprolol

(D) Onabotulinum toxin A

(E) Rizatriptan

Item 17

A 29-year-old woman is evaluated before attempting pregnancy. Juvenile myoclonic epilepsy was diagnosed 11 years ago, at which time she started taking valproic acid; she has had no symptoms for 10.5 years. Her only other medication is an oral contraceptive agent. She is concerned about taking her medications if she becomes pregnant.

All physical examination findings are normal, as was her most recent electroencephalogram.

A plan is made to discontinue the oral contraceptive, start folic acid, and then taper the valproic acid.

Which of the following is the most appropriate additional step in treatment?

(A) Gabapentin

(B) Levetiracetam

(C) Oxcarbazepine

(D) Topiramate

(E) No additional treatment is necessary

Item 18

A 58-year-old man is evaluated in the emergency department for a 3-week history of worsening pain in the middle back and a 2-day history of increasing leg weakness that has made ambulation difficult. He has metastatic prostate cancer treated with leuprolide.

On physical examination, vital signs are normal. Muscle strength testing shows 4/5 weakness in the hip flexors. Reflexes are 3+ in both legs.

An MRI of the thoracic spine shows a contrast-enhancing mass originating in the T8 vertebral body with invasion into the epidural space that causes moderate cord compression.

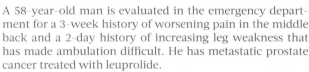

CONT. **After administration of high-dose glucocorticoids, which of the following is the most appropriate next step in management?**

(A) Decompressive surgery with radiation

(B) Laminectomy

(C) Radiation only

(D) Spinal angiography

 Item 19

A 47-year-old woman is evaluated in the hospital for a 4-month history of increasingly frequent falls and episodes of confusion. She was fired from her job 3 months ago because of poor performance. Since that time, she also has had occasional anxiety, problems sleeping, and visual hallucinations. For the past 2 weeks, she has had repeated falls, exhibited erratic behavior, and been unable to prepare even a cup of coffee.

On physical examination, vital signs are normal. The patient is agitated and disoriented to place and time. She exhibits word-finding difficulty and intermittent myoclonic movements of the arms and legs. She scores 8/30 (normal, ≥24) on the Mini–Mental State Examination.

Results of laboratory studies are normal, including cerebrospinal fluid findings of a normal leukocyte count and normal glucose and protein levels.

An electroencephalogram shows periodic sharp wave complexes. Diffusion-weighted brain MRIs show high-signal changes in the basal ganglia and cerebral cortex.

Which of the following is the most likely diagnosis?

(A) Creutzfeldt-Jakob disease

(B) HIV encephalopathy

(C) Lyme disease

(D) Wernicke encephalopathy

Item 20

A 49-year-old-man is evaluated 1 day after having an episode of right arm weakness without pain that lasted 5 minutes. He is now asymptomatic. The patient has type 2 diabetes mellitus and dyslipidemia. Medications are aspirin, metformin, and atorvastatin.

On physical examination, blood pressure is 126/68 mm Hg, pulse rate is 86/min and regular, and respiration rate is 12/min. No carotid bruits or cardiac murmurs are heard on cardiac auscultation. All other physical examination findings are normal.

An electrocardiogram shows normal sinus rhythm with no ST-segment or T-wave changes.

Which of the following is the most appropriate initial imaging test?

(A) Carotid duplex ultrasonography

(B) CT angiography of the neck

(C) MRI of the brain

(D) Transesophageal echocardiography

Item 21

A 64-year-old man is evaluated for an abnormal gait and twitching. He is brought to the office by his wife, who reports that the patient has depression and that he has abused drugs and alcohol for the past 15 years; she further states that within the past year, he has developed impulsivity, imbalance, and incoordination and often appears restless. His father had major depressive disorder and committed suicide at age 60 years.

On physical examination, vital signs are normal. Orientation, language, memory, and attention are intact. Speech is dysarthric. The patient cannot perform multistep tasks and cannot sit still on command. He exhibits frequent and variable flowing movements of the limbs and trunk that he incorporates into purposeful gestures. Reflexes are brisk, and gait is rapid, wide based, and uncoordinated.

Which of the following is the most likely diagnosis?

(A) Creutzfeldt-Jakob disease

(B) Frontotemporal dementia

(C) Huntington disease

(D) Parkinson disease

Item 22

A 62-year-old man is evaluated in the emergency department after being struck by a vehicle while crossing the street 3 hours earlier and hitting his head on the pavement. He did not lose consciousness. The patient now reports a moderate headache. He describes the headache as global, dull, and aching without photophobia or phonophobia. He has had no nausea, visual changes, or neurologic symptoms since the incident.

On physical examination, vital signs are normal, as are findings from a neurologic examination.

Which of the following is the most appropriate initial step in management?

(A) Head CT with contrast

(B) Head CT without contrast

(C) Hospital observation

(D) Prochlorperazine administration

Item 23

A 71-year-old woman is evaluated for difficulty holding her head upright. She notes that her head feels heavy and reports intermittent difficulty with swallowing and speech that is worse in the evening. She has had no pain, sensory changes, weakness in the extremities, or cognitive or visual symptoms. She has no other medical problems and takes no medication.

On physical examination, vital signs are normal. Speech is mildly dysarthric. Cervical extension is weak. No ptosis, ophthalmoplegia, sensory deficit, or weakness in the extremities is noted.

Results of laboratory studies show a normal serum creatine kinase level; no acetylcholine receptor antibodies are detected.

Findings from routine nerve conduction and needle electromyography studies of the limbs are unremarkable, but a repetitive stimulation protocol reveals a decremental response. An MRI of the brain is normal.

Which of the following is the most likely diagnosis?

(A) Bulbar amyotrophic lateral sclerosis
(B) Inclusion body myositis
(C) Multiple sclerosis
(D) Myasthenia gravis
(E) Polymyositis

Item 24

A 72-year-old woman is evaluated for a 12-month history of increasing forgetfulness. The patient is retired from her position as a professor of economics at a local university. She takes no medication and drinks no alcoholic beverages. Her husband says that his wife's occasional forgetfulness has caused no major problems and that she is able to function normally.

On physical examination, vital signs are normal. Her Geriatric Depression Scale score is normal and Montreal Cognitive Assessment score is 25/30 (normal, ≥26), with a score of 1/5 on the delayed recall section and 5/6 on the orientation section. All other physical and neurologic examination findings are normal.

Results of laboratory studies show normal vitamin B_{12}, thyroid-stimulating hormone, and 25-hydroxyvitamin D levels.

Complete neuropsychological testing findings indicate normal global cognition, language function, and attention, but verbal learning and memory performance are 2 SDs below that of an age- and education-matched control population.

An MRI of the brain shows a slight loss of hippocampal volume that is greater on the right than the left but is otherwise normal.

Which of the following is the most likely diagnosis?

(A) Alzheimer disease
(B) Depression
(C) Mild cognitive impairment
(D) Normal aging

Item 25

A 59-year-old woman comes to the office for a follow-up evaluation of a 2-year history of worsening urinary urgency and frequency. Episodes of urinary incontinence have occurred more often in the past 6 months because she cannot walk fast enough to get to the bathroom in time. Recently, she also has experienced intermittent urinary hesitancy and a frequent feeling of incomplete emptying, sometimes requiring changing body position or manual pelvic pressure. The patient has a 5-year history of secondary progressive multiple sclerosis. She takes no disease-modifying therapy. Her only medication is a vitamin D supplement.

Physical examination findings are unremarkable.
Urinalysis results are normal.

Which of the following is the most appropriate next step in management?

(A) Dalfampridine administration
(B) Oxybutynin administration
(C) Solifenacin administration
(D) Urodynamic testing

Item 26

A 55-year-old woman is evaluated in the hospital after diagnosis of pulmonary embolism. She was admitted to the hospital 3 days ago for evaluation of a brain mass with imaging features characteristic of glioblastoma. Twenty-four hours after brain biopsy, the patient developed chest pain and dyspnea. Imaging confirmed a filling defect in the right pulmonary artery.

On physical examination, blood pressure is 110/60 mm Hg, pulse rate is 100/min, respiration rate is 18/min, and oxygen saturation is 93% with the patient receiving 2 L/min of nasal oxygen. Cardiopulmonary examination shows mild tachycardia but is otherwise normal. Right upper and lower facial numbness and right arm weakness and numbness are noted. Biceps, triceps, and brachioradialis reflexes are increased on the right, as is right-sided hyperreflexia. An extensor plantar response is present on the right.

Results of laboratory studies show a serum creatinine level of 1.7 mg/dL (150 μmol/L).

Which of the following is the most appropriate treatment?

(A) Apixaban
(B) Inferior vena cava filter placement
(C) Intravenous alteplase
(D) Intravenous heparin
(E) Subcutaneous low-molecular-weight heparin

Item 27

A 52-year-old man is evaluated for a 1-year history of progressive weakness that began as right foot drop and bilateral tingling in the feet. Within the past 2 months, the patient has developed progressive weakness, which makes walking difficult; he also notes weakness in the hands and burning below the knees but no autonomic symptoms. He has hypothyroidism treated with levothyroxine.

On physical examination, vital signs are normal. Motor strength is 4/5 in the intrinsic hand and quadriceps muscles and 3/5 in the tibialis anterior and gastrocnemius muscles; bulbar and facial muscle strength is normal. Deep tendon reflexes are absent in the lower extremities. Sensory perception of vibration is severely impaired at the knees. Pinprick testing shows reduced sensation below the ankles. Splenomegaly is present, as are patchy areas of hyperpigmentation and scattered angiomas on the trunk. Gait is broad based and wobbly, and a Romberg test has positive results.

Serum immunofixation reveals a λ light chain monoclonal protein.

Needle electromyography reveals a demyelinating sensorimotor polyneuropathy.

Which of the following is the most likely diagnosis?

(A) Amyotrophic lateral sclerosis
(B) Chronic inflammatory demyelinating polyradiculo-neuropathy
(C) Mitochondrial myopathy
(D) POEMS syndrome

Item 28

A 19-year-old woman is evaluated for a 6-month history of recurrent episodes of confusion that occur approximately once monthly. Her boyfriend says she has periods of wide-eyed staring, chewing motions, and repetitive grabbing of her clothes with the right hand. The patient sometimes experiences a strange but familiar feeling before the episodes but does not remember the episodes themselves, which last approximately 45 to 60 seconds and are followed by exhaustion and sleepiness for 20 minutes.

All physical examination findings are normal.

Which of the following is the most likely diagnosis?

(A) Absence seizures
(B) Atonic seizures
(C) Focal seizures
(D) Myoclonic seizures

Item 29

A 42-year-old man comes to the office for a follow-up evaluation 4 weeks after undergoing laparoscopic abdominal surgery. Two days after the operation, he developed severe, unrelenting pain of the right shoulder and arm lasting 1 week followed by progressive weakness of the right shoulder and proximal arm. He currently has no pain but cannot maintain the right arm above his head. The patient reports numbness affecting the right arm and says that his grip has become weak. He has had no problem with speech, swallowing, or moving the lower extremities. He has hyperlipidemia treated with atorvastatin.

On physical examination, vital signs are normal. Motor examination reveals moderate weakness of arm abduction, forearm extension, and hand grip on the right side. Winging of the right scapula is present. Trapezius and deltoid muscle bulk is reduced on the right side compared with the left. Right biceps and brachioradialis reflexes are absent, but other deep tendon reflexes are intact. Patchy areas of sensory loss are noted over the right shoulder, forearm, and palm. The cranial nerves are intact, the lower extremities have normal strength bilaterally, and gait and balance are both normal.

Results of laboratory studies show an erythrocyte sedimentation rate of 18 mm/h, a serum creatine kinase level of 150 U/L, and a hemoglobin A_{1c} value of 5.7%.

MRI of cervical spine is unremarkable.

Which of the following is the most likely diagnosis?

(A) Compressive polyradiculopathy
(B) Idiopathic brachial plexopathy
(C) Lambert-Eaton myasthenic syndrome
(D) Statin myopathy

Item 30

An 18-year-old woman is evaluated for a 2-year history of repetitive fast movements of the neck that tilt the head to the right side. She reports that these movements are preceded by a feeling of discomfort in the right shoulder and that if she concentrates and taps the right foot immediately after this sensory cue, she usually can avoid the neck movements. She is a senior in high school and says she has not been able to use this method successfully in the classroom, especially during examinations, when she often experiences a cluster of movements that exhaust and distract her. Her mother notes that before onset of the neck symptoms, the patient used to roll her eyes and clear her throat frequently. She has obsessive-compulsive disorder treated with sertraline.

On physical examination, vital signs are normal. During the examination, the patient displays rapid tilting movements of the head followed by rolling of the head and shoulder; these movements repeat several times in a stereotyped manner. The patient can suppress these movements on request.

Which of the following is the most appropriate treatment?

(A) Botulinum toxin injection
(B) Clonidine administration
(C) Cognitive behavioral therapy
(D) Haloperidol administration

Item 31

A 38-year-old man is evaluated for a 6-month history of increasingly frequent episodes of migraine with aura. The patient has had migraine with aura since age 23 years. Auras involve 15 to 20 minutes of twinkling lights and visual blurring in either hemifield. On occasion, he has noted ipsilateral numbness and paresthesia of the face, tongue, and hand lasting another 15 to 20 minutes after the visual blurring has resolved. Migraine episode frequency has increased from once to twice monthly. Acetaminophen, ibuprofen, and naproxen were each discontinued after becoming ineffective, with headaches now lasting 24 hours.

On physical examination, all findings, including vital signs and results of a neurologic examination, are unremarkable.

Which of the following is the most appropriate next step in treatment?

(A) Hydrocodone
(B) Sumatriptan
(C) Topiramate
(D) Verapamil

Item 32

A 27-year-old woman is evaluated in the emergency department after a sudden, first-time episode of loss of consciousness while standing in line to board a tour bus. She had warning symptoms of tunnel vision and palpitations, after which she lost consciousness and fell. According to her father, who witnessed the episode, she was limp and unconscious for approximately 20 to 30 seconds, during which

CONT.

time she displayed intermittent twitching of all four limbs, with the limbs shaking independently at separate times. After the patient regained consciousness, she was confused about why she was on the ground but answered questions appropriately and was oriented to self and place.

All physical examination findings are normal.

Which of the following is the most likely diagnosis?

(A) Atonic seizure

(B) Convulsive syncope

(C) Generalized tonic-clonic seizure

(D) Myoclonic seizure

(E) Tonic seizure

Item 33

A 66-year-old woman comes to the office for a follow-up evaluation 1 month after being hospitalized with an ischemic stroke of the pons. Neurologic deficits have improved steadily in the intervening weeks, but the patient now reports having difficulty with outpatient rehabilitation because of a diminished energy level and fatigue in the absence of depressed mood, anhedonia, or loss of interest. She also has hypertension, dyslipidemia, and depression. Medications are aspirin, amlodipine, chlorthalidone, atorvastatin, and citalopram.

On physical examination, vital signs are normal; BMI is 36. Right facial weakness and dysarthria are noted. Muscle strength is 4/5 in the right arm, 5/5 in the right leg, and 4/5 in the right ankle. The patient scores in the normal range on a two-point depression scale.

Results of laboratory studies, including a basic metabolic panel, liver chemistry and thyroid function studies, and serum creatine kinase measurement, are normal.

Which of the following is the most appropriate next step in management?

(A) Discontinuation of atorvastatin

(B) Fluoxetine initiation

(C) MRI of the brain

(D) Polysomnography

Item 34

A 38-year-old man comes to the office to discuss treatment of his recently diagnosed multiple sclerosis. The patient also has diabetes mellitus and nonalcoholic steatohepatitis. Medications are metformin and atorvastatin.

On physical examination, vital signs are normal; BMI is 30. All remaining physical examination findings are unremarkable.

A T2-weighted MRI of the brain obtained just before diagnosis shows three hyperintense lesions in the periventricular white matter, a hyperintense lesion in the pons, and three juxtacortical hyperintense lesions. The pontine lesion was enhanced with administration of intravenous contrast.

Which of the following is the most appropriate treatment?

(A) Fingolimod

(B) Glatiramer acetate

(C) Interferon beta

(D) Natalizumab

Item 35

A 70-year-old man is evaluated for a 6-month history of right upper extremity weakness, intermittent painful spasms in both calves, and occasional brief muscle twitches. The patient reports right arm and hand weakness and says that for the past 2 weeks, his right foot drags when he walks quickly. He has had no numbness, sensory loss, paresthesia, or problems with swallowing, sphincter control, or coordination.

On physical examination, vital signs are normal. Weakness and muscle wasting is noted in the thumb abductor and intrinsic hand muscles on the right side. Spontaneous muscle twitches are present in the bilateral thumb adductor, gastrocnemius, and paraspinal muscles. Minor weakness of right ankle dorsiflexion, a right Hoffman sign, and right foot clonus is noted. Deep tendon reflexes are brisk throughout. Cranial nerves are intact, as is sensory perception.

Electromyography and nerve condition studies reveal evidence of lower motor neuron involvement in the upper and lower extremities and paraspinal muscles. MRIs of the brain and cervical spine are unremarkable.

Which of the following is the most likely diagnosis?

(A) Amyotrophic lateral sclerosis

(B) Charcot-Marie-Tooth disease

(C) Granulomatosis with polyangiitis

(D) Miller Fisher variant of Guillain-Barré syndrome

Item 36

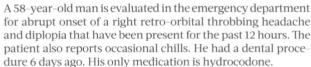

A 58-year-old man is evaluated in the emergency department for abrupt onset of a right retro-orbital throbbing headache and diplopia that have been present for the past 12 hours. The patient also reports occasional chills. He had a dental procedure 6 days ago. His only medication is hydrocodone.

On physical examination, temperature is 38.9 °C (102.0 °F), blood pressure is 138/90 mm Hg, and pulse rate is 88/min; BMI is 28. Right proptosis with lid edema is noted. The right pupil is dilated and sluggishly reactive. Oculomotor nerve (cranial nerve III), trochlear nerve (cranial nerve IV), and abducens nerve (cranial nerve VI) palsies are present on the right. Other findings from the physical examination are unremarkable.

Results of laboratory studies show an erythrocyte sedimentation rate of 60 mm/h and a leukocyte count of 13,400/μL (13.4×10^9/L), with 85% polymorphonuclear leukocytes.

Which of the following is the most likely diagnosis?

(A) Carotid artery dissection

(B) Cavernous sinus thrombosis

(C) Posterior communicating artery aneurysm

(D) Vertebral artery dissection

Item 37

A 51-year-old woman is evaluated in the hospital after having an ischemic stroke. She has hypertension treated with

CONT.
candesartan and dyslipidemia treated with rosuvastatin. The patient is otherwise in good health.

On physical examination, blood pressure is 168/76 mm Hg. A right carotid bruit is heard. Left-sided weakness (including the face) is present.

An electrocardiogram shows sinus rhythm. A CT scan of the head shows a hypodensity in the right parietal lobe. A carotid duplex ultrasound shows greater than 80% stenosis in the right internal carotid artery. A magnetic resonance angiogram of the neck without contrast confirms greater than 80% stenosis.

Which of the following is the most appropriate next step in management?

(A) Carotid endarterectomy
(B) Carotid stenting
(C) Diagnostic cerebral angiography
(D) 30-Day outpatient telemetry

Item 38

A 68-year-old man is evaluated for increasing cognitive deficits, walking difficulties with occasional falls, and depression. He has become more forgetful over the past 5 years, has a 1-year history of shuffling his feet when walking, awakens three to four times each night to urinate (sometimes becoming incontinent), and generally has become more withdrawn and irritable. He also has difficulty remembering names and appointments, and his wife now manages their finances and his medications, which consist of hydrochlorothiazide for hypertension and metformin for type 2 diabetes mellitus.

On physical examination, vital signs are normal. The patient is slow to rise from a seated position. Gait examination reveals slow, short steps and difficulty turning. He scores 22/30 (normal, ≥24) on the Mini–Mental State Examination, losing four points in the orientation sections, one point in the registration section, and three points in the attention/calculation section.

An MRI of the brain shows moderate generalized atrophy and prominent cerebral ventricles.

Which of the following is most likely to be diagnostic in this patient?

(A) Amyloid PET scan
(B) Fluorodeoxyglucose PET scan
(C) Lumbar puncture
(D) Neuropsychological testing

Item 39

A 33-year-old man is evaluated in the emergency department for a 10-week history of worsening confusion, memory loss, and difficulty speaking. He has become progressively more disorganized at work and can no longer complete routine tasks. His medical history is otherwise unremarkable, and he takes no medication.

On physical examination, vital signs are normal. The patient exhibits decreased attention, is able to follow only simple commands, and is oriented only to person. Speech is

dysarthric. Intermittent myoclonic jerking of varying limbs also is noted.

Results of laboratory studies show a serum sodium level of 128 mEq/L (128 mmol/L) but are otherwise unremarkable, including a normal complete blood count, comprehensive metabolic panel, serum thyroid-stimulating hormone level, and free thyroxine (T_4) level.

An urgent electroencephalogram shows evidence of nonconvulsive status epilepticus with focal seizures arising independently from both temporal lobes. A contrast-enhanced brain MRI is normal.

Which of the following is the most likely diagnosis?

(A) Autoimmune limbic encephalitis
(B) Lyme disease
(C) Progressive multifocal leukoencephalopathy
(D) Rapidly progressive dementia

Item 40

A 79-year-old woman is evaluated for persistent depression, declining function, and memory changes. According to family members, she has been depressed ever since her husband died 3 years ago. They further report that the patient's memory has gotten much worse in the past year and that she no longer cooks or cleans her home, despite previously preparing lavish weekly family meals and keeping a meticulous house. The patient says she feels healthy but "just no longer cares" or sometimes "forgets." She started taking paroxetine at the time of her husband's death and switched to venlafaxine 1 year later because of no improvement in her depression; although symptoms are now slightly less severe, they have not abated.

On physical examination, vital signs are normal. The two-question depression screening test is positive, and her score on the Patient Health Questionnaire (PHQ)-9 is 11/30 (moderate depression). The patient scores 23/30 (normal, ≥24) on a Mini–Mental State Examination; an evaluation for reversible causes of memory impairment is unrevealing.

An MRI obtained 1 year ago was normal.

Which of the following is the most appropriate next step?

(A) Addition of mirtazapine
(B) Cerebrospinal fluid analysis
(C) Neuropsychological testing
(D) Repeat MRI of the brain

Item 41

A 35-year-old man is evaluated for a 3-year history of epilepsy. Seizures typically occur twice monthly, last 2 minutes, and are characterized by staring, lip smacking, and confusion; approximately once every 6 months, the patient experiences a whole-body convulsion marked by incontinence and prolonged confusion for several hours. Treatment with oxcarbazepine and lamotrigine, although initially reducing seizure frequency, has been largely ineffective. He no longer drives or works because of the seizures. He also has migraines, which are well controlled by sumatriptan.

On physical examination, vital signs are normal. All other physical examination findings, including those from a neurologic examination, are unremarkable.

Results of routine outpatient electroencephalography (EEG) are normal. An MRI of the brain shows right hippocampal atrophy.

Which of the following is the most appropriate next step in management?

(A) Levetiracetam

(B) Topiramate

(C) Vagus nerve stimulation

(D) Video EEG monitoring

Item 42

A 38-year-old woman is evaluated for recent onset of visual blurriness when looking straight ahead or reading. She has a 4-mm right posterior communicating artery aneurysm that was first detected 1 year ago. She has not had any recent headaches and is otherwise well. The patient's only medication is an oral contraceptive agent.

On physical examination, blood pressure is 138/78 mm Hg; other vital signs are normal. The neck is supple. Findings from funduscopic examination are normal. On neurologic examination, the right pupil is 5-millimeters in diameter and unreactive; left lateral gaze results in diplopia. The left pupil and right lateral gaze are normal.

A magnetic resonance angiogram (MRA) of the brain shows that her aneurysm has grown in size to 8 millimeters.

Which of the following is the most appropriate next step in management?

(A) Lisinopril administration

(B) MRA of the neck

(C) Neurosurgical intervention

(D) Repeat MRA of the brain in 6 months

Item 43

A 75-year-old man comes to the office for a follow-up evaluation of Parkinson disease, which was diagnosed 12 years ago. Worsening motor symptoms have been controlled with a combination of carbidopa-levodopa and pramipexole for the past 3 years. According to family members, the patient becomes rigid and slow before taking his next dose of Parkinson medications, but these symptoms resolve after he has taken them. He reports recent visual hallucinations that have been distressing, occasionally seeing small animals and unfamiliar people mostly at night, which sometimes frightens him. He has had no recent illness, fever, anhedonia, or depressive symptoms.

On physical examination, vital signs are normal. The patient performs well on screening cognitive testing. He reports no active hallucinations. Masked facies, mild dysarthria, resting tremor, bradykinesia, and cogwheel rigidity are noted. Gait is narrow based and shuffling. Other physical examination findings are unremarkable.

Results of laboratory studies, including a complete blood count, comprehensive metabolic panel, serum creatine kinase measurement, and urinalysis, are normal.

Which of the following is the most appropriate next step in treatment?

(A) Add aripiprazole

(B) Add pimavanserin

(C) Add risperidone

(D) Discontinue pramipexole

Item 44

A 37-year-old man is evaluated in the emergency department 12 hours after sudden onset of a global, severe headache with associated neck stiffness. The patient has a 5-year history of migraine treated with sumatriptan. He says that his current headache feels different from previous headaches and did not respond to sumatriptan.

On physical examination, temperature is normal, blood pressure is 148/72 mm Hg, heart rate 86/min and regular, respiration rate is 12/min, and oxygen saturation is 96% with the patient breathing ambient air. The patient has discomfort and appears restless. Funduscopic examination is normal. The left pupil is 2 millimeters larger than the right and poorly reactive to light. Neck stiffness is noted with passive movement.

A CT scan of the head is normal.

Which of the following is the most appropriate next diagnostic test?

(A) Lumbar puncture

(B) Magnetic resonance angiography of the neck

(C) MRI of the brain

(D) No further testing is necessary

Item 45

A 79-year-old man is evaluated for a 2-month history of progressively worsening headaches, nausea, visual disturbance, and difficulty speaking. He also has hypertension and gastroesophageal reflux disease. Medications are lisinopril and omeprazole.

On physical examination, vital signs are normal. Right oculomotor nerve (cranial nerve III) and bilateral abducens nerve (cranial nerve VI) palsies are noted, as is right upper and lower facial weakness.

An MRI of the brain shows a well-demarcated, homogeneously enhancing, hyperintense lesion that is suspicious for primary central nervous system lymphoma in the brainstem extending from the left pons to the medulla. Mass effect but no edema is present. The lesion obstructs the cerebral aqueduct, and hydrocephalus with enlargement of the lateral and third ventricles is noted.

Which of the following is the most appropriate next step in management?

(A) Brain biopsy

(B) Intravenous dexamethasone

(C) Lumbar puncture

(D) Vitreous fluid sampling

Item 46

A 56-year-old woman is evaluated for a 6-month history of nocturnal leg movements. According to her husband, she frequently kicks her legs during sleep but does not exhibit vocalizations or complex movements while asleep. The patient is unaware of these movements and has not had any sensory discomfort or urge to move the legs. She snores at night but has had no sudden loss of consciousness, sleep attacks, or excessive daytime sleepiness.

Results of physical examination and laboratory studies are unremarkable.

A polysomnogram shows good sleep efficiency, a low apnea-hypopnea index, and absence of motor activity during the rapid eye movement phase of sleep; no sleep fragmentation is evident, despite frequent leg movements. A video recording of her movements reveals slow flexion movements of the ankles, knees, and hips that repeat every 20 seconds in a stereotyped manner.

Which of the following is the most appropriate next step in management?

(A) Clonazepam administration
(B) Electroencephalography
(C) Ferritin level measurement
(D) No further testing or treatment is necessary

H Item 47

A 25-year-old woman is evaluated in the emergency department (ED) 90 minutes after being struck in the right temple by a foul ball at a baseball game. Although knocked from her seat and initially dazed by the blow, the patient continued to watch the game for another 45 minutes until she developed a worsening headache with nausea and vomiting. On arrival in the ED, the patient was stuporous and became unresponsive during subsequent CT of the head.

On physical examination, blood pressure is 140/90 mm Hg, pulse rate is 100/min, and respiration rate is 14/min. The right pupil is dilated. Right occulomotor nerve (cranial nerve III) palsy and left hemiparesis are noted. A plantar extensor response is present on the left.

A CT scan of the head is shown (see top of next column).

Which of the following is the most likely diagnosis?

(A) Epidural hematoma
(B) Lobar hemorrhage
(C) Subarachnoid hemorrhage
(D) Subdural hematoma

Item 48

A 36-year-old man is evaluated for severe muscle cramping. The patient reports occasional painful muscle cramps, sometimes associated with brownish urine discoloration, after intense physical activity since he was a teenager and intermittent proximal muscle pain; he has had no stiffness, rigidity, or other muscle weakness or pain. He says that if he briefly interrupts his exercise routine after onset of cramping, he can continue further exercise without difficulty; eating carbohydrate-rich food also increases his exercise tolerance.

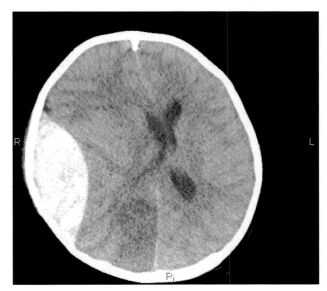

ITEM 47

On physical examination, vital signs are normal. "Mild" muscle weakness (inability to hold a limb against full resistance) and pain is present in the shoulder and limb girdle muscles. Muscle tone and bulk are normal, as are all reflexes. Results of sensory examination are unremarkable. Normal relaxation after hand grip is noted.

Results of laboratory studies show a serum creatine kinase level of 500 U/L and a serum creatinine level of 1.8 mg/dL (159 µmol/L); urinalysis results are normal.

Which of the following is the most likely diagnosis?

(A) Acute intermittent porphyria
(B) Limb-girdle muscular dystrophy
(C) McArdle disease (metabolic myopathy)
(D) Myotonic dystrophy
(E) Polymyositis

Item 49

A 59-year-old man is evaluated for recent cognitive problems resulting in worsening performance in his work as an electrician. He reports having increasing difficulty "running the numbers" when determining the materials needed for a job and increasing problems understanding the layout of plans when working on a new construction. He also notes occasional hand tremors when he works. According to his wife, his gait has slowed somewhat and he seems to have less of a response to things occurring around him in the past few weeks, stating that he "doesn't show any emotion in his face anymore." The patient also has a 5-year history of erectile dysfunction, a 4-year history of constipation, and episodes of lightheadedness when standing for long periods at work.

On physical examination, vital signs are normal. A general paucity of movements is noted, as are slowness of movement in the upper and lower extremities and a mildly stooped posture when walking. He scores 20/30 (normal, ≥26) on the

Montreal Cognitive Assessment, having significant difficulty with the cube drawing, clock drawing, and sustained attention portions of the test.

Which of the following additional clinical findings would be most helpful in establishing the diagnosis in this patient?

(A) Delusions

(B) Depression

(C) Rapid eye movement sleep behavior disorder

(D) Repeated falls

Item 50

A 71-year-old woman is evaluated in the emergency department 1 hour after acute onset of a severe headache and left-sided weakness. The patient had a myocardial infarction 3 years ago that was treated with a bare metal stent in the right coronary artery. She also has hypertension. Medications are carvedilol, atorvastatin, and aspirin.

On physical examination, blood pressure is 200/110 mm Hg, pulse rate 78/min, respiration rate is 20/min, and oxygen saturation is 98% with the patient breathing ambient air. The patient is awake and attentive to both sides and has normal language function. Funduscopic examination shows no papilledema or hemorrhage. Pupils are both 3 millimeters in size and reactive. Left facial weakness, dysarthria, and flaccid paralysis in the left arm and leg with loss of sensation are noted.

An emergent noncontrast CT scan shows an acute intracerebral hemorrhage, 1 centimeter in diameter, in the right basal ganglia without intraventricular hemorrhage or midline shift.

Which of the following is the most appropriate treatment?

(A) Hematoma evacuation

(B) Intravenous nicardipine

(C) Intravenous nitroprusside

(D) Platelet transfusion

Item 51

A 34-year-old man is evaluated for recurrent right-sided severe, sharp periorbital headache. Episodes have been occurring nocturnally for the past 2 weeks, typically last 90 minutes, and are associated with ipsilateral nasal congestion, tearing, nausea, and photophobia. He reports having had a similar series of headaches over a 2-month period 6 months ago. The patient has been taking combination acetaminophen, aspirin, and caffeine as needed for pain. He takes no other medication and has a 10-pack-year smoking history.

On physical examination, vital signs and all other physical examination findings, including those from a neurologic examination, are unremarkable.

An MRI of the brain is normal.

Which of the following is the most appropriate preventive treatment?

(A) Carbamazepine

(B) Fexofenadine

(C) Indomethacin

(D) Propranolol

(E) Verapamil

Item 52

A 47-year-old man is evaluated for recent weakness and loss of balance during ambulation, multiple episodes of orthostatic syncope, and a 2-year history of burning paresthesia in the lower extremities. He also reports dry mouth and dry eyes. The patient has glaucoma, erectile dysfunction, constipation, and carpal tunnel syndrome. His father had sensory neuropathy, and his father and paternal uncle died of restrictive cardiomyopathy. Medications are gabapentin, sildenafil, and docusate sodium.

On physical examination, blood pressure is 130/70 mm Hg sitting and 110/64 standing, and pulse rate is 110/min. Weakness in the distribution of the bilateral median nerves and in the proximal lower extremities is noted. Loss of sensation to pinprick is present in both hands and below the knees. Deep tendon reflexes are reduced in the lower extremities.

Electromyography, including nerve conduction studies and needle electrode examination, reveals diffuse axonal sensorimotor polyneuropathy.

Which of the following is the most likely diagnosis?

(A) Amyotrophic lateral sclerosis

(B) Cervical myelopathy

(C) Chronic inflammatory demyelinating polyradiculo-neuropathy

(D) Familial amyloidosis

(E) West Nile virus infection

Item 53

A 65-year-old man is evaluated in the ICU for a 24-hour history of altered mental status with a fluctuating level of consciousness. He was admitted to the hospital 5 days ago for urosepsis and acute kidney injury and developed acute respiratory distress syndrome on hospital day 3. The patient is currently intubated, mechanically ventilated, and receiving continuous hemodialysis. Medications are cefepime, norepinephrine, and fentanyl.

On physical examination, temperature is 38.4 °C (101.1 °F), blood pressure is 105/71 mm Hg, pulse rate is 108/min, and respiration rate is 12/min; FIO$_2$ is 0.9. The patient opens his eyes to voice but does not fixate on the examiner or follow commands. Pupils are reactive, and gag and corneal reflexes are present. All limbs move intermittently but not on command. The patient withdraws from painful stimuli in all four limbs. Intermittent twitching of the shoulders and eyelids is noted.

Results of laboratory studies show a serum creatinine level of 5.4 mg/dL (477 µmol/L). Glucose, calcium, and electrolyte levels are within normal limits.

A 20-minute electroencephalogram shows generalized slow activity, a nonspecific finding compatible with encephalopathy, but no evidence of seizure activity.

A head CT scan is normal.

Which of the following is the most appropriate next step in management?

CONT.

(A) Continuous (24-hour) electroencephalography

(B) Intravenous fosphenytoin

(C) Intravenous lorazepam

(D) No treatment

Item 54

A 52-year-old man is evaluated for a 9-month history of progressively worsening gait, ataxia, and paresthesia in the legs. He is a dentist who was recently barred from practice because of chronic illicit drug use, specifically amphetamines and nitrous oxide.

On physical examination, vital signs are normal. Decreased vibration and position sense is noted in both feet. Reflexes are 3+ in both legs. Muscle strength is 4/5 in both hips.

A complete blood count is normal, as is a routine chemistry panel.

A T2-weighted MRI of the thoracic spinal cord shows hyperintensity in the posterior columns and throughout the cord. There is no associated contrast enhancement.

Measurement of which of the following serum levels is the most appropriate next diagnostic test?

(A) 25-Hydroxyvitamin D

(B) Thiamine

(C) Vitamin A

(D) Vitamin B_6

(E) Vitamin B_{12}

Item 55

A 51-year-old woman is evaluated for increasingly poor ambulation ever since having a relapse of multiple sclerosis 20 months ago. She was diagnosed with MS 4 years ago and has been tasking natalizumab, baclofen, and a vitamin D supplement since that time.

On physical examination, vital signs are normal. Muscle strength is 4/5 in the left hip flexor, knee flexor, and ankle dorsiflexor. Gait is slow and deliberate with the assistance of a cane; left leg swing is noted. All other physical examination findings are unremarkable.

Which of the following medications is the most appropriate treatment?

(A) Dalfampridine

(B) Dextromethorphan-quinidine

(C) Gabapentin

(D) Memantine

(E) Modafinil

Item 56

A 56-year-old man is evaluated for a 10-day history of pain in a patchy region to the right of the umbilicus. He says that the area is sensitive to light touch. He reports no recent systemic illness, weakness, or fever. The patient has

hypertension and hyperlipidemia. Medications are losartan, aspirin, and atorvastatin.

On physical examination, vital signs are normal; BMI is 36. Sensory examination reveals a patchy area of paresthesia and allodynia on the right side of the abdomen that extends posteriorly but does not cross the midline. Abdominal swelling is noted on the right. No abdominal mass or tenderness is present. There is no skin rash. Results of cranial nerve, motor strength, coordination, and gait testing are normal, and deep tendon reflexes are preserved.

Results of laboratory studies show a serum creatinine level of 2.1 mg/dL (186 µmol/L) and a hemoglobin A_{1c} value of 7.8% (0.078).

Results of serum and urine protein electrophoresis and serum light chain measurement are unremarkable.

An MRI of the thoracic spine is normal.

Which of the following is the most likely diagnosis?

(A) Diabetic mononeuropathy

(B) Paraproteinemic neuropathy

(C) Uremic neuropathy

(D) Vitamin B_{12} deficiency

Item 57

A 78-year-old man is evaluated in the emergency department for a 2-day history of bilateral leg weakness and urinary retention. He has atrial fibrillation and hypertension. Medications are warfarin, lisinopril, and hydrochlorothiazide.

On physical examination, vital signs are normal. Muscle strength is 4/5 in both legs. Decreased sensation in the groin, medial buttocks, and rectal area is noted, as is decreased rectal tone. No spinal sensory level is detected in the abdomen or chest region. Gait is wide based.

Results of laboratory studies show an INR level of 5.3.

Which of the following is the most appropriate management?

(A) Administration of intravenous glucocorticoids

(B) CT myelogram

(C) MRI of the lumbosacral spine

(D) Radiograph of the lumbosacral spine

Item 58

A 19-year-old woman is evaluated in the emergency department for a 6-month history of headaches that initially were intermittent but have been occurring daily for the past 6 weeks. She describes the pain as bilateral, frontotemporal, and a steady pressure. Neck stiffness has been present for 8 weeks. Vision intermittently darkens for seconds. For the past 3 nights, she has noted pulsatile tinnitus. The patient has inflammatory acne treated with minocycline and topical benzoyl peroxide gel.

On physical examination, vital signs are normal; BMI is 22. Papilledema and left abducens nerve (cranial nerve VI) palsy are noted, but all other findings are normal.

Results of brain MRI and magnetic resonance venography are normal.

CONT.

Which of the following is the most appropriate management?

(A) Amitriptyline
(B) Indomethacin
(C) Lumbar puncture
(D) Magnetic resonance angiography
(E) Temporal artery biopsy

Item 59

A 67-year-old man is evaluated for a carotid bruit detected on routine medical examination. He reports no history of previous focal neurologic symptoms or visual loss. He has type 2 diabetes mellitus and hyperlipidemia treated with metformin, moderate-intensity pravastatin, and aspirin.

On physical examination, blood pressure is 128/64 mm Hg, pulse rate is 78/min and regular, and respiration rate is 16/min. A left carotid bruit is heard on cardiac examination. All other physical examination findings, including those from a neurologic examination, are unremarkable.

Results of laboratory studies show an LDL cholesterol level of 82 mg/dL (2.12 mmol/L).

The carotid ultrasound report describes a mixed-density plaque at the origin of the left internal carotid artery with stenosis estimated to be 60% to 80%.

Which of the following is the most appropriate next step in management?

(A) Carotid endarterectomy
(B) Carotid stenting
(C) Magnetic resonance angiography of the neck
(D) Replacement of aspirin with clopidogrel
(E) No further treatment or intervention

Item 60

A 52-year-old woman is hospitalized for rapidly progressive weakness in the arms and respiratory muscle weakness that necessitates ventilatory support. Cerebrospinal fluid analysis reveals a cell count of 3/µL (3 × 10⁶/L) and a protein level of 190 mg/dL (1900 mg/L). Electromyographic findings, including those from a nerve conduction study, reveal slowing of nerve conduction. Guillain-Barré syndrome is diagnosed and treated with a standard 10-day course of plasma exchange; at the end of treatment, motor strength is improved by 50%, and she is extubated.

On subsequent physical examination, vital signs are normal. There is full range of motion in all extremities. The patient's strength has improved in the upper and lower extremities, but residual weakness persists. Ambulation is possible only with assistance because of weakness. Deep tendon reflexes are absent throughout. The cranial nerves are intact.

Which of the following is the most appropriate next step in management?

(A) Continue hospital monitoring for another week
(B) Discharge to rehabilitation

(C) Repeat plasma exchange
(D) Treat with intravenous glucocorticoids
(E) Treat with intravenous immune globulin

Item 61

A 35-year-old man is evaluated for two breakthrough focal seizures in the past week. He started having focal and generalized tonic-clonic seizures 20 years ago. The seizures previously had been well controlled by phenytoin, which he has taken since age 16 years, but he missed three doses of medication this week. He has had no recent illnesses or fevers.

On physical examination, all findings, including vital signs, are normal.

Results of bone densitometry show osteoporosis (T-score of –2.8).

In addition to starting the patient on alendronate, which of the following drugs should be substituted for the phenytoin?

(A) Carbamazepine
(B) Lamotrigine
(C) Phenobarbital
(D) Valproic acid

Item 62

A 61-year-old woman is admitted to the ICU 1 hour after having a subarachnoid hemorrhage (SAH). An emergent CT scan of the head showed an SAH, and a cerebral angiogram revealed a 6-mm rupture of the anterior communicating artery. The patient has hypertension treated with amlodipine.

On physical examination, vital signs are stable, and oxygen saturation is 96% with the patient breathing ambient air. She is somnolent. Nuchal rigidity is present. Subhyaloid hemorrhages are seen on funduscopic examination. No motor or sensory deficits are present.

Administration of which of the following medications is the most appropriate treatment?

(A) Dexamethasone
(B) Magnesium sulfate
(C) Nimodipine
(D) Nitroglycerin
(E) Verapamil

Item 63

A 76-year-old man is evaluated for recent worsening of balance. He has no dizziness or lightheadedness. The patient has an 8-year history of Parkinson disease treated with carbidopa-levodopa and entacapone.

On physical examination, vital signs are normal; no orthostatic decrease in blood pressure is noted. The patient has masked facies, a resting tremor, and bradykinesia. Gait assessment reveals mild shuffling without freezing. Findings from cognitive, cerebellar, and sensory examinations are unremarkable.

Which of the following is the most appropriate test to determine the patient's risk of falling backward?

(A) Head impulse test
(B) Pull test
(C) Romberg test
(D) Tandem gait test

Item 64

A 30-year-old man is evaluated for a 6-week history of repeated episodes of sharp pain isolated to the right parietal region lasting less than 10 seconds. The pain is intense, begins and ends spontaneously without a clear trigger, and can recur multiple times each day, sometimes in series. The patient has a history of migraine with aura from age 6 through 12 years but has had no headaches since that time. He has had no associated autonomic features and no symptoms of migraine. He has a family history of migraine with aura. The patient takes no medication.

All physical examination findings, including vital signs and those from a neurologic examination, are unremarkable.

An MRI of the brain is normal.

Which of the following is the most likely diagnosis?

(A) Cluster headache
(B) New daily persistent headache
(C) Primary stabbing headache
(D) Trigeminal neuralgia

Item 65

A 71-year-old man is evaluated for a 2-year history of episodes of staring, confusion, and repetitive left-arm movements (grabbing at his clothes or face). These events occur every 2 to 3 months, last approximately 2 minutes, and typically are followed by a 15-minute period of disorientation and fatigue. On one occasion, the episode was followed immediately by the patient's falling down, experiencing shaking of the entire body, and having urinary incontinence. He also has hypertension, nephrolithiasis, and mild cognitive impairment. Medications are hydrochlorothiazide and metoprolol.

All physical examination findings, including vital signs, are normal.

A routine electroencephalogram and brain MRI are normal.

Which of the following is the most appropriate treatment?

(A) Lamotrigine
(B) Oxcarbazepine
(C) Phenytoin
(D) Topiramate
(E) Valproic acid

Item 66

A 56-year-old man is evaluated for worsening memory and increasing behavioral problems. He was fired from his job as an accountant 6 months ago after forgetting to file necessary forms, making repeated calculation errors, and sending inappropriate emails to coworkers. He developed compulsive spending habits 3 years ago and completely depleted his retirement savings account; he has shown little concern about his financial losses. The patient was previously very physically active but now spends most of the day obsessively watching television. His wife says he eats high-calorie, nonnutritional food constantly and has gained 27.3 kg (60.1 lb) in the past 2 years. No other symptoms, including visual hallucinations, are reported.

On physical examination, the patient has a blunted affect and provides little information spontaneously. Vital signs are normal. He scores 18/30 (normal, ≥26) on the Montreal Cognitive Assessment and has significant difficulty with letter and number sequencing, word fluency, and memory, recalling only two of five items. Remaining physical examination findings are normal.

Which of the following is the most likely diagnosis?

(A) Alzheimer disease
(B) Dementia with Lewy bodies
(C) Frontotemporal dementia
(D) Parkinson disease

Item 67

A 56-year-old woman is evaluated for a 1-year history of tremor that is most notable on the right. She also has developed increasing problems with balance resulting in several falls, especially when she stands from a seated position or turns abruptly. The patient exhibits occasional shouting and arm flailing during sleep.

On physical examination, blood pressure is 128/75 mm Hg sitting and 105/70 mm Hg standing, pulse rate is 65/min sitting and 75/min standing, and respiration rate is 22/min. Decreased facial expression, full range of extraocular movements with dysmetric saccades, and hypophonic speech are noted. A low-amplitude resting tremor is more prominent on the right; the patient also has a more symmetric bilateral postural and kinetic tremor. On finger-to-nose testing, movements are slow and usually miss the target. Repetitive finger tapping movements become progressively smaller in amplitude. Gait is wide based, with frequent veering to the side, and the patient comes close to falling whenever she turns; gait speed is normal, but arm swing is decreased. The pull test results in the patient falling backward, and she is unable to walk a straight line.

An MRI of the brain is unremarkable.

Which of the following is the most likely diagnosis?

(A) Corticobasal degeneration
(B) Multiple system atrophy
(C) Parkinson disease
(D) Progressive supranuclear palsy
(E) Vascular parkinsonism

Item 68

A 64-year-old woman is evaluated in the emergency department 45 minutes after sudden onset of right-sided

CONT.

weakness and the loss of the ability to speak. An emergent noncontrast CT of the head shows no hemorrhage or early signs of infarct. The patient also has hypertension and atrial fibrillation. Medications are hydrochlorothiazide and warfarin.

On physical examination, blood pressure is 158/78 mm Hg, and pulse rate is 72/min and irregularly irregular. Global aphasia, left-gaze preference, right hemiparesis, and loss of pain sensation on the right side are noted.

Results of laboratory studies show an INR of 1.3.

The patient receives intravenous recombinant tissue plasminogen activator (alteplase) 1 hour after symptom onset. Blood pressure is now 168/86 mm Hg, but other vital signs are unchanged, as are results of repeat neurologic examination.

Which of the following is the most appropriate next step in management?

(A) Aspirin administration
(B) CT angiography of the head
(C) Intravenous labetalol administration
(D) MRI of the brain

Item 69

A 62-year-old man is evaluated in the emergency department because of progressive confusion. After his vital signs are obtained (normal temperature, blood pressure of 169/95 mm Hg, pulse rate of 44/min, and respiration rate of 12/min), he suddenly becomes unresponsive and comatose, with irregular respirations, and is emergently intubated.

On further physical examination, oxygen saturation is 93% with the patient receiving 100% oxygen. The pupils are large and unreactive bilaterally. The corneal reflex and oculocephalic reflex are absent on the right. The patient displays no spontaneous movements and withdraws his upper and lower limbs from noxious stimuli on the right but not on the left.

An emergent CT scan of the head without contrast shows a right temporal 4.1-cm heterogenous lesion with significant surrounding edema that is most consistent with a high-grade glioma. Mass effect and compression of the upper brainstem are noted without evidence of hemorrhage.

Which of the following is the most appropriate next step in management?

(A) Brain MRI
(B) Immediate brain biopsy
(C) Intravenous dexamethasone
(D) Intravenous levetiracetam

Item 70

A 54-year-old man is evaluated in the hospital for respiratory distress. The patient has well-controlled generalized epilepsy and was admitted 5 days earlier for a cervical discectomy, laminectomy, and fusion. On hospital day 4, he developed a productive cough, chills, and dyspnea. Medications are oxycodone, levetiracetam, and docusate sodium.

On physical examination, temperature is 38.4 °C (101.1 °F), blood pressure is 125/84 mm Hg, pulse rate is 108/min, respiration rate is 22/min, and oxygen saturation with the patient breathing ambient air is 93%. Crackles are heard in the right posterior thorax on pulmonary auscultation.

Results of laboratory studies show a leukocyte count of 18,400/µL (18.4 × 10⁹/L).

A chest radiograph shows a right lower lobe infiltrate.

Which of the following is the most appropriate treatment?

(A) Cefepime
(B) Imipenem
(C) Levofloxacin
(D) Piperacillin-tazobactam

Item 71

A 39-year-old woman is evaluated for a 4-year history of headaches that typically occur twice weekly and last 8 to 12 hours when not treated early. The pain is bilateral, frontotemporal, vice-like, and aggravated by physical activity. Approximately half of the episodes have become severe and are associated with combined photophobia and phonophobia. She has had no associated nausea, vomiting, or visual or neurologic symptoms and reports no cranial autonomic features. Stress is the only clear trigger. Naproxen resolves the headache when administered early in the headache course. She takes no other medication.

On physical examination, vital signs are normal; BMI is 23. All other physical examination findings, including those from a neurologic examination, are unremarkable.

Which of the following is the most likely diagnosis?

(A) Medication-overuse headache
(B) Migraine
(C) Sinus headache
(D) Tension-type headache

Item 72

A 49-year-old woman is evaluated in the emergency department for a 12-hour history of new-onset right-sided visual loss. The patient has type 2 diabetes mellitus treated with metformin.

On physical examination, blood pressure is 138/72 mm Hg, and pulse rate is 102/min and irregularly irregular. Cardiac auscultation reveals no carotid bruits or cardiac murmurs. A visual field deficit is present on the right side of both eyes. No weakness or sensory loss is noted.

A CT scan of the head shows a hypodensity in the left occipital lobe, and a carotid duplex ultrasound shows less than 60% stenosis of both internal carotid arteries with normal vertebral artery flow. An electrocardiogram shows atrial fibrillation.

Which of the following medications should be administered now?

(A) Apixaban
(B) Aspirin
(C) Clopidogrel
(D) Intravenous heparin

Item 73

A 20-year-old woman comes to the office for follow-up evaluation 2 weeks after being involved in a head-to-head collision in a soccer game. She lost consciousness for several seconds on the field and was removed from play. On the sidelines, she reported a severe occipital headache, dizziness, "brain fog," and nausea. Subsequent neurologic examination and head CT findings were unremarkable. She was started on a 1-week course of ibuprofen and prochlorperazine, which she took regularly. Besides mild cognitive slowing and short-term memory issues, she has been completely asymptomatic without medication for 1 week.

On physical examination, blood pressure is 96/66 mm Hg and pulse rate is 62/min. All other physical examination findings, including those from a neurologic examination, are normal.

Which of the following is the most appropriate next step in management?

(A) Amantadine
(B) Brain MRI
(C) Neuropsychological testing
(D) Return to play

Item 74

An 85-year-old woman is evaluated for declining function. According to her son, her memory has been failing, her gait has slowed, she has fallen four times, and she often cries without apparent reason. He further reports that he does most of her cooking and has assumed responsibility for her finances. The patient had a right basal ganglia infarct 5 years ago and left cerebellar infarct 2 years ago. She also has atrial fibrillation and hypertension. Medications are rivaroxaban, hydrochlorothiazide, and metoprolol.

On physical examination, blood pressure is 155/80 mm Hg in both arms, and pulse rate is irregularly irregular at 90/min; other vital signs are normal. Cardiac examination shows findings consistent with atrial fibrillation. All other physical examination findings are normal. The patient says she has not been depressed but becomes tearful when discussing her medications. Depression screening has normal findings. She scores 20/30 (normal, ≥26) on the Montreal Cognitive Assessment. Bradykinesia with normal strength is noted in the legs bilaterally, as are increased deep tendon reflexes and an extensor plantar response on the left. Gait examination reveals a shuffling pattern.

Results of laboratory studies show normal thyroid-stimulating hormone and vitamin B$_{12}$ levels.

An MRI shows diffuse white matter hyperintensities bilaterally and lacunar infarcts in the bilateral basal ganglia and left cerebellum.

Which of the following is most appropriate for this patient's cognitive impairment?

(A) Citalopram
(B) Donepezil
(C) Ginkgo biloba
(D) Methylphenidate

Item 75

A 65-year-old man comes to the office for follow-up evaluation of progressive weakness in the proximal muscles that has been present for the past 4 months. One month after symptom onset, an electromyogram showed myopathic changes without active denervation, and subsequent measurement of the serum creatine kinase level was 1500 U/L. The simvastatin he was taking to treat hyperlipidemia was stopped at that time, but his symptoms have persisted. He is otherwise well. He has no family history of neuromuscular disease.

On physical examination, vital signs are normal. Muscle strength is 5/5 in the facial, bulbar, and neck muscles and 3/5 in the proximal muscles of the upper and lower extremities. The proximal limbs are tender to palpation. Results of sensory and reflex examinations are normal.

Serum creatine kinase level is 4200 U/L.

Examination of a muscle biopsy specimen reveals evidence of muscle necrosis without inflammation.

Which of the following is the most appropriate next step in management?

(A) Azathioprine administration
(B) Clinical monitoring
(C) Coenzyme Q10 supplementation
(D) Prednisone administration

Item 76

A 52-year-old woman is evaluated for a 3-week history of new-onset daily headaches. The pain is absent nocturnally and on awakening but starts within 15 minutes of the patient's arising from bed and becomes progressively severe throughout the day. The headache is global, steady, and (when severe) associated with photophobia and mild nausea. Intermittent bilateral tinnitus and brief episodes of horizontal diplopia also have occurred. The pain improves within 15 to 20 minutes of the patient's lying down. Analgesic agents have been unhelpful. She has no other medical problems.

On physical examination, vital signs are normal; BMI is 26. Partial right abducens nerve (cranial nerve VI) palsy is noted.

An MRI of the brain shows diffuse nonnodular pachymeningeal enhancement, a cerebellar tonsillar descent of 3 mm, and clinically insignificant bilateral subdural fluid collections.

Which of the following is the most appropriate first step in management?

(A) Acetazolamide administration
(B) Epidural blood patch
(C) Lumbar puncture
(D) Subdural evacuation

Item 77

A 39-year-old woman is evaluated in the emergency department for a 2-day history of bilateral lower extremity weakness and numbness. The patient has no other symptoms and no relevant medical history. She takes no medication.

On physical examination, temperature is 36.7 °C (98.1 °F); all other vital signs are normal. Muscle strength testing shows 4/5 weakness in hip flexion bilaterally and in foot dorsiflexion. Temperature sensation is partially reduced below spinal cord level T5. All other physical examination findings are normal.

A T2-weighted MRI of the thoracic spine shows a hyperintense lesion at the T4 level.

Which of the following is the most appropriate next test to evaluate for multiple sclerosis?

(A) Cerebrospinal fluid (CSF) analysis for antibodies to myelin basic protein
(B) CSF analysis for oligoclonal bands
(C) Erythrocyte sedimentation rate
(D) MRI of the brain
(E) Visual evoked potentials

Item 78

A 56-year-old man is hospitalized 8 hours after developing difficulty speaking and left-sided weakness. An emergent CT scan of the head shows an acute right thalamic hemorrhage with no hydrocephalus or intraventricular hemorrhage; a follow-up CT scan obtained 48 hours later shows no changes. The patient also has hypertension and type 2 diabetes mellitus. Medications before admission were lisinopril, aspirin, and glipizide. On hospital admission, hydrochlorothiazide and lisinopril are continued, aspirin and glipizide are discontinued, and insulin is initiated.

On physical examination, blood pressure is 186/94 mm Hg, pulse rate is 74/min and regular, and respiration rate is 12/min. Left facial weakness with dysarthria and left-sided body weakness with no discernible movement are noted.

An electrocardiogram shows sinus rhythm without acute changes.

Which of the following is the most appropriate next step in management?

(A) Administration of low-molecular-weight heparin
(B) Administration of warfarin
(C) Application of thigh-high graduated compression stockings
(D) Resumption of aspirin

Item 79

A 68-year-old woman is evaluated for a 1-year history of neck stiffness and dull, achy neck pain. She also notes intermittent difficulty with dexterity while performing fine motor tasks at the hair salon where she works. Medications are ibuprofen as needed.

On physical examination, vital signs are normal. Range of motion of the neck is limited because of pain and stiffness. Fine finger movements exhibit subtle slowness. Reflex examination findings are normal, including a plantar flexor response. Muscle strength is 5/5 throughout. Gait is normal.

An MRI of the cervical spine shows multilevel cervical stenosis that is worst at C4/5 and C6/7. There is moderate deformation of the cord, but no signal change in the cord is noted.

Which of the following is the most appropriate next step in management?

(A) Gabapentin
(B) Neck immobilization in a hard cervical collar
(C) Neurosurgical intervention
(D) Physical therapy

Item 80

An 84-year-old woman is evaluated for dementia. She lives alone and is brought to the office by her son, who reports first noticing gradually progressive symptoms 4 years ago when his mother began having episodes of memory loss and a tendency to repeat herself excessively. He also notes increasing hygiene-related problems and says his mother recently called him several times in the middle of the night and asked him to pick her up "so she can go home." She can no longer manage her finances, keep appointments, or remember to take her medications; she stopped driving 1 year ago after getting lost several times. She has sick sinus syndrome and hypothyroidism treated with levothyroxine.

On physical examination, blood pressure is 155/60 mm Hg and pulse rate is 55/min and intermittently irregular. She scores 17/30 (normal, ≥24) on the Mini–Mental State Examination, but all other findings from neurologic examination are unremarkable.

Results of laboratory studies and brain imaging are normal.

Which of the following is the most appropriate treatment at this time?

(A) Alprazolam
(B) Donepezil
(C) Memantine
(D) Paroxetine
(E) Risperidone

Item 81

A 72-year-old man is evaluated for a 6-month history of headaches that have gradually increased in frequency and have been daily and constant for the past 6 weeks. The pain is bilateral, occipital, and described as a steady "pulling" sensation of mild to moderate intensity. Fatigue and neck discomfort are present. He has had no associated nausea, photophobia, phonophobia, or neurologic symptoms. The patient has atrial fibrillation treated with warfarin and verapamil and no other personal or family history of headache.

On physical examination, blood pressure is 128/88 mm Hg and pulse rate is 88/min and irregular. Decreased cervical range of motion is noted. Neurologic examination findings are unremarkable.

Results of laboratory studies show a normal erythrocyte sedimentation rate and complete blood count, a therapeutic INR, a normal comprehensive metabolic profile, and a normal serum level of C-reactive protein.

Which of the following is the most appropriate next step in management?

(A) Amitriptyline administration
(B) Brain MRI
(C) Cervical spine MRI
(D) Head CT
(E) Temporal artery biopsy

Item 82

A 40-year-old woman is evaluated after having two relapses of multiple sclerosis, which was diagnosed 3 years ago. She works as a human resource manager and has no other medical issues. The patient has been taking once-weekly interferon beta-1a by intramuscular injection and a vitamin D supplement since diagnosis and has been adherent to the drug regimen. After reviewing her options, she elects to change her disease-modifying therapy to the oral medication fingolimod.

All physical examination findings, including vital signs, are normal.

Which of the following should now be a part of her drug monitoring program?

(A) JC virus antibody testing
(B) Ophthalmologic examinations
(C) Serum creatinine measurement
(D) Tuberculin skin testing

Item 83

A 63-year-old woman is evaluated for increasing difficulties with communication at work. She teaches mathematics at a local high school. Her most recent work evaluation cited a growing inability to provide clear instructions when assigning homework. She continues to manage the home finances and to drive, cook, and shop without difficulty.

On physical examination, vital signs are normal. The patient's speech pattern is fluent, but she has frequent problems with word finding and often repeats herself. She has difficulty understanding and following two-step commands. On the Montreal Cognitive Assessment, she scores 0/3 in the object-naming section, 0/1 in the letter-fluency section, and 4/5 in the recall section. All other physical examination findings are unremarkable.

An MRI of the brain is shown.

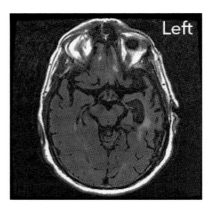

Which of the following is the most likely diagnosis?

(A) Alzheimer disease
(B) Behavioral-variant frontotemporal dementia
(C) Dementia with Lewy bodies
(D) Primary progressive aphasia

Item 84

A 62-year-old woman comes to the office for a follow-up evaluation of involuntary movements. She has a history of type 2 diabetes mellitus and gastroparesis for which she was taking long-term metoclopramide; the medication was stopped 6 months ago after she developed shuffling gait, involuntary facial movements, and a pill-rolling tremor. Since then, the gait problems and tremor have resolved, but she continues to experience persistent choreiform involuntary movements involving the face, lips, and hands. Medications are now metformin, insulin glargine, atorvastatin, and low-dose aspirin.

On physical examination, constant choreiform movements of the face, lips, and hands are noted. Vital signs and the remaining neurologic examination findings are unremarkable.

Which of the following is the most likely diagnosis?

(A) Akathisia
(B) Dystonic reaction
(C) Tardive dyskinesia
(D) Withdrawal emergent syndrome

Item 85

A 56-year-old man comes to the office for a follow-up evaluation after hospitalization for an intracerebral hemorrhage in the right thalamus. He reports feeling generally fatigued but has had no symptoms, such as depressed mood, since discharge. The patient has hypertension. His only medication is chlorthalidone.

On physical examination, blood pressure is 136/78 mm Hg, pulse rate is 68/min, and respiration rate is 12/min; BMI is 32. Neurologic examination reveals a left-sided loss of sensation and 4/5 muscle strength with mildly increased tone throughout the left side.

Results of laboratory studies show a serum creatinine level of 1.1 mg/dL (97.2 µmol/L), an LDL cholesterol of 86 mg/dL (2.23 mmol/L), and a hemoglobin A_{1c} value of 5.9%.

His calculated 10-year atherosclerotic heart disease risk for a major cardiovascular event is 4.3%.

Initiation of which of the following medications is the most appropriate next step?

(A) Aspirin
(B) Fluoxetine
(C) Lisinopril
(D) Rosuvastatin

Item 86

A 48-year-old woman is evaluated for an 8-hour history of facial paralysis. She reports having "droopiness" on the right side of the face when she awoke this morning. She further says that her lunch tasted "odd" and that sounds on her right seem louder than usual.

On physical examination, vital signs are normal. A right facial droop associated with difficulty closing the eye and elevating the eyebrow is noted on the right side. Hearing is intact to whispering, but noises are more pronounced on the right side. The palate is symmetrically elevated, and the tongue protrudes at the midline. Taste is impaired on the right side of the tongue and intact on the left side. Muscle strength is intact on the left side of the face and in both extremities. Shoulder shrug and head turning are normal bilaterally. Facial sensation is intact bilaterally, as are all deep tendon reflexes. The neck is supple, no skin rash is visible, and coordination and gait are normal.

Which of the following is the most appropriate initial step in management?

(A) Brain MRI

(B) Intracranial magnetic resonance angiography

(C) Oral prednisone

(D) Oral valacyclovir

Item 87

A 37-year-old woman is evaluated for a 3-day history of recurrent episodes of severe, piercing right maxillary pain lasting several seconds. Attacks have become progressively more frequent, now occurring several times per hour, and can either arise spontaneously or be triggered by washing the face, chewing, or applying facial cosmetics. She has had no associated conjunctival injection, tearing, or nasal congestion or drainage. The patient has multiple sclerosis. Medications are glatiramer acetate and an oral contraceptive.

On physical examination, vital signs are normal; BMI is 22. A left afferent pupillary defect is noted, as is unsteadiness of tandem gait. All other physical examination findings are unremarkable, including normal facial sensation bilaterally.

A fluid-attenuated inversion recovery MRI reveals periventricular and brainstem hyperintensities that are not seen with contrast enhancement.

Which of the following is the most appropriate treatment?

(A) Acetazolamide

(B) Carbamazepine

(C) Indomethacin

(D) Lamotrigine

Item 88

A 19-year-old man is evaluated in the hospital after admission for subacute onset of bilateral lower extremity paraplegia, urinary incontinence, and sensory deficits. His initial treatment was a 5-day course of high-dose intravenous methylprednisolone. Four days after completion of the infusions, no clinical improvement has occurred. The patient had flu-like symptoms for several days before onset of neurologic symptoms but otherwise has been healthy.

On physical examination, vital signs are normal. Muscle strength is 0/5 in both legs and 5/5 in both arms. Reflexes are absent in the lower extremities and normal in the upper extremities. Moderate sensory loss is noted below T3 bilaterally.

Cerebrospinal fluid analysis:

Erythrocyte count	$2/\mu L$ ($2 \times 10^6/L$)
Leukocyte count	$38/\mu L$ ($38 \times 10^6/L$), with a predominance of lymphocytes
Glucose	Normal
Protein	62 mg/dL (620 mg/L)

A T2-weighted MRI of the thoracic spine shows a hyperintense lesion in the thoracic cord at T2 with peripheral contrast enhancement. An MRI of the brain is normal.

Which of the following is the most appropriate next step in treatment?

(A) Antituberculosis drug regimen

(B) Inpatient rehabilitation only

(C) Intravenous immunoglobulin therapy

(D) Plasma exchange therapy

Item 89

A 41-year-old woman comes to the office for follow-up evaluation of relapsing-remitting multiple sclerosis, which was diagnosed 1 year ago. She has been taking the maximum dose of interferon beta-1a in three-times-weekly injections as disease-modifying therapy since that time. The patient currently has no symptoms and takes no other medication or supplement.

On physical examination, all findings are unremarkable.

A routine surveillance MRI of the brain shows two new lesions in the periventricular white matter, both of which enhance with contrast.

Which of the following is the most appropriate next step in management?

(A) Add dalfampridine

(B) Add glatiramer acetate

(C) Evaluate for cerebrospinal fluid JC virus antibody

(D) Measure serum 25-hydroxyvitamin D level

Item 90

A 64-year-old man comes to the office for a follow-up evaluation of mild cognitive impairment (MCI), which was diagnosed 6 months earlier after he scored 25/30 (normal, ≥26) on the Montreal Cognitive Assessment. The patient reports no worsening of symptoms. He now scores 24/30 on a repeat Montreal Cognitive Assessment, scoring 0/5 on the recall section. The patient wants to know if there are additional tests that would indicate whether his symptoms are caused by Alzheimer disease. A brain MRI obtained at the time of diagnosis was reported as normal.

Which of the following diagnostic studies is most likely to establish a diagnosis?

(A) Cerebrospinal fluid analysis

(B) Electroencephalography

(C) Fluorodeoxyglucose PET scan

(D) Repeat MRI

(E) Serum apolipoprotein E (*ApoE*) allele testing

Item 91

A 47-year-old man is evaluated in the emergency department 2 hours after sudden onset of right-sided face, arm, and leg weakness and numbness. He has a history of hypertension. Medications are amlodipine and hydrochlorothiazide.

On physical examination, blood pressure is 166/72 mm Hg, pulse rate is 82/min, and respiration rate is 12/min. Right facial weakness, dysarthria, and loss of pinprick sensation in the right arm and leg are noted. The patient can lift the right arm and leg off the bed. The National Institutes of Health Stroke Scale score is 8 (moderate stroke).

A CT scan of the head without contrast shows no hemorrhage or early signs of infarct.

The patient receives intravenous recombinant tissue plasminogen activator (alteplase) 3 hours after symptom onset. One hour after treatment, blood pressure is 170/86 mm Hg; other physical examination findings are unchanged. A CT angiogram shows 80% stenosis of the left internal carotid artery and no intracranial arterial occlusion.

Administration of which of the following is the most appropriate next step in treatment?

(A) Amlodipine

(B) Clopidogrel

(C) Intravenous nitroprusside

(D) No further treatment is necessary

Item 92

A 52-year-old man is evaluated for a 3-year history of slowly progressive worsening gait, left leg weakness, spasticity, and fatigue without periods of improvement. Relapsing-remitting multiple sclerosis was diagnosed 20 years ago after an episode of optic neuritis from which he recovered fully. He takes interferon beta-1a as disease-modifying therapy. His disease was well controlled until symptom onset 3 years ago.

On physical examination, vital signs are normal. Muscle strength testing shows 3/5 left hip flexion and ankle dorsiflexion and 4/5 right hip flexion. Finger-to-nose testing elicits dysmetria on the right. The patient ambulates with the assistance of a cane and cannot perform tandem walking.

A T2-weighted MRI of the brain obtained 2 weeks ago showed a new lesion in the periventricular white matter that enhanced with gadolinium administration.

Which of the following best describes the current status of this patient's multiple sclerosis?

(A) Primary progressive, with progression but without activity

(B) Primary progressive, without progression but with activity

(C) Relapsing remitting, with activity

(D) Secondary progressive, with progression and activity

(E) Secondary progressive, without progression but with activity

Item 93

A 38-year-old man comes to the office for a routine follow-up evaluation of generalized tonic-clonic seizures, which he has experienced for the past year. He has had no improvement in seizures despite treatment with maximal doses of valproic acid. The patient also has depression with psychotic features. He attempted suicide 3 years ago. He has no additional medical problems. His only other medication is citalopram.

In addition to discontinuing the valproic acid, which of the following is the most appropriate treatment?

(A) Ethosuximide

(B) Lamotrigine

(C) Levetiracetam

(D) Topiramate

Item 94

A 49-year-old man is evaluated for a 6-month history of difficulty walking and frequent falls. He first noticed these symptoms after a prolonged hospitalization for pneumonia that was complicated by sepsis and cardiopulmonary arrest requiring intubation and antibiotic therapy. The patient also has hypothyroidism treated with levothyroxine.

On physical examination, vital signs are normal; BMI is 35. Muscle strength is normal in all limbs. At rest, few rapid jerky movements are noted in various limbs. On standing, rapid, nonrhythmic, shock-like movements are noted in the trunk and lower extremities, and there are brief lapses of muscle tone in the legs, which lead to loss of balance. These movements are not suppressible. Cognition, cranial nerves, reflexes, and sensation are normal. Plantar response is flexor bilaterally, and clonus is absent.

An MRI of the brain is unremarkable.

Which of the following most accurately describes this patient's abnormal movements?

(A) Ataxia

(B) Chorea

(C) Dystonia

(D) Myoclonus

(E) Orthostatic tremor

Item 95

A 51-year-old man is evaluated for morning headaches and increasing difficulty with focus and memory. He reports growing problems at work, including making occasional mistakes when updating spreadsheets, missing three recent appointments, and occasionally falling asleep during staff meetings. The patient has no other medical problems. He does not drink alcoholic beverages, smoke, or have a family history of dementia.

On physical examination, blood pressure is 150/90 mm Hg but other vital signs are normal; BMI is 33. He scores 25/30 (normal, ≥26) on the Montreal Cognitive Assessment, scoring 2/5 in the recall section, 0/1 in word generation, and 0/1 in letter identification. He scores normally on several clinical depression scales. Other physical examination findings, including those from a neurologic examination, are unremarkable.

Which of the following is the most appropriate next step in evaluating this patient?

(A) Cerebrospinal fluid analysis
(B) Fluorodeoxyglucose PET scanning
(C) MRI of the brain
(D) Polysomnography

Item 96

A 55-year-old man is evaluated for increasing difficulty keeping track of tasks and performing his job adequately. The patient works as an accountant and lately has been making frequent calculation errors. He also has noticed some word-finding difficulties and marked difficulty with short-term memory. Symptoms have progressed over the past 18 months but recently have become more prominent. The patient has a 15-year history of multiple sclerosis and also has depression, which has been in remission. Medications are glatiramer acetate, vitamin D_3, and fluoxetine.

On physical examination, vital signs are normal. On neurologic examination, the patient can recall only one of three objects at 3 minutes, skips "August" when reciting the months backward, and makes one error when subtracting serial sevens.

Which of the following is the most appropriate treatment?

(A) Cognitive rehabilitation
(B) Increased dosage of fluoxetine
(C) Memantine
(D) Methylphenidate

Answers and Critiques

Item 1   Answer: D

Educational Objective: Diagnose a psychogenic nonepileptic spell/event.

This patient most likely is experiencing psychogenic nonepileptic spells/events (PNES). Although event capture during video electroencephalographic monitoring usually is required to confirm the diagnosis, the history is strongly suggestive of PNES because of the variability of symptoms (events not entirely stereotyped), eyes being closed, facial redness due to intermittent breath holding, shaking that starts with retained posture, long duration of shaking that waxes and wanes, limpness after falling, variable limb involvement, and rapid breathing without postictal confusion afterward.

Convulsive status epilepticus (CSE) is unlikely in this patient. The (relatively) long duration of symptoms without subsequent confusion or altered mental status places doubt on the diagnosis of CSE, which is not associated with a return to baseline mental status after seizures cease.

Unlike this patient's episodes, a generalized tonic-clonic seizure is characterized by stereotyped movements (essentially the same from one event to the next), eyes being open, cyanosis due to cessation of breathing, a duration of 2 to 5 minutes, stiffness and falling before symptoms of shaking, shaking that initially is fast but gradually slows and stops, and postictal confusion.

Myoclonic seizures are typically very brief (<1 second) and characterized by synchronous jerking or shaking of the limbs with retained awareness and no postictal confusion afterward. Given the duration and variable nature of this patient's seizures, they are not myoclonic.

KEY POINT

- Historical features that suggest the diagnosis of psychogenic nonepileptic spells/events include variability of symptoms, closing of eyes, long duration of shaking that waxes and wanes, and lack of postictal confusion; confirmation with video electroencephalographic monitoring usually is required.

Bibliography

LaFrance WC Jr, Baker GA, Duncan R, Goldstein LH, Reuber M. Minimum requirements for the diagnosis of psychogenic nonepileptic seizures: a staged approach: a report from the International League Against Epilepsy Nonepileptic Seizures Task Force. Epilepsia. 2013;54:2005-18. [PMID: 24111933] doi:10.1111/epi.12356

Item 2   Answer: C

Educational Objective: Treat a patient who has dementia with Lewy bodies and acute agitation with donepezil.

This patient should be treated with donepezil. Delirium is a potentially preventable syndrome associated with other medical disorders, the adverse effects of medication, or drug withdrawal. Preexisting cognitive impairment is the major predisposing factor for delirium. With treatment, delirium typically resolves within days. Environmental interventions include orienting strategies (reliance on calendars, clocks, and familiar objects in the room), promoting a normal sleep-wake cycle (having no or limited interruptions during nocturnal sleeping hours, minimizing light and noise at night, and opening curtains and encouraging activity during the daytime), identifying and correcting sensory impairments, avoiding physical restraints, and early discontinuation of catheters and intravenous lines. This patient has dementia with Lewy bodies (DLB) and has developed acute agitation and delirium associated with a concurrent urinary tract infection (UTI). He should continue to receive therapy for the UTI until it resolves. The treatment of acute agitation in patients with dementia is challenging, and no medications are FDA approved for the treatment of delirium. Atypical and typical antipsychotic agents have a black-box safety warning when used in patients with underlying dementia. Although not formally approved for DLB, donepezil can be effective in treating the behavioral and cognitive symptoms associated with the disorder; controlled clinical trials, however, remain inconclusive. Because donepezil (or any other medication) has not been shown to be efficacious for DLB in high level, well-conducted trials, its use is based on expert opinion at this time. Nevertheless, donepezil is likely the safest and most efficacious medication for this patient.

Benzodiazepines (such as alprazolam) and diphenhydramine have a strong potential for worsening delirium symptoms in an older population and thus should be avoided in this patient.

Haloperidol is absolutely contraindicated in DLB because of the risk of significant worsening of the dementia syndrome. In addition, the patient is not aggressive at this point and is unlikely to harm himself or others, so antipsychotic agents are unnecessary, as are medications with a strong sedating effect (such as diphenhydramine).

KEY POINT

- Haloperidol is absolutely contraindicated in dementia with Lewy bodies; donepezil is a safer alternative and may improve the behavioral and cognitive symptoms associated with dementia.

Bibliography

Cummings J, Lai TJ, Hemrungrojn S, Mohandas E, Yun Kim S, Nair G, et al. Role of donepezil in the management of neuropsychiatric symptoms in Alzheimer's disease and dementia with Lewy bodies. CNS Neurosci Ther. 2016;22:159-66. [PMID: 26778658] doi:10.1111/cns.12484

Item 3   Answer: B

Educational Objective: Treat advanced Parkinson disease.

This patient should have deep brain stimulation, which is indicated for patients with advanced Parkinson disease who derive a continued benefit from carbidopa-levodopa but experience medication-related complications. The patient has two common levodopa-related complications: motor fluctuations (caused by the wearing off of the beneficial effects of the medication before the next dose is administered) and medication-induced dyskinesia (involuntary choreic movements). Attempting to increase the dose of levodopa to mitigate the "wearing-off" phenomenon resulted in dyskinesia, nausea, and hypotension. Deep brain stimulation enables a persistent motor benefit and reduction of the total levodopa dosage, which would diminish the levodopa-induced adverse effects, including dyskinesia, nausea, and orthostatic hypotension.

Apomorphine is a fast-acting subcutaneous dopamine agonist that is indicated for rapid relief of symptoms caused by sudden wearing off of a Parkinson medication. It is inappropriate for this patient, who experiences predictable episodes of wearing off of the carbidopa-levodopa benefit before she takes the next dose. Apomorphine also does not address the dyskinesia or nausea.

Droxidopa has been approved for management of neurogenic orthostatic hypotension in Parkinson disease. This treatment, however, would not improve the wearing off of the dopaminergic medication before the next dose or the patient's other symptoms of gait freezing, dyskinesia, and medication-induced nausea.

Rotigotine, a dopamine agonist, can worsen both nausea and orthostatic hypotension. Additionally, an overall increase in dopaminergic medication dosing is likely to aggravate dyskinesia.

KEY POINT

- Deep brain stimulation is appropriate for patients with Parkinson disease who derive a continued benefit from carbidopa-levodopa but experience medication-related complications.

Bibliography
Okun MS. Deep-brain stimulation for Parkinson's disease. N Engl J Med. 2012;367:1529-38. [PMID: 23075179] doi:10.1056/NEJMct1208070

Item 4   Answer: A

Educational Objective: Treat severe traumatic brain injury.

This patient should be treated with acetaminophen. The patient has symptoms and signs of a severe head injury. Severe headache combined with nausea and focal neurologic symptoms, such as tinnitus and hearing loss, raises concerns of a major cranial injury. Bilateral periorbital bruising ("raccoon eyes"), mastoid bruising ("Battle sign"), and hemotympanum suggest the presence of a basilar skull fracture. Cerebrospinal fluid (CSF) rhinorrhea, epistaxis, and cranial nerve palsies also can be noted with these fractures, and fractures of the temporal bone occur in 75% of affected patients. Maintenance of an arterial P_{O_2} level of greater than 60 mm Hg (8.0 kPa) and a systolic blood pressure of greater than 90 mm Hg have been shown to improve outcomes in these patients. Fever worsens outcomes after stroke and possibly after severe head injury, most likely by promoting secondary brain injury, and acetaminophen is the most appropriate treatment at this time.

Prophylactic antibiotics, such as ceftriaxone, are inappropriate for this patient. Fever is a common complication of severe head injury and should be managed aggressively with antipyretic agents. There is no evidence of focal infection or sepsis. Although rhinorrhea in this patient most likely represents CSF drainage, no evidence supports the use of antibiotics without evidence of meningitis.

Dexamethasone is contraindicated in severe head injury because glucocorticoids have been shown to worsen its prognosis.

Naloxone is inappropriate for this patient. Although the urine drug screen was positive for opiates, there were no signs of central nervous system or respiratory depression. Naloxone also can worsen nausea and dizziness and occasionally cause sedation.

Norepinephrine is not required in this patient. Although blood pressure normalization in the presence of significant systolic hypotension (<90 mm Hg) has been shown to improve outcomes in severe closed head injury, this patient's systolic blood pressure does not require vasopressor support.

KEY POINT

- In patients with severe head injury, fever must be controlled aggressively with an agent such as acetaminophen.

Bibliography
Sheriff FG, Hinson HE. Pathophysiology and clinical management of moderate and severe traumatic brain injury in the ICU. Semin Neurol. 2015 Feb;35(1):42-9. [PubMed: 25714866] doi: 10.1055/s-0035-1544238

Item 5   Answer: A

Educational Objective: Treat intracranial atherosclerosis.

This patient should receive high-intensity statin therapy with atorvastatin. The use of atorvastatin for secondary stroke prevention is associated with a reduced long-term risk of ischemic stroke, regardless of the baseline LDL cholesterol level. In addition to lowering the cholesterol level, high-intensity statin therapy has other benefits that are important in secondary stroke prevention, including plaque stabilization, anti-inflammatory properties, and slowing the progression of carotid arterial disease. A secondary-prevention randomized trial of high-dose statins established their efficacy among patients with LDL cholesterol levels greater than 100 mg/dL (2.59 mmol/L), irrespective of stroke subtype. Although this trial enrolled patients who were 30 days past stroke onset,

CONT.

statins are recommended to be part of a standardized hospital discharge order set for patients with ischemic stroke because this approach enhances patient adherence to medications. Standardized order sets, which also include antithrombotic agents and smoking cessation, focus on quality metrics of designated stroke centers.

Data have shown that stenting in patients with symptomatic intracranial atherosclerotic disease is associated with a nearly two-fold higher risk of stroke when compared with best medical therapy. Therefore, stenting is not routinely recommended or indicated for patients with intracranial atherosclerosis.

No clinical trial data support the use of methylphenidate, amphetamines, amantadine, bromocriptine, or similar agents for stroke recovery or prevention of stroke recurrence. Although these medications are not routinely recommended, they can be used on an individual basis in patients with behavioral syndromes, such as diminished wakefulness.

Compared with aspirin, warfarin has an increased risk of mortality when used for prevention of recurrence in patients with stroke due to intracranial atherosclerosis. Warfarin is indicated in patients with other stroke subtypes, such as those resulting from atrial fibrillation.

KEY POINT

- In ischemic stroke due to intracranial atherosclerosis, the use of high-intensity atorvastatin therapy for secondary stroke prevention is associated with a reduced long-term risk of ischemic stroke.

Bibliography

Kernan WN, Ovbiagele B, Black HR, Bravata DM, Chimowitz MI, Ezekowitz MD, et al; American Heart Association Stroke Council, Council on Cardiovascular and Stroke Nursing, Council on Clinical Cardiology, and Council on Peripheral Vascular Disease. Guidelines for the prevention of stroke in patients with stroke and transient ischemic attack: a guideline for healthcare professionals from the American Heart Association/ American Stroke Association. Stroke. 2014;45:2160-236. [PMID: 24788967] doi:10.1161/STR.0000000000000024

Item 6   Answer: C

Educational Objective: Treat fatigue in multiple sclerosis.

This patient should receive modafinil. Chronic fatigue is a common symptom in multiple sclerosis (MS). The fatigue associated with MS can have various causes, such as depression, insomnia, or other comorbid conditions. However, patients with MS without these conditions also can experience significant fatigue, which is often described as a sensation of mental exhaustion, frequently occurring in the midafternoon. Lifestyle adjustments, such as improving sleep hygiene, getting regular exercise, and treating depression, can sometimes resolve this symptom. For those with refractory fatigue, stimulant medications can be used. The most common medications of this type used (off-label) in MS are modafinil, armodafinil, and amantadine. For fatigue that is refractory to these medications, amphetamine stimulants, such as methylphenidate, also can be considered.

Spasticity is a frequent consequence of damage to the corticospinal tract in MS. This symptom manifests clinically as increased muscle tone, painful muscle cramps, spasms, and contractures. Spasticity can be reduced by using muscle relaxants, such as baclofen, tizanidine, or cyclobenzaprine. Antispasticity drugs, such as baclofen, are not effective agents for the management of fatigue.

Memantine has been evaluated as a means of treating MS-related cognitive deficits but has proved ineffective for this purpose. There is no reported benefit for MS-related fatigue with memantine.

Substituting an interferon beta for the glatiramer acetate would not be an appropriate step. Her fatigue is not an adverse effect of glatiramer acetate (which might necessitate a therapeutic switch), but rather a treatable symptom of an MS relapse.

Cannabinoids, such as tetrahydrocannabinol-cannabidiol, have been tested in clinical trials for a number of MS-related symptoms but have not improved outcomes. Trials have included the treatment of disease progression, spasticity, pain, and muscle stiffness. There are no data on the effect of cannabinoids on fatigue.

KEY POINT

- Multiple sclerosis–related fatigue is most appropriately treated with a stimulant medication, such as modafinil.

Bibliography

Tur C. Fatigue management in multiple sclerosis. Curr Treat Options Neurol. 2016;18:26. [PMID: 27087457] doi:10.1007/s11940-016-0411-8

Item 7   Answer: A

Educational Objective: Evaluate a first-time unprovoked seizure.

This patient should have CT of the head. Neuroimaging is indicated in all patients with a first-time seizure to rapidly exclude conditions requiring emergent intervention, including hemorrhage. Head CT is the most appropriate initial study because it typically is readily available in most emergency departments and can be performed rapidly. The patient will later require both MRI and electroencephalography, but CT is the best initial study.

Levetiracetam and other antiepileptic drugs are not recommended for first-time seizures until the results of further testing, such as head CT, brain MRI, and electroencephalography (EEG), are known and the recurrence risk of seizures can be determined. He had an unprovoked seizure but does not meet criteria for the diagnosis of epilepsy (at least two unprovoked seizures more than 24 hours apart, or one unprovoked seizure with a high risk of recurrence on the basis of abnormalities found on testing). The 2-year recurrence risk after a single generalized tonic-clonic seizure in patients with normal findings on clinical examination, no epilepsy risk factors, and a normal head CT scan is approximately 40%; that number decreases to about 20% if MRI and

CONT.

EEG are normal. In the setting of two unprovoked seizures or one unprovoked seizure with significant EEG or MRI abnormalities, recurrence risk is at least 60% and treatment is recommended

Although this seizure lasted 5 minutes and thus would meet the definition of convulsive status epilepticus (CSE) if seizure activity were ongoing, the patient has recovered completely and has normal findings on clinical examination. Therefore, he does not have CSE, and intravenous lorazepam is not indicated.

In adults, lumbar puncture is appropriate when meningitis is clinically suspected (for example, in the presence of neck stiffness, altered mental status, or fever) or when a patient has symptoms highly suggestive of subarachnoid hemorrhage in conjunction with normal noncontrast head CT findings. It otherwise is not indicated after a seizure in adults.

KEY POINT

- In a patient with an unprovoked, first-time seizure, head CT is the most appropriate initial study to rapidly exclude emergent pathologic issues.

Bibliography

Gavvala JR, Schuele SU. New-onset seizure in adults and adolescents: a review. JAMA. 2016;316:2657-68. [PMID: 28027373] doi:10.1001/jama.2016.18625

Item 8   **Answer:**   **A**

Educational Objective: Treat the symptoms of behavioral-variant frontotemporal dementia.

This patient should be given the selective serotonin reuptake inhibitor citalopram to control her obsessive-compulsive behaviors. Early changes in social behavior and personality are the defining characteristics of behavioral-variant frontotemporal dementia (FTD). Apathy, diminished interest, loss of empathy, lack of initiative, increased emotionality, disinhibition, euphoria, impulsivity, changes in eating behaviors, hyperorality, and compulsiveness are the most common symptoms reported by families. Other changes include irritability, aggression, verbal abuse, hypomania, and restlessness. The treatment of behavioral-variant FTD is symptom based and should target the most troubling manifestations of the disorder. This patient's obsessive-compulsive tendencies not only have had embarrassing consequences but have resulted in a confrontation with family members. Selective serotonin reuptake inhibitors, such as citalopram, have the potential to alleviate these symptoms. Tricyclic antidepressants may also have this effect.

The acetylcholinesterase inhibitor donepezil is approved by the FDA to treat mild to moderate Alzheimer disease. This class of drug has shown modest benefit in improving cognitive performance in patients with this type of dementia without clear improvements in daily functioning. The body of evidence does not support acetylcholinesterase inhibitors as being beneficial in behavioral-variant FTD.

Similarly, the N-methyl-D-aspartate receptor antagonist memantine, which is approved for moderate to severe dementia in patients with Alzheimer disease associated with significant functional impairment, has shown no benefit in in patients with behavioral-variant FTD and may, in fact, worsen symptoms.

In patients with severe apathy, which can be a common and sometimes debilitating symptom of behavioral-variant FTD, stimulant medications, such as methylphenidate, are sometimes used. This patient has not exhibited apathy. More importantly, referral to a psychiatrist or neurologist is generally recommended before dispensing these medications.

Atypical antipsychotic agents (such as olanzapine) can be effective in treating agitation, aggression, delusions, and hallucinations. However, these drugs are not FDA approved for this clinical indication and have an associated black-box warning due to increased cerebrovascular events and mortality rates in patients with dementia. Olanzapine can be considered if there are psychotic symptoms, such as hallucinations or psychotic delusions. This patient has exhibited no psychotic symptoms. In general, antipsychotic agents should be avoided in patients with dementia.

KEY POINT

- Because there are currently no disease-modifying treatments for behavioral-variant frontotemporal dementia, treatment is symptom based and should target the disease's most troublesome manifestations.

Bibliography

Tsai RM, Boxer AL. Treatment of frontotemporal dementia. Curr Treat Options Neurol. 2014;16:319. [PMID: 25238733] doi:10.1007/s11940-014-0319-0

Item 9   **Answer:**   **B**

Educational Objective: Evaluate a patient who has a cryptogenic stroke for atrial fibrillation.

This patient should have outpatient cardiac telemetry. She has a cryptogenic infarct with no clear source identified on arterial imaging, no evidence of atrial fibrillation (AF) or other high-risk embolic cause, and a stroke location that is not typical for lacunar infarcts. Accumulating data on patients with cryptogenic stroke indicate that an evaluation for AF with an outpatient rhythm monitor may yield a new diagnosis of AF in almost one third of patients. Given the high risk of recurrent stroke associated with AF, additional outpatient evaluation is warranted. The various options available for monitoring include mobile outpatient cardiac telemetry, 24-hour electrocardiographic monitoring, transtelephonic and event monitors, and implantable subcutaneous devices. Longer monitoring results in a higher diagnostic yield. In one study comparing 30-day monitoring to 24-hour monitoring, atrial fibrillation lasting for at least 30 seconds was found in 16.1% of patients monitored for 30 days vs. 3.2% of patients monitored for 24 hours, and AF lasting for at least 2.5 minutes

CONT.

was found in 9.9% of patients with prolonged monitoring vs. 2.5% of patients with 24-hour monitoring.

The combination of clopidogrel and aspirin is associated in the long term with a higher risk of hemorrhagic complications compared with a single antiplatelet agent only. This combination additionally provides no reduction in the risk of ischemic stroke.

Apixaban and similar anticoagulants have not been shown to be effective for the routine prevention of cryptogenic stroke. Warfarin and aspirin have similar rates of recurrent stroke in patients with noncardioembolic stroke; warfarin is not indicated as first-line therapy for stroke prevention in cryptogenic stroke.

Transesophageal echocardiography is unnecessary because the patient is in sinus rhythm and already has had structural imaging of the valves and chamber sizes, which makes a transesophageal echocardiogram likely to be of low yield. This diagnostic test also is invasive and costly and is of higher yield when used to evaluate for unusual causes of cardiac emboli, such as valvular endocarditis or intracardiac tumors.

> **KEY POINT**
>
> - Evaluation of cryptogenic stroke with prolonged outpatient rhythm monitoring may yield a new diagnosis of atrial fibrillation in almost one third of patients.

Bibliography

Kernan WN, Ovbiagele B, Black HR, Bravata DM, Chimowitz MI, Ezekowitz MD, et al; American Heart Association Stroke Council, Council on Cardiovascular and Stroke Nursing, Council on Clinical Cardiology, and Council on Peripheral Vascular Disease. Guidelines for the prevention of stroke in patients with stroke and transient ischemic attack: a guideline for healthcare professionals from the American Heart Association/ American Stroke Association. Stroke. 2014;45:2160-236. [PMID: 24788967] doi:10.1161/STR.0000000000000024

 Item 10   Answer: B

Educational Objective: Treat reversible cerebral vasoconstriction syndrome.

This patient should undergo magnetic resonance angiography of the brain. Her recent history of thunderclap headache is characteristic of reversible cerebral vasoconstriction syndrome (RCVS). The term thunderclap headache is applied to severe headaches that reach maximum intensity within 1 minute. Although subarachnoid hemorrhage (SAH) is the most frequent cause of thunderclap headache, and some patients may experience an isolated sentinel leak before aneurysmal rupture, three episodes within 4 days would be highly unusual for SAH. Normal results of head CT scans and lumbar puncture (LP) effectively exclude this diagnosis. RCVS is the second most frequent source of thunderclap headaches. Head CT and LP findings are both typically normal. Diagnosis is confirmed by documentation of multifocal constriction of intracranial vessels that normalizes within 3 months of onset. Brain magnetic resonance angiography or head CT angiography are the diagnostic procedures of choice. Predisposing factors include vasoactive drugs (such as sympathomimetic

agents, triptans, cocaine, and cannabis) and antidepressants (such as sertraline). The headaches may be triggered by exertion, Valsalva maneuvers, emotion, or showering/bathing. Although some patients develop focal deficits, encephalopathy, or seizures, most have normal findings on clinical examination. Calcium channel blockers, such as verapamil and nimodipine, are the treatments of choice.

Digital subtraction angiography in patients with RCVS has been associated with transient neurologic deficits and is typically avoided.

Because glucocorticoids are associated with a worse clinical course in RCVS, methylprednisolone sodium succinate has no role in its management. This drug can be appropriate therapy for other headache disorders, such as giant cell arteritis, optic neuritis, cerebral vasculitis, or pituitary apoplexy, but none of these is compatible with the patient's clinical presentation and normal results on a head CT scan and LP.

Sumatriptan is an appropriate treatment for acute migraine headache but should be avoided in RCVS. Triptans may predispose patients to RCVS and potentially worsen cerebral vasospasm.

Valproic acid has been shown to be effective in the prevention of episodic migraine. The International Classification of Headache Disorders, third edition, (ICHD-3) criteria for all primary headaches, including migraine, include the requirement that headache is "not better accounted for by another ICHD-3 diagnosis." The clinical picture of recurrent thunderclap headache over a span of days or weeks is much more likely to represent RCVS than migraine.

> **KEY POINT**
>
> - Brain magnetic resonance angiography or head CT angiography are the diagnostic procedures of choice for reversible cerebral vasoconstriction syndrome, the second most frequent source of thunderclap headache.

Bibliography

Ducros A, Wolff V. The typical thunderclap headache of reversible cerebral vasoconstriction syndrome and its various triggers. Headache. 2016 Apr;56(4):657-73. Epub 2016 Mar 26. [PMID: 27015869] doi: 10.1111/head.12797

Item 11   Answer: A

Educational Objective: Treat a multiple sclerosis exacerbation.

This patient should receive high-dose oral prednisone, 1250 mg/d for 5 days. She is experiencing an acute exacerbation, or relapse, of multiple sclerosis (MS). Administration of high-dose glucocorticoids is the standard treatment for MS exacerbations. This treatment approach derives from the landmark Optic Neuritis Treatment Trial, in which high-dose intravenous methylprednisolone (1 g/d for 5 days) was compared to prednisone (1 mg/kg/d for 2 weeks) and placebo. Intravenous methylprednisolone was associated with a more rapid recovery of visual function. Subsequent studies have

CONT.

shown that use of a bioequivalent oral high-dose regimen (such as oral prednisone, 1250 mg, or oral methylprednisolone, 1 g) is as efficacious as intravenous methylprednisolone and has no significant differences in adverse effects. Because of their ease of administration and reduced costs, high-dose oral regimens are beginning to replace intravenous methylprednisolone, although either approach is valid.

Low-dose oral prednisone, 1 mg/kg/d for 2 weeks, is inappropriate. In fact, low-dose oral prednisone was inferior to high-dose intravenous glucocorticoids and actually resulted in worse outcomes than placebo in the Optic Neuritis Treatment Trial. Although this dose of oral prednisone is used for some other neuroinflammatory conditions (such as Bell palsy), it potentially can harm patients with MS experiencing a flare and should be avoided.

A randomized control trial has documented that plasmapheresis may result in clinical improvement in patients with acute exacerbations of MS who do not respond to glucocorticoid therapy. Plasmapheresis is not considered primary, or first-line, therapy for patients with an acute relapse of MS.

The links between vitamin D deficiency and MS pathophysiology have been clearly established, with reduced levels of serum vitamin D predicting future accumulation of new lesions on MRI. Administration of vitamin D supplementation has been shown to provide additional disease activity control, with a recent trial finding less MRI activity in patients taking interferon plus vitamin D versus interferon alone. However, there is no role for vitamin D in the management of an acute relapse of MS. Chronic supplementation with vitamin D is reasonable for most patients with MS, especially if vitamin D levels are low.

KEY POINT

- Administration of high-dose glucocorticoids is the standard treatment for multiple sclerosis exacerbations.

Bibliography
Burton JM, O'Connor PW, Hohol M, Bevene J. Oral versus intravenous steroids for treatment of relapses in multiple sclerosis. Cochrane Database Syst Rev. 2012 Dec 12;12:CD006921. [PMID: 23235634]

Item 12   Answer: B

Educational Objective: Diagnose dystonic tremor.

This patient has a dystonic tremor, which occurs both at rest and with action and is characterized by associated dystonic posturing and the presence of a null point at which change in the position of the affected limb resolves the tremor. The null point is the position at which the trajectories of the forces caused by dystonic coactivation of agonist and antagonist muscles neutralize each other, which leads to resolution of the tremor. In addition, the action component of tremor has task specificity in that it is worse with use of scissors but spares the handwriting.

Cerebellar tremor is characterized by increasing tremor amplitude as the limb approaches the target (terminal intention tremor) and the presence of associated cerebellar symptoms. These features are absent in this patient.

Essential tremor is the most common movement disorder and often presents with a bilateral upper extremity postural and action tremor. It is not associated with dystonic features. Additional features include bilateral involvement and a positive family history. Amelioration of the tremor by ethanol is typical and did not occur in this patient.

Parkinsonian tremor is prominent at rest and can reemerge after a brief delay when the arms are held in an outstretched position. Although dystonia can be seen secondary to Parkinson disease, the absence of other associated features, especially the bradykinesia required for a diagnosis of Parkinson disease, excludes this diagnosis.

Rubral tremor is caused by focal injury to cerebellar outflow pathways and is characterized by a coarse tremor that is present at rest but most severe during action. This type of tremor has a prominent proximal component and interferes with various actions, such as feeding, typing, and writing, in a nonselective way. Also, MRIs of the brain reveal a focal causative lesion that is not present in this patient.

KEY POINT

- Dystonic tremor occurs both at rest and with action and is characterized by associated dystonic posturing and the presence of a null point at which a change in the position of the affected limb resolves the tremor.

Bibliography
Fasano A, Deuschl G. Therapeutic advances in tremor. Mov Disord. 2015;30:1557-65. [PMID: 26293405] doi:10.1002/mds.26383

Item 13   Answer: E

Educational Objective: Treat convulsive status epilepticus in a patient allergic to phenytoin.

The patient should now receive intravenous valproic acid. He is in generalized convulsive status epilepticus (CSE). A medical emergency that can lead to significant morbidity and mortality, CSE is defined as persistent tonic-clonic activity with impaired mental status that lasts longer than 5 minutes. Initial management of CSE requires rapidly assessing airways, breathing, and circulation; checking the blood glucose level; and administering thiamine with glucose, if needed. These steps should be performed simultaneously with initiation of drug treatment. According to a guideline from the American Epilepsy Society, intramuscular midazolam, intravenous (IV) lorazepam, and IV diazepam have been judged to be equivalent and are the first-line agents for the initial treatment of CSE. Phenytoin, a longer-acting antiseizure drug, should then be administered; if available, fosphenytoin, a prodrug of phenytoin, is preferable to phenytoin for initial treatment of CSE because it can be administered faster and does not carry the risk of thrombophlebitis or skin necrosis (purple glove syndrome) that is associated with phenytoin extravasation. Valproic acid is an alternative to phenytoin or fosphenytoin, particularly in patients with an allergy to phenytoin or

CONT.

primary generalized epilepsy. Therefore, intravenous valproic acid should be administered to this patient as a second-line therapy.

CSE usually is diagnosed clinically. Obtaining an MRI of the brain is an unnecessary time-consuming process and would delay treatment. Once CSE is controlled, head CT usually is indicated because it takes less time and is more readily available in the acute setting.

Electroencephalography could eventually be considered, but, again, the diagnosis of CSE is primarily clinical, and treatment should not be postponed.

Lacosamide, which is available intravenously, sometimes is considered in the management of convulsive status epilepticus. However, evidence is insufficient to recommend it as part of the standard guidelines for initial treatment of generalized CSE, which makes it inappropriate for this patient.

KEY POINT

- According to current guidelines, valproic acid is an appropriate second-line therapy for convulsive status epilepticus for patients allergic to phenytoin.

Bibliography

Glauser T, Shinnar S, Gloss D, Alldredge B, Arya R, Bainbridge J, et al. Evidence-based guideline: treatment of convulsive status epilepticus in children and adults: report of the Guideline Committee of the American Epilepsy Society. Epilepsy Curr. 2016;16:48-61. [PMID: 26900382] doi: 10.5698/1535-7597-16.1.48

Item 14   Answer: B

Educational Objective: Treat depression as a cause of memory difficulties in an older patient.

This patient should undergo treatment for depression. Depression is common in older adults, although it is both under-recognized and undertreated. In these patients, depression can frequently masquerade as cognitive impairment or multiple somatic complaints, which often results in delayed diagnosis. The patient expresses concern about subjective cognitive changes. However, given his age, the fact that he recently assumed new responsibilities after losing his wife, the limited evidence of memory loss, and the normal findings on cognitive and neurologic examination, a significant cognitive disorder is not likely. His recent decreased appetite, problems falling asleep, and withdrawal from social activities suggest onset of a depressive disorder that is most likely associated with the loss of his wife. Depression is further suggested by the positive Geriatric Depression Scale (GDS) score of 9. The GDS has been validated in the older population. The GDS relies less on somatic symptoms and has a simplified yes-or-no format, which may be more conducive to screening those with possible cognitive impairment. Treatment of his depression with close follow-up evaluations is thus most advisable.

Because Alzheimer disease is an unlikely diagnosis in this patient and is unsupported by results of cognitive testing, treatment with an acetylcholinesterase inhibitor is premature and unwarranted at this point.

An MRI without contrast is similarly unwarranted in this patient who has normal scores on screening cognitive evaluation and lacks concerning findings in his history or examination findings.

Although often helpful in patients with cognitive impairment, a complete neuropsychological evaluation is unnecessary in this situation, given the normal findings of the screening examination. This patient's symptoms, including his memory difficulty, are most likely due to depression, and this reversible contributor should be treated first. If treatment results in no alleviation of the symptoms, then further testing can be pursued.

KEY POINT

- In older patients, depression can frequently masquerade as cognitive impairment; screening and treatment is appropriate in these patients.

Bibliography

Knopman DS, DeKosky ST, Cummings JL, Chui H, Corey-Bloom J, Relkin N, et al. Practice parameter: diagnosis of dementia (an evidence-based review). Report of the Quality Standards Subcommittee of the American Academy of Neurology. Neurology. 2001;56:1143-53. [PMID: 11342678]

Item 15   Answer: C

Educational Objective: Diagnose teratoma-associated anti–N-methyl-D-aspartate receptor antibody encephalitis.

This patient most likely has an ovarian teratoma. An autoimmune condition termed anti–N-methyl-D-aspartate receptor (anti-NMDAR) antibody encephalitis has emerged as an increasingly common cause of encephalitis. Anti-NMDAR antibody encephalitis is associated with ovarian teratomas in more than 50% of patients with the disease because of production of an antibody to a tumor protein that cross-reacts with neuronal tissue. The diagnosis is suggested by the presence of choreoathetosis, psychiatric symptoms, seizures, and autonomic instability and is confirmed by detection of anti-NMDAR antibody in serum. This patient has developed new-onset psychiatric disease and a movement disorder. These symptoms raise suspicion of paraneoplastic or autoimmune encephalitis, and testing confirms the presence of the anti-NMDAR antibody in the serum. Patients are evaluated with CT and/or transvaginal ultrasound. Treatment includes removal of the teratoma to eradicate the immune stimulus and immunosuppression with glucocorticoids or intravenous immune globulin.

Paraneoplastic syndromes associated with breast adenocarcinoma can present as ataxia, brainstem encephalitis, ophthalmoplegia, and parkinsonism. They are most often associated with anti-Ri and anti–glutamic acid decarboxylase antibodies rather than anti-NMDAR antibody.

Unlike small cell lung cancer, non–small cell lung cancer (NSCLC) typically is not associated with neurologic paraneoplastic syndromes. NSCLC, however, may be associated with other paraneoplastic syndromes, including hypercalcemia and hypertrophic osteoarthropathy.

CONT.

Small cell lung cancer is associated with a host of neurologic paraneoplastic syndromes, including dementia, chorea, ataxia, brainstem encephalitis, and neuropathies, among others. The antibodies associated with these syndromes include anti-Hu, anti-LGI1 (voltage-gated potassium channel), and anti-CRMP5 antibodies but not the anti-NMDAR antibody.

KEY POINT

- Ovarian teratoma–associated anti–*N*-methyl-D-aspartate receptor antibody encephalitis is suggested by the presence of choreoathetosis, psychiatric symptoms, seizures, and autonomic instability.

Bibliography

Titulaer MJ, McCracken L, Gabilondo I, Armangué T, Glaser C, Iizuka T, et al. Treatment and prognostic factors for long-term outcome in patients with anti-NMDA receptor encephalitis: an observational cohort study. Lancet Neurol. 2013;12:157-65. [PMID: 23290630] doi:10.1016/S1474-4422(12)70310-1

Item 16   Answer: C

Educational Objective: Prevent migraine.

This patient should be treated with metoprolol. Her headaches meet the criteria for episodic migraine without aura. Pharmacologic prevention should be considered for migraine occurring at a frequency of at least 5 days per month. According to guidelines, metoprolol, propranolol, timolol, divalproex sodium, and topiramate all have Level A evidence for prevention of episodic migraine, with atenolol, amitriptyline, and venlafaxine having level B evidence. Approximately a third of patients with episodic migraine meet criteria for pharmacologic prevention, yet only 3% to 13% receive this treatment. The goal of prevention is an at least 50% reduction in headache frequency; reductions in migraine intensity, disability, and cost are other established outcomes. Drug tapering or elimination should be considered after a period of 6 to 12 months of adequate control.

No data support the use of citalopram or other selective serotonin reuptake inhibitor antidepressants in migraine prevention.

Insufficient evidence about the effectiveness of gabapentin in migraine prevention is available; therefore, its use for this purpose is inappropriate.

Onabotulinum toxin A has an FDA indication for the prevention of chronic migraine but is not approved and has no established efficacy in the prevention of episodic migraine. Chronic migraine is defined as headache occurring 15 or more days per month with at least 8 days meeting full criteria for migraine or responding to migraine-specific medication.

Rizatriptan is an effective treatment option for acute migraine. However, this patient is responding well to an NSAID, and no adjustment in acute therapy is warranted. Escalation in headache frequency requires migraine-preventive measures.

KEY POINT

- Metoprolol, propranolol, timolol, divalproex sodium, and topiramate all have Level A evidence for prevention of episodic migraine and should be considered for migraine occurring at a frequency of at least 5 days per month.

Bibliography

Silberstein SD, Holland S, Freitag F, Dodick DW, Argoff C, Ashman E; Quality Standards Subcommittee of the American Academy of Neurology and the American Headache Society. Evidence-based guideline update: pharmacologic treatment for episodic migraine prevention in adults: report of the Quality Standards Subcommittee of the American Academy of Neurology and the American Headache Society (erratum appears in Neurology. 2013 Feb 26;80(9):871). Neurology. 2012 Apr 24;78(17):1337-45. [PMID: 22529202] doi:10.1212/WNL.0b013e3182535d20

Item 17   Answer: B

Educational Objective: Treat juvenile myoclonic epilepsy in a woman with childbearing potential.

Besides discontinuing the oral contraceptive, starting folic acid, and then tapering off valproic acid, this patient should begin taking levetiracetam for her juvenile myoclonic epilepsy (JME). This type of generalized epilepsy requires a history of myoclonic seizures for diagnosis but is also usually associated with generalized tonic-clonic seizures. In a woman with childbearing potential, levetiracetam and lamotrigine are the most appropriate treatment options because of their relatively low risk of teratogenicity. Levetiracetam is often preferred because lamotrigine can worsen myoclonus in some patients.

Valproic acid is strongly associated with neural tube defects and lower IQ in offspring and should be avoided in women with childbearing potential, unless absolutely necessary. In this patient, who has been seizure free for 10.5 years and has never taken another antiepileptic drug, replacing valproic acid with another medication should be attempted. In patients whose epilepsy is difficult to control with other medications, valproic acid may be continued during pregnancy.

Gabapentin and oxcarbazepine also have a relatively favorable profile in terms of lower fetal risk, but both are known to worsen generalized epilepsy and thus should be avoided in patients with JME.

Maternal topiramate use is associated with cleft lip/palate in offspring. This teratogenic drug should be avoided by women with childbearing potential.

JME most often requires lifelong treatment, even if patients have normal results on testing and are seizure free for many years. Therefore, providing this patient no additional treatment is inappropriate.

KEY POINT

- In a woman with childbearing potential, levetiracetam and lamotrigine are the most appropriate treatment options because of their relatively low risk of teratogenicity.

Bibliography

Crespel A, Gelisse P, Reed RC, Ferlazzo E, Jerney J, Schmitz B, et al. Management of juvenile myoclonic epilepsy. Epilepsy Behav. 2013;28 Suppl 1:S81-6. [PMID: 23756489] doi:10.1016/j.yebeh.2013.01.001

 Item 18   **Answer: A**

Educational Objective: Treat spinal cord metastases.

This patient should undergo decompressive surgery followed by radiation. This patient most likely has a metastatic extra-dural lesion from the prostate cancer that has resulted in cord compression. Spinal cord compression due to metastatic disease from most tumor types requires emergent use of high-dose glucocorticoids (dexamethasone, 20 mg) followed by maintenance glucocorticoids until definitive therapy with urgent surgical decompression followed by radiation is possible. Certain radiosensitive tumor types, such as leukemia, lymphoma, myeloma, and germ cell tumors, may not require initial surgical decompression and may be treated urgently with radiation therapy followed by chemotherapy. Surgical intervention sometimes is deferred in patients with a poor prognosis for long-term survival or with a low functional status. However, in appropriate patients, clinical trials have shown the superiority of surgical decompression followed by radiation compared with radiation alone in optimizing ambulation in patients younger than 65 years.

Laminectomy, in which the lamina (the back part of the vertebra covering the spinal canal) is removed to create more space, is not preferable to decompressive surgery, in which regions of the vertebra infiltrated by tumor are removed and reconstructed. In fact, radiation alone is superior to laminectomy in this patient because it would address the metastatic lesion.

Spinal angiography is appropriate to use in the diagnosis and treatment of a spinal dural arteriovenous fistula (AVF) or a spinal arteriovenous malformation (AVM) but not for a T8 vertebral body with invasion into the epidural space. An AVF or an AVM would result in vascular-appearing lesions (usually associated with flow voids) on T2-weighted imaging.

KEY POINT

- Spinal cord compression from metastatic disease requires emergent use of high-dose glucocorticoids and urgent surgical decompression followed by radiation.

Bibliography

George R, Jeba J, Ramkumar G, Chacko AG, Tharyan P. Interventions for the treatment of metastatic extradural spinal cord compression in adults. Cochrane Database Syst Rev. 2015:CD006716. [PMID: 26337716] doi:10.1002/14651858.CD006716.pub3

 Item 19   **Answer: A**

Educational Objective: Diagnose Creutzfeldt-Jakob disease.

This patient most likely has Creutzfeldt-Jakob disease (CJD). CJD is the most common form of prion disease in humans, with most cases being sporadic. Iatrogenic transmission of CJD is possible and has resulted mainly from receipt of growth hormone prepared from cadaveric pituitaries and contaminated cadaveric dura mater allografts. Contaminated surgical instruments have also been documented to transmit CJD in rare instances. Sporadic CJD does not appear to be transmissible by blood. Brain MRIs typically show a pattern of increased intensity in the diffusion-weighted sequence in the basal ganglia and various cortical regions.

Periodic sharp wave complexes are often seen on electroencephalography. Elevated levels of tau and 14-3-3 proteins in the cerebrospinal fluid (CSF) also are typical but not necessary for diagnosis. Although rapidly progressive dementia has a broad differential diagnosis, CJD is very likely if it is accompanied by myoclonus, sleep problems, and other psychiatric symptoms. Progressive neurologic decline resulting in death occurs rapidly, typically within 6 to 12 months.

HIV encephalopathy is characterized by a subacute syndrome of cognitive and motor dysfunction. Although HIV screening is standard for rapid-onset dementia, the electroencephalographic and MRI findings are inconsistent with a diagnosis of acute HIV encephalopathy.

Lyme disease can be responsible for a seldom-reported inflammatory encephalomyelitis. The disease often mimics multiple sclerosis, with MRI abnormalities of the brain or spinal cord and abnormal CSF findings, including increased total immunoglobulin and oligoclonal bands. The patient's rapidly progressive dementia, myoclonus, psychiatric symptoms, and normal CSF findings are not compatible with this diagnosis.

Wernicke encephalopathy is an acute neuropsychiatric syndrome characterized by the triad of nystagmus and ophthalmoplegia, mental status changes, and ataxia. It is caused by thiamine deficiency, most often in patients who abuse alcohol, but can be seen in patients being treated for cancer, those with chronic vomiting or malnutrition, or those who have had gastrointestinal surgery, in particular bariatric surgery. The patient's findings are not compatible with Wernicke encephalopathy.

KEY POINT

- Creutzfeldt-Jakob disease is a transmissible prion-related disorder characterized by rapidly progressive dementia, myoclonus, sleep problems, and other psychiatric symptoms; typical imaging findings include an increased signal in the cortex and subcortical structures on diffusion-weighted MRI sequences.

Bibliography

Geschwind MD. Rapidly Progressive Dementia. Continuum (Minneap Minn). 2016;22:510-37. [PMID: 27042906] doi:10.1212/CON.0000000000000319

Item 20   **Answer: A**

Educational Objective: Evaluate a transient ischemic attack.

This patient should have carotid duplex ultrasonography. He most likely has had a transient ischemic attack (TIA) referable to the left hemisphere and is at risk of ischemic stroke within the next 90 days, with the highest risk occurring within the first 2 days. Although his ABCD^2 score (based on patient Age, Blood pressure, Clinical presentation, Duration of symptoms, and presence of Diabetes mellitus) of 3 indicates a predicted stroke risk of 1.3% and the need for hospitalization and rapid evaluation, these scores are neither sensitive nor specific enough to identify patients at highest risk of stroke. Several studies have identified extracranial symptomatic internal carotid artery stenosis as an indicator of stroke risk of greater than 70% after TIA; this risk can be modified with carotid revascularization. Several modalities are available for imaging the internal carotid artery and identifying extracranial symptomatic stenosis, including duplex ultrasonography, CT angiography, and magnetic resonance angiography (MRA). Duplex ultrasonography has the benefit of being inexpensive, readily available, low risk, and noninvasive and thus is an appropriate early study. If the carotid duplex ultrasound shows high-grade stenosis, confirmation of this finding by CT angiography or MRA is required before surgical intervention. If the carotid duplex ultrasound is unrevealing, then additional vessel imaging of the neck is unnecessary.

CT angiography of the neck is more costly and less widely available than carotid duplex ultrasonography. Additionally, the radiation exposure makes CT angiography less desirable as an initial imaging test.

Brain MRI is not the initial test of choice because the presence or absence of a cerebral infarct will not immediately change medical management or affect the patient's stroke risk. Cerebral imaging with either CT or MRI eventually may be required in this patient but should occur after an evaluation of the internal carotid artery that may lead to hospitalization and surgical intervention.

In patients with risk factors for stroke after a TIA, transesophageal echocardiography is (TEE) is unlikely to immediately change management, is invasive, and has low yield for finding an embolic source of stroke in patients who are in sinus rhythm. TEE can be considered in certain patients with stroke if they are young and have no apparent risk factors for stroke or if unusual causes are suspected, such as cardiac tumor, patent foramen ovale, aortic arch atherosclerosis, or endocarditis.

KEY POINT

- In a patient with a transient ischemic attack, carotid duplex ultrasonography is an inexpensive, readily available, and noninvasive imaging modality for identifying high-grade stenosis and the possible need for surgery.

Bibliography
Yaghi S, Willey JZ, Khatri P. Minor ischemic stroke: Triaging, disposition, and outcome. Neurol Clin Pract. 2016;6:157-163. [PMID: 27104067]

Item 21   Answer: C

Educational Objective: Diagnose Huntington disease.

The most likely diagnosis is Huntington disease. His history of psychiatric disease, impulsivity, and substance abuse

and clinical examination findings of executive dysfunction, dysarthria, incoordination, and ataxia are consistent with Huntington disease. His nonsuppressible flowing and variable movements are consistent with chorea, a major manifestation of Huntington disease. A positive family history is common in patients affected by this autosomal dominant disorder, but in its absence, a family history of associated conditions is suggestive. His father's prominent psychiatric disease may have led to suicide before onset of the motor features of Huntington disease; young-onset parkinsonism is a common presentation in younger patients with the disease. Tetrabenazine and deutetrabenazine are the most appropriate treatments of chorea in this disorder.

Creutzfeldt-Jakob disease (CJD) is the most common form of prion disease in humans. Onset usually occurs in the seventh decade of life. The most prominent neurologic sign is disordered cognition. Typically, patients also have motor signs, such as ataxia or spasticity, vague sensory problems, or changes in visual perception. Myoclonus is common. Progressive neurologic decline resulting in death occurs rapidly, typically within 6 to 12 months. This patient's duration of symptoms is likely too long for CJD.

Behavioral-variant frontotemporal dementia (FTD) is associated with prominent changes in behavior, personality, or executive function. Apathy, diminished interest, loss of empathy, lack of initiative, increased emotionality, disinhibition, euphoria, impulsivity, changes in eating behaviors, hyperorality, and compulsiveness are the most common symptoms. Motor neuron disease, including amyotrophic lateral sclerosis, is seen in approximately 15% of patients preceding, simultaneous with, or after the diagnosis of FTD. Chorea is not typical.

The four cardinal signs of Parkinson disease are resting tremor, bradykinesia, cogwheel rigidity, and gait/postural impairment. Resting tremor is characteristically unilateral at onset and remains asymmetric. This patient's clinical features, including impulsivity, ataxia, hyperreflexia, and unprovoked chorea, are not consistent with Parkinson disease.

KEY POINT

- Huntington disease is an autosomal dominant disorder characterized by psychiatric disease, impulsivity, and clinical examination findings of executive dysfunction, dysarthria, incoordination, and ataxia; chorea is a major manifestation of Huntington disease.

Bibliography
Dayalu P, Albin RL. Huntington disease: pathogenesis and treatment. Neurol Clin. 2015;33:101-14. [PMID: 25432725] doi:10.1016/j.ncl.2014.09.003

Item 22   Answer: B

Educational Objective: Manage a mild traumatic brain injury.

This patient should have CT of the head without contrast. He sustained a mild traumatic brain injury (TBI), defined as head injury due to contact and/or acceleration or deceleration

CONT.

forces, and now reports headache. Guidelines recommend imaging with noncontrast CT for patients exposed to mechanisms of injury perceived to be dangerous. These include falls from greater than 3 feet or 5 stairs, vehicular ejection, or vehicle-pedestrian motor vehicle collisions. Age greater than 60 years also is considered an indication for imaging, as are severe headache, vomiting, Glasgow Coma Scale score less than 15, focal deficit(s), posttraumatic seizure, coagulopathy, or persistent drowsiness or amnesia. Most patients with mild TBI will not require brain imaging.

Contrast administration with CT is helpful in the evaluation of malignant, vascular, and some inflammatory disorders of the nervous system. However, the addition of contrast to head CT adds nothing to the evaluation of acute head injury. Visualization of skull fracture and acute intracranial hemorrhage is best accomplished through noncontrasted head CT.

Hospital observation of patients with mild TBI may be indicated for those with intractable headache or vomiting, focal neurologic deficits, or persistent impairment of memory or consciousness but not for this patient with less severe symptoms. In all of these settings, however, patients should first undergo head CT to exclude intracranial hemorrhage. Hospital admission without imaging would be inappropriate for patients with TBI.

Intravenous prochlorperazine is indicated in the management of acute migraine in the emergency department. This patient describes neither nausea nor headache compatible with migraine.

KEY POINT

- Guidelines recommend imaging with noncontrast CT for patients with mild traumatic brain injury (TBI) who are exposed to dangerous mechanisms of injury, such as falls from greater than 3 feet or 5 stairs, vehicular ejection, or vehicle-pedestrian motor vehicle collisions; other indications for head CT in mild TBI include age older than 60 years, severe headache, vomiting, Glasgow Coma Scale score of less than 15, focal deficit(s), posttraumatic seizure, coagulopathy, or persistent drowsiness or amnesia.

Bibliography

Jagoda AS, Bazarian JJ, Bruns JJ, et al; American College of Emergency Physicians; Centers for Disease Control and Prevention. Clinical policy: neuroimaging and decision making in adult mild traumatic brain injury in the acute setting. Ann Emerg Med. 2008;52(6):714-48. [PMID: 19027497] doi: 10.1016/j.annemergmed.2008.08.021

Item 23   Answer: D

Educational Objective: Diagnose myasthenia gravis.

Myasthenia gravis can present with pronounced weakness of cervical or bulbar muscles. Fluctuation in weakness, with a fatigable pattern that worsens later in the day, suggests this neuromuscular junction disorder. In the setting of probable myasthenia gravis, seronegative status for acetylcholine receptor antibodies should trigger testing for muscle-specific kinase (MuSK) antibodies, which are positive in half of seronegative patients. Weakness of cervical extension, such as this patient exhibits, is a hallmark of MuSK antibody–positive myasthenia gravis. Although nerve conduction studies using a special protocol for repetitive stimulation can reveal a pattern of decrementing weakness in neuromuscular junction disorders, this protocol is not part of routine electromyography. Therefore, if suspicion for myasthenia gravis is high, a repetitive stimulation protocol should be specifically requested.

Although amyotrophic lateral sclerosis can present with prominent bulbar and cervical weakness, the fluctuating nature of the weakness, the absence of tongue weakness or fasciculations and of upper motor neuron signs, and the negative electromyography (EMG) findings make this an unlikely diagnosis.

Inclusion body myositis is a progressive inflammatory myopathy that can present with bulbar, forearm flexor, and quadriceps weakness. The absence of additional muscle involvement, the normal creatine kinase level, and the normal limb findings on needle EMG rule out this entity.

Multiple sclerosis (MS) can cause bulbar weakness secondary to central demyelination. Focal neck extensor weakness is atypical. The patient's history and normal MRI exclude MS.

Polymyositis also can present with head drop, but often proximal limb muscles are involved. In addition, a normal creatine kinase level and normal results on routine limb EMG rule out this entity.

KEY POINT

- In a patient with fluctuating weakness of the cervical muscles that worsens in the evening, myasthenia gravis should be suspected; weakness of cervical extension is a hallmark of muscle-specific kinase antibody–positive myasthenia gravis.

Bibliography

Sanders DB, Guptill JT. Myasthenia gravis and Lambert-Eaton myasthenic syndrome. Continuum (Minneap Minn). 2014;20:1413-25. [PMID: 25299290] doi:10.1212/01.CON.0000455873.30438.9b

Item 24   Answer: C

Educational Objective: Diagnose mild cognitive impairment.

The patient's symptoms of subjective cognitive problems, near-normal function, and objective cognitive impairment (score of 1/5 on the delayed recall section of the Montreal Cognitive Assessment) are most consistent with a diagnosis of mild cognitive impairment (MCI), amnestic type. MCI is a cognitive state between normal aging and dementia characterized by a decline in cognitive functioning that is greater than what is expected with normal aging but has not resulted in significant functional disability. The suggestive MRI evidence of minimal hippocampal atrophy is a biomarker conferring a risk of symptom progression. Given her objective performance on cognitive tests and the noted MRI changes, the patient has an annual risk of developing Alzheimer disease of 5% to 15%.

In contrast to MCI, dementia is a progressive deterioration of cognitive function severe enough to impair occupational or social functioning. Alzheimer disease is the most common type of dementia (60%-80%). Whereas typical Alzheimer disease presents with the insidious development of recent memory loss, as this patient has experienced, she lacks the functional impairment that is a hallmark of dementia.

Multiple relationships between depression and cognitive impairment have been reported in the literature: late-life depression may lead to prodromal Alzheimer disease; depression may be a risk factor for future development of cognitive impairment, dementia, and Alzheimer disease; cerebrovascular disease can precipitate late-life depression; and cognitive impairment itself can lead to depression. More than half of patients with late-life major depression exhibit clinically significant cognitive impairment, most frequently affecting processing speed, executive function, and visuospatial ability. However, this patient's depression screening was negative, and thus depression is unlikely to account for her symptoms.

Normal aging can be associated with memory problems, but cognitive testing shows functioning within the normal range. In contrast, this patient's verbal learning and memory performance are 2 SDs below that of an age- and education-matched control population and are not consistent with normal aging.

KEY POINT

- Mild cognitive impairment is a cognitive state between normal aging and dementia characterized by a decline in cognitive functioning that is greater than what is expected with normal aging but has not resulted in significant functional disability.

Bibliography

Petersen RC. Clinical practice. Mild cognitive impairment. N Engl J Med. 2011;364:2227-34. [PMID: 21651394] doi:10.1056/NEJMcp0910237

Item 25   Answer: D

Educational Objective: Evaluate urinary symptoms in patients with multiple sclerosis.

This patient should undergo urodynamic testing. Her symptoms and history of multiple sclerosis (MS) suggest the presence of a neurogenic bladder. Given the mix of symptoms of urgency and frequency (symptoms of an overactive, spastic bladder) plus hesitancy and retention (symptoms of a hypotonic bladder or overactive sphincter), the patient has aspects of both hypertonic and hypotonic bladder. She also may have bladder-sphincter dyssynergia, in which the contraction of the bladder wall is not properly timed with relaxation of the urinary sphincter. Management of complicated forms of neurogenic bladder involves proper diagnosis through urodynamic testing (which will guide medication choices), potential use of urinary catheterization, and monitoring of postvoid residuals while the patient is treated to avoid urinary retention. Involvement of a urologist is often required.

Dalfampridine has been shown to improve walking speed in patients with MS. Although the patient says that incontinence occurs when she is unable to get to the bathroom fast enough, use of this medication would not address the underlying cause of her urinary symptoms. Further, frequent urinary tract infections are a common adverse effect of this medication, and thus using it without first addressing her current urinary symptoms would be counterproductive.

Urinary frequency and urgency are more readily managed than other patterns of bladder dysfunction and are often amenable to abstinence from caffeine, timed voids, and anticholinergic medications, such as oxybutynin or tolterodine. Patients with urinary hesitancy or retention, such as this patient, should not be treated with anticholinergic agents because these medications can worsen retention and lead to predisposition to urinary tract infections. This patient with mixed bladder symptoms should be evaluated with urodynamic testing.

Solifenacin has been shown to reduce symptoms of overactive bladder in patients with MS. However, this patient's mixed bladder symptoms suggest that she is prone to urinary retention. Use of this medication without concurrent use of catheterization and monitoring of postvoid residuals would result in worsened urinary retention and predispose the patient to more frequent urinary tract infections and, possibly, bladder cancer.

KEY POINT

- In a patient with multiple sclerosis and mixed urinary symptoms that suggest both a hypertonic and a hypotonic bladder, urodynamic testing to guide medication choices is appropriate, as are the potential use of urinary catheterization and monitoring of postvoid residuals while the patient is treated.

Bibliography

Phé V, Chartier-Kastler E, Panicker JN. Management of neurogenic bladder in patients with multiple sclerosis. Nat Rev Urol. 2016;13:275-88. [PMID: 27030526] doi:10.1038/nrurol.2016.53

Item 26   Answer: D   H

Educational Objective: Treat pulmonary embolism in patients with primary brain tumors.

This patient should receive intravenous heparin. Venous thromboembolism (VTE) is a common complication in patients with brain tumors, occurring in up to 30% of patients with high-grade glioma. Risk of VTE is correlated with higher-grade malignancies and is associated with release of the potent procoagulant tissue factor. Other factors, including immobilization and recent surgery, increase the risk. The risk of intracranial hemorrhage with the use of anticoagulants

CONT.

complicates the management of VTE in patients with brain tumor, including patients undergoing brain surgery. Although brain tumors have a risk of hemorrhage, therapeutic anticoagulation is generally considered safe. Intravenous heparin is the best choice for this patient because it has a short half-life and is reversible should hemorrhage occur. Although evidence does not support routine use of preanticoagulation neuroimaging to assess for hemorrhage, noncontrast head CT can be considered and is the most cost-effective test in this situation.

Apixaban is not indicated. Although non–vitamin K oral anticoagulants are a recommended therapy for VTE, evidence is insufficient to support their use in the setting of central nervous system tumors.

Inferior vena cava (IVC) filter placement is not indicated. IVC filters incur an increased risk of subsequent deep venous thrombosis and should be reserved for patients with an absolute contraindication to anticoagulation. The presence of a primary brain tumor and recent biopsy do not absolutely preclude anticoagulation.

Alteplase, a tissue plasminogen activator, is contraindicated in most CNS tumors. This class of drugs can be considered in low-risk tumors, such as meningioma, but not high-risk tumors, such as glioblastoma multiforme.

Subcutaneous low-molecular-weight heparin (LMWH) is an effective treatment for VTE but should be avoided in this patient because of her kidney dysfunction. LMWH also lacks an effective reversal agent and has a prolonged duration of action, making it a less optimal choice in a patient at increased risk of bleeding.

KEY POINT

- In patients with glioblastoma multiforme and pulmonary embolism, anticoagulation with heparin is the most appropriate treatment.

Bibliography
Jo JT, Schiff D, Perry JR. Thrombosis in brain tumors. Semin Thromb Hemost. 2014;40:325-31. [PMID: 24599439] doi:10.1055/s-0034-1370791

Item 27   Answer: D
Educational Objective: Diagnose POEMS syndrome.

The most likely diagnosis is POEMS syndrome (polyneuropathy, organomegaly, endocrinopathy, monoclonal gammopathy, and skin changes). POEMS syndrome is characterized by the presence of a monoclonal plasma cell disorder, peripheral neuropathy, and one or more of the following: osteosclerotic myeloma, Castleman disease (angiofollicular lymph node hyperplasia), elevated serum vascular endothelial growth factor, organomegaly, endocrinopathy, edema, typical skin changes, and papilledema. His clinical presentation, including splenomegaly, skin lesions (hyperpigmentation and angiomas), endocrine disease (hypothyroidism), peripheral neuropathy, and λ monoclonal gammopathy support the diagnosis of POEMS syndrome. POEMS syndrome is typically secondary to an underlying cancer; identification and treatment of the underlying cancer leads to improvement of the neuropathy.

Amyotrophic lateral sclerosis (ALS) is characterized by upper motor neuron signs (such as hyperreflexia, spasticity, and an extensor plantar response) coexistent with lower motor neuron findings (such as atrophy and fasciculation). Sensory deficits are characteristically absent, and sensory nerve conduction studies are often normal in ALS. These findings are not consistent with this patient's presentation.

The classic presentation of chronic inflammatory demyelinating polyradiculoneuropathy (CIDP) is generalized areflexia and progressive or relapsing symmetric sensory and motor neuropathy. CIDP resembles POEMS syndrome in its neurologic manifestations, but the presence of monoclonal gammopathy, splenomegaly, and skin changes makes this diagnosis unlikely.

Mitochondrial myopathy can present with significant variability and may cause fatigue, myalgia, ophthalmoplegia, and various extramuscular manifestations. Mitochondrial myopathies should be suspected in the presence of multiorgan involvement and maternal transmission. In this patient, the presence of sensory deficits and neuropathic findings on needle electromyography are not consistent with a myopathy.

KEY POINT

- POEMS syndrome is characterized by the presence of a monoclonal plasma cell disorder, peripheral neuropathy, and one or more of the following: osteosclerotic myeloma, Castleman disease (angiofollicular lymph node hyperplasia), elevated serum vascular endothelial growth factor, organomegaly, endocrinopathy, edema, typical skin changes, and papilledema.

Bibliography
Rison RA, Beydoun SR. Paraproteinemic neuropathy: a practical review. BMC Neurol. 2016;16:13. [PMID: 26821540] doi:10.1186/s12883-016-0532-4

Item 28   Answer: C
Educational Objective: Diagnose focal seizures.

The patient is experiencing focal seizures with altered awareness (formerly known as complex partial seizures or focal dyscognitive seizures). These seizures typically are infrequent, are associated with "warning" symptoms (aura, which may consist of an epigastric rising sensation or a feeling of déjà vu), last more than 30 seconds, have associated mouth or limb automatisms (semipurposeful repetitive movements), and are followed by confusion and/or exhaustion. Patients who experience this type of seizure often have no memory of the episode itself.

Absence seizures may also present with staring and confusion but typically are more frequent (occurring multiple times per day), last less than 15 seconds, and are associated with immediate recovery, to the point that patients and witnesses may not realize a seizure has occurred. Absence seizures are most characteristic of childhood absence epilepsy, which typically resolves by puberty but also can occur in adults with idiopathic generalized epilepsy syndromes.

Atonic seizures involve the abrupt loss of muscle tone and typically are associated with falling down and a brief loss of consciousness lasting only a few seconds. Atonic seizures are one cause of "drop attacks" in which the patient will suddenly, and without warning symptoms, drop to the ground. Individuals with drop attacks can get themselves up and typically will deny loss of consciousness. Other causes of drop attacks include cataplexy, vertebrobasilar transient ischemic attack, and vestibular pathologies. The patient's seizures do not match the description of atonic seizures.

Myoclonic seizures generally consist of a single jerk of the entire body, usually last less than 1 second, and are associated with retained awareness and no postictal confusion. In contrast, this patient's seizures last at least 45 seconds and are characterized by staring, chewing motions, repetitive grabbing of her clothes, and a 20-minute postseizure period of exhaustion and sleepiness.

KEY POINT

- Focal seizures with altered awareness typically are infrequent, are associated with warning symptoms (aura), last more than 30 seconds, have associated mouth or limb automatisms (semipurposeful repetitive movements), and are followed by confusion and/or exhaustion.

Bibliography

Dobrin S. Seizures and epilepsy in adolescents and adults. Dis Mon. 2012;58:708-29. [PMID: 23149523] doi:10.1016/j.disamonth.2012.08.011

Item 29   Answer: B

Educational Objective: Diagnose idiopathic brachial plexopathy.

Idiopathic brachial plexopathy (also known as neuralgic amyotrophy and Parsonage-Turner syndrome) is characterized by subacute severe pain followed by resolution of pain and progressive weakness and atrophy involving the shoulder girdle and upper extremity muscles. This syndrome often is triggered by a preceding event, such an infection or surgery. In this patient, motor and sensory involvement in the territory of multiple nerves and roots is consistent with a process involving the brachial plexus. Imaging rules out a pathologic process at the level of the cervical spine. An iatrogenic traumatic plexopathy caused by surgery is unlikely, given the absence of weakness immediately after the procedure and the abdominal location of the procedure.

Although compressive polyradiculopathy secondary to degenerative spinal disease can simulate plexopathy, with a presentation consisting of mixed motor, sensory, and pain symptoms in multiple nerve root distributions, negative cervical imaging rules out this entity in this patient.

Lambert-Eaton syndrome is associated with neuromuscular junction dysfunction. Sensory deficits, prominent pain, and focal weakness are atypical.

Statins can cause a toxic myopathy, but sensory deficits are not expected findings in myopathies, and asymmetry also is atypical. Moreover, in this patient, rapid weakness appeared after resolution of pain, whereas in statin myopathy, pain often persists along with muscle necrosis–induced weakness.

KEY POINT

- Idiopathic brachial plexopathy is characterized by subacute severe pain followed by resolution of pain and progressive weakness and atrophy involving the shoulder girdle and upper extremity muscles; this syndrome often is triggered by a preceding event, such as an infection or surgery.

Bibliography

Van Eijk JJ, Groothuis JT, Van Alfen N. Neuralgic amyotrophy: an update on diagnosis, pathophysiology, and treatment. Muscle Nerve. 2016;53:337-50. [PMID: 26662794] doi:10.1002/mus.25008

Item 30   Answer: B

Educational Objective: Treat Tourette syndrome.

This patient should be treated with clonidine. The suppressible stereotyped neck movements and premonitory sensory cues are consistent with motor tics, and the history of other motor (eye rolling) and vocal (throat clearing) tics, childhood onset, duration of greater than 1 year, and comorbidity of obsessive-compulsive disorder (OCD) are consistent with the diagnosis of Tourette syndrome. Clonidine is a first-line agent used to treat Tourette syndrome. Anti-tic medications should be considered when tics interfere with education, daily function, or work. Other first-line medications include guanfacine, topiramate, and the dopamine-depleter agent tetrabenazine. Second-line treatments include antipsychotic agents (such as haloperidol), but their benefit should be weighed against risk of tardive dyskinesia.

Although botulinum toxin can be considered as an off-label option in the treatment of severe refractory cervical tics, this patient has not yet tried medication to control her tics. Botulinum toxin also is indicated in the treatment of cervical dystonia, but this disorder is not consistent with her clinical findings of suppressibility and the absence of sustained motor activity.

Treatment of mild tics includes reassurance, treatment of psychiatric comorbidities (such as the sertraline she already takes for OCD), and cognitive behavioral therapy to teach patients about tic diversion techniques (such as the foot taps she initiates after sensory premonitory cues). Given that this patient's symptoms have persisted, pharmacologic therapy for Tourette syndrome is appropriate.

Haloperidol should not be considered before a trial of first-line anti-tic medications is attempted. Clonidine appears to be better tolerated than antidopaminergic drugs, such as haloperidol or risperidone. Additionally, the tardive dyskinesia that can result from neuroleptic agents may take months to years to resolve after discontinuation of the culprit drug.

- First-line agents used to treat Tourette syndrome when the associated tics interfere with education, daily function, or work are clonidine, guanfacine, topiramate, and tetrabenazine.

Bibliography

Kurlan RM. Treatment of Tourette syndrome. Neurotherapeutics. 2014; 11:161-5. [PMID: 24043501] doi:10.1007/s13311-013-0215-4

Item 31   Answer: B

Educational Objective: Treat migraine with aura.

This patient should be treated with sumatriptan. He has a history of episodic migraine with typical aura that is no longer responsive to appropriate NSAIDs. Guidelines recommend the use of triptans in patients with moderate to severe migraine for whom NSAID therapies are not effective. Triptans (5-hydroxytryptamine receptor 1B [5-HT1B] and 5-hydroxytryptamine receptor 1D [5-HT1D] agonists) are migraine-specific agents with a direct impact on the trigeminovascular activation associated with migraine attacks. Activation of the 5-HT1B receptor reverses vasodilation. Binding to the 5-HT1D receptors on trigeminal nerve terminals blocks release of vasoactive and inflammatory mediators, such as calcitonin gene–related peptide. This second action is likely more important in the interruption of nociceptive transmission. Unless medication overuse headache is a concern, patients should be advised to treat at the first sign of pain. Because migraine intensity is highly variable, occasional attacks that are less responsive to medication are to be expected. Contraindications include coronary, cerebral, or peripheral vascular disease; uncontrolled hypertension; and migraine with brainstem or hemiplegic auras.

Guidelines recommend against the use of opioid agents, such as hydrocodone, in migraine management. Concerns include the potential for dependence or addiction and, more importantly, an increased risk of transformation from episodic to chronic migraine. In patients with migraine, opioids are associated with a 44% increase in risk of headache progression over 1 year and butalbital compounds with a 70% increase. Both drug classes should be used cautiously and only when more appropriate acute therapies are contraindicated.

Level A evidence exists for migraine prevention with topiramate. Because this patient has only two episodes of migraine per month, prophylactic medication is not indicated.

Verapamil has no established benefit in the acute treatment or prevention of migraine.

- For patients with a history of episodic migraine with typical aura that no longer responds to appropriate NSAIDs, guidelines recommend the use of triptans.

Bibliography

Marmura MJ, Silberstein SD, Schwedt TJ. The acute treatment of migraine in adults: the American Headache Society evidence assessment of migraine pharmacotherapies. Headache. 2015;55(1):3-20. [PMID: 25600718] doi: 10.1111/head.12499

Item 32   Answer: B

Educational Objective: Diagnose convulsive syncope.

The patient most likely had an episode of convulsive syncope. Syncope is nontraumatic, complete transient loss of consciousness and loss of postural tone. Onset is abrupt and recovery is spontaneous, rapid, and complete. Neurally mediated syncope, the most common type of syncope, generally occurs with standing and is associated with a prodrome of nausea, lightheadedness, and warmth. It may follow cough, urination, defecation, pain, or laughing. This patient's tunnel vision, palpitations, short duration of loss of consciousness (<1 minute), and immediate and complete neurologic recovery is typical of syncope. Movements and shaking (in this instance, nonepileptic myoclonus) are common with syncope. In fact, syncope without any movements is the exception rather than the rule.

Atonic seizures can be associated with falling and brief loss of consciousness with decreased tone, but their duration is much briefer (a few seconds only) than that of syncope, and they usually do not have warning symptoms, such as tunnel vision or palpitations.

Generalized tonic-clonic seizures have increased tone at the onset (tonic phase), followed by rhythmic, synchronous jerking of all limbs (clonic phase), typically for more than 1 minute. These seizures are followed by confusion, lethargy, and (sometimes) combativeness. This patient's seizure, especially her normal neurologic state after regaining consciousness, does not match this description.

Myoclonic seizures are very brief, typically lasting less than 1 second, and usually involve synchronous limb jerking (all limbs shaking together at the same time). The duration of this patient's seizure and her asynchronous limb jerking are not consistent with myoclonic seizure.

Tonic seizures may involve brief loss of consciousness and falling, but there is no associated aura (prodrome or warning symptoms). Additionally, patients generally have increased tone that leads to the fall.

- Convulsive syncope is a seizure type typically associated with tunnel vision, palpitations, short duration of loss of consciousness (<1 minute), movements and shaking, and immediate and complete neurologic recovery.

Bibliography

Lempert T, Bauer M, Schmidt D. Syncope: a videometric analysis of 56 episodes of transient cerebral hypoxia. Ann Neurol. 1994;36:233-7. [PMID: 8053660] doi: 10.1002/ana.410360217

Item 33   Answer: D

Educational Objective: Evaluate for stroke-related sleep-disordered breathing with polysomnography.

This patient should undergo polysomnography. Sleep-disordered breathing is highly prevalent in patients with any form of stroke and is a leading cause of fatigue, headaches, and difficult-to-control hypertension in these patients. Given her recent stroke and elevated BMI, she is at particularly high risk for sleep-disordered breathing, which is best detected by polysomnography. Measurement tools, such as the Epworth Sleepiness Scale, also may help in patients with stroke but have not been well validated in this population. Treatment of sleep-disordered breathing can improve this patient's energy level, fatigue, and blood pressure.

Discontinuation of atorvastatin would be reasonable only if the patient were experiencing significant adverse effects, such as myalgia, rhabdomyolysis, or persistently elevated liver transaminase levels. Atorvastatin is effective in reducing the risk of recurrent ischemic stroke and is a key component of secondary risk reduction in this patient. Fatigue may be a side effect of atorvastatin but would not prompt discontinuation of the medication.

Fluoxetine should not be initiated in this patient, who already is taking another antidepressant medication and has no symptoms of depression other than fatigue. Although fluoxetine has been studied as an agent to promote motor recovery independent of its effect on depression in the acute stroke setting, the current evidence supporting this indication is lacking.

An MRI of the brain may be indicated if there is concern for a specific intracranial structural process, such as a new stroke or an underlying intracranial mass. These processes, however, are usually associated with specific neurologic symptoms or focal neurologic findings on examination. Fatigue is a nonspecific symptom that is not attributable to a specific region of the brain and is unlikely to be the sole clinical manifestation of a new stroke or mass.

KEY POINT

- Sleep-disordered breathing is highly prevalent in patients with any form of stroke, and the best diagnostic test is polysomnography.

Bibliography

Kernan WN, Ovbiagele B, Black HR, Bravata DM, Chimowitz MI, Ezekowitz MD, et al; American Heart Association Stroke Council, Council on Cardiovascular and Stroke Nursing, Council on Clinical Cardiology, and Council on Peripheral Vascular Disease. Guidelines for the prevention of stroke in patients with stroke and transient ischemic attack: a guideline for healthcare professionals from the American Heart Association/American Stroke Association. Stroke. 2014;45:2160-236. [PMID: 24788967] doi:10.1161/STR.0000000000000024

Item 34   Answer: B

Educational Objective: Treat multiple sclerosis in a patient with hepatic disease.

This patient should receive glatiramer acetate. He has newly diagnosed multiple sclerosis (MS) and should begin a disease-modifying therapy. Definitive treatment of MS relies less on addressing relapses as they occur than on preventing relapse occurrence (and the associated accrual of disability) in the first place. This prevention is achieved with MS disease-modifying therapies, a series of immunomodulatory or immunosuppressive medications that have been shown to reduce the risk of relapse, disability progression, and new lesion formation on MRI. Several disease-modifying therapies have been approved by the FDA for use in relapsing-remitting MS, each differing in their route of administration, mechanism of action, and potential adverse effects. Generally, most physicians recommend self-injection medications (one of the interferon beta preparations or glatiramer acetate) as first-line agents, given their favorable risk profiles. Glatiramer acetate, a copolymer of four amino acids, is administered daily or several times weekly by subcutaneous injection. Glatiramer acetate and high-dose interferon beta formulations exhibit similar reductions in relapse rates compared with placebo and are equivalent in head-to-head studies. In choosing which therapy is most appropriate to recommend, the clinician should consider all comorbid conditions. Given the patient's history of liver disease, the most appropriate treatment is glatiramer acetate. This medication has no known adverse effects on liver function.

Liver dysfunction is a potential adverse effect of fingolimod, the interferon beta preparations, and natalizumab. Therefore, none of these drugs would be the best choice for this patient. Additionally, natalizumab is recommended for patients who have not responded to previous disease-modifying therapy. Because this patient has not yet been treated for his MS, use of natalizumab as a first-line agent would be inappropriate.

KEY POINT

- Interferon beta preparations or glatiramer acetate are considered first-line agents for relapsing-remitting multiple sclerosis given their favorable risk profiles; glatiramer acetate is preferred in patients with liver disease.

Bibliography

Wingerchuk DM, Weinshenker BG. Disease modifying therapies for relapsing multiple sclerosis. BMJ. 2016;354:i3518. [PMID: 27549763] doi:10.1136/bmj.i3518

Item 35   Answer: A

Educational Objective: Diagnose amyotrophic lateral sclerosis.

This patient most likely has amyotrophic lateral sclerosis (ALS). Diagnosis requires fulfillment of positive diagnostic criteria and exclusion of mimics. Positive diagnostic criteria for ALS include the presence of clinical upper (hyperreflexia, Hoffman sign, clonus) and lower (atrophy, fasciculation, weakness) motor neuron signs and electromyographic lower motor neuron signs in two (probable ALS) or more (definitive ALS) body regions (upper and lower limbs, paraspinal, bulbar). Because hyperthyroidism can lead to a combination of upper and lower motor neuron findings that may mimic ALS, it must be excluded before diagnosis. Other important mimics include structural brain and cervical spinal lesions, vitamin B_{12} and copper deficiency, Lyme disease, and hyperparathyroidism.

Charcot-Marie-Tooth (CMT) disease is an inherited neuropathy arising from mutations in several genes encoding for myelin formation, structure, and function. The two most common forms are demyelinating (CMT1) and axonal (CMT2). Both share the clinical features of numbness, distal extremity weakness, unsteady gait, areflexia, high arches, hammer toes, and atrophy of distal extremity muscles and foreleg muscles ("stork leg" deformity). This patient's findings are not consistent with CMT disease.

Granulomatosis with polyangiitis is an antineutrophil cytoplasmic antibody–associated vasculitis. Areas most commonly affected by the vasculitis include the airways, lung parenchyma, kidneys, skin, eyes, and nervous system. The vasculitic neuropathy can present as mononeuropathy multiplex and are associated with focal or multifocal weakness. However, these entities are associated with pain and sensory deficits and not with upper motor neuron signs.

The Miller Fisher variant of Guillain-Barré syndrome typically presents with subacute ataxia, areflexia, and ophthalmoplegia, with or without diffuse weakness. Antibodies to GQ1b (a ganglioside component of nerve) are present in more than 85% of patients. The patient's findings are not compatible with the Miller Fisher variant.

KEY POINT

- Amyotrophic lateral sclerosis is characterized by upper motor neuron signs (hyperreflexia, spasticity, and an extensor plantar response) coexistent with lower motor neuron findings (atrophy and fasciculation); sensory deficits are characteristically absent.

Bibliography

Kiernan MC, Vucic S, Cheah BC, Turner MR, Eisen A, Hardiman O, et al. Amyotrophic lateral sclerosis. Lancet. 2011;377:942-55. [PMID: 21296405] doi:10.1016/S0140-6736(10)61156-7.

 Item 36   Answer: B

Educational Objective: Diagnose cavernous sinus thrombosis.

This patient has right cavernous sinus thrombosis. Painful ophthalmoplegia affecting multiple nerves involved with extraocular movement indicates a pathologic process in the superior orbital fissure or cavernous sinus. Proptosis and chemosis are typical because of marked venous congestion. Thrombosis of the cavernous sinus most commonly arises from contiguous spread of infection, most likely from nasal, sinus, and dental sites. *Staphylococcus aureus* is the most common organism and is found in 70% of affected patients. Progression to bilateral involvement of the cavernous sinuses may be seen within 1 to 2 days of presentation. Brain MRI

is more sensitive than head CT in confirming the diagnosis; magnetic resonance venography also is frequently helpful. Lumbar puncture is required to exclude meningeal involvement. This condition is life-threatening and requires immediate administration of antibiotics and consideration of surgical drainage.

Dissection of the carotid artery can present with orbital pain, partial Horner syndrome (ptosis and miosis only), and ipsilateral signs of cerebral or retinal ischemia. Ptosis with Horner syndrome is partial, whereas that seen with oculomotor nerve palsy is complete. Ophthalmoplegia would be highly unusual and proptosis and chemosis unexpected in carotid artery dissection.

Aneurysms of the posterior communicating artery may expand and present with ipsilateral third nerve palsy but not fourth or sixth nerve palsies. Even without aneurysmal rupture, aneurysmal expansion can provoke ipsilateral or global headache. A fixed dilated pupil, ptosis, and inability to elevate or adduct the globe are noted. Diabetic third nerve palsy may present in a similar fashion but typically spares the pupil.

Vertebral artery dissection often presents with occipital and neck pain and posterior fossa symptoms, such as dysarthria, dysphagia, ataxia, and hemifield visual loss. Ophthalmoplegia, chemosis, and proptosis are not features of this type of dissection.

KEY POINT

- Painful ophthalmoplegia affecting multiple nerves involved with extraocular movement indicates a pathologic process in the superior orbital fissure or cavernous sinus.

Bibliography

Sparaco M, Feleppa M, Bigal M. Cerebral venous thrombosis and headache– a case-series. Headache. 2015 Jun;55(6):806-14. doi: 10.1111/head.12599 [PubMed 26084237] doi:10.1111/head.12599

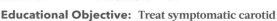

Item 37   Answer: A

Educational Objective: Treat symptomatic carotid artery stenosis.

Carotid endarterectomy is the most appropriate next step in management. This patient has an ischemic stroke due to symptomatic extracranial internal carotid artery stenosis, which is associated with a high short-term risk of recurrent stroke despite best medical therapy. Guidelines recommend carotid endarterectomy for patients with symptomatic carotid artery stenosis within 2 weeks of transient ischemic attack or nondisabling stroke. The procedure is safe and reduces the risk of ischemic stroke. The choice of revascularization procedure is largely driven by medical comorbidities and by the expertise of locally available surgeons. However, a consistent finding has been a higher risk of perioperative stroke with stenting. In a clinical trial that enrolled symptomatic patients with carotid stenosis in Europe, endarterectomy was associated with a lower risk of recurrent stroke risk than was stenting.

CONT.

Carotid stenting may be considered in patients with significant cardiac comorbidities that would preclude surgery under general anesthesia because of safety considerations; this patient has no such comorbidities. Patients should be counseled that stenting is associated with a higher risk of perioperative stroke, according to randomized clinical trials of symptomatic patients.

Diagnostic angiography is not routinely indicated to confirm the degree of stenosis before carotid revascularization, given the associated risk of vessel injury. Additionally, sufficient information is available from both the magnetic resonance angiogram and the carotid duplex ultrasound.

A 30-day period of outpatient telemetry is not required to diagnose the stroke subtype in this patient with established high-grade stenosis in the carotid artery. Evaluation for occult atrial fibrillation is recommended for patients in whom the cause of stroke has not been identified, especially if an embolic cause (suggested by infarcts involving the brain surface or in the distribution of more than one cerebral artery) is suspected.

KEY POINT

- Carotid endarterectomy within 2 weeks of transient ischemic attack or nondisabling stroke is safe and reduces the risk of ischemic stroke in patients with symptomatic carotid artery stenosis.

Bibliography

Kernan WN, Ovbiagele B, Black HR, Bravata DM, Chimowitz MI, Ezekowitz MD, et al; American Heart Association Stroke Council, Council on Cardiovascular and Stroke Nursing, Council on Clinical Cardiology, and Council on Peripheral Vascular Disease. Guidelines for the prevention of stroke in patients with stroke and transient ischemic attack: a guideline for healthcare professionals from the American Heart Association/ American Stroke Association. Stroke. 2014;45:2160-236. [PMID: 24788967] doi:10.1161/STR.0000000000000024

Item 38   Answer: C

Educational Objective: Diagnose normal pressure hydrocephalus.

This patient most likely has normal pressure hydrocephalus (NPH) and should undergo lumbar puncture with removal of a large volume of cerebrospinal fluid (CSF) and subsequent measurement of CSF opening pressure. Because NPH is reversible, detecting it early is essential. The triad of gait changes, urinary incontinence, and cognitive impairment is most characteristic of NPH, with gait impairment being the most prominent feature. The MRI shows ventricular dilation typical of normal pressure hydrocephalus. The diagnosis is suggested by an expansion of the entire ventricular system in the absence of sulcal atrophy or an obstruction. A timed gait evaluation performed just before CSF removal and again before 60 minutes have passed since removal is appropriate to confirm the diagnosis. If gait improves after CSF removal, then NPH likely is present and reversal is possible.

Amyloid PET scanning is approved for clinical use in patients with suspected Alzheimer disease. The most prominent early symptom of Alzheimer disease is memory disturbance, not gait disturbance or urinary incontinence. More importantly, however, this imaging test would delay the diagnosis of NPH, a potentially reversible cause of his symptoms.

Although a fluorodeoxyglucose PET scan can be used for pattern recognition of certain dementias, it is a nonspecific test and is unlikely to definitively establish the diagnosis in this patient.

Neuropsychological testing is most helpful in patients with mild symptoms of cognitive impairment, especially in localizing these symptoms. It also can help establish or exclude malingering as the reason for the symptoms. It likely would have limited utility for this patient who had good results on the memory portion of the Mini–Mental State Examination and whose other symptoms are gait impairment and urinary incontinence.

KEY POINT

- In patients with normal pressure hydrocephalus (NPH), lumbar puncture with removal of a large volume of cerebrospinal fluid (CSF) and subsequent measurement of CSF opening pressure can help confirm the diagnosis and determine if the NPH is reversible.

Bibliography

Halperin JJ, Kurlan R, Schwalb JM, Cusimano MD, Gronseth G, Gloss D. Practice guideline: Idiopathic normal pressure hydrocephalus: response to shunting and predictors of response: report of the Guideline Development, Dissemination, and Implementation Subcommittee of the American Academy of Neurology. Neurology. 2015;85:2063-71. [PMID: 26644048] doi:10.1212/WNL.0000000000002193

Item 39   Answer: A

Educational Objective: Diagnose autoimmune limbic encephalitis.

This patient most likely has autoimmune limbic encephalitis. New-onset status epilepticus in a previously healthy person suggests the presence of a neurologic autoimmune disorder. This patient has a rapidly progressive neurologic syndrome that is most consistent with autoimmune encephalitis, with antibodies directed against the voltage-gated potassium channel receptor complex (the most common target being the LGI1 antibody). This condition is marked by the presence of hyponatremia, myoclonus, and limbic encephalitis (amnesia, temporal lobe seizures, and confusion). Although many neurologic autoimmune disorders are paraneoplastic, primary autoimmune disorders with no accompanying cancer may occur.

Lyme disease with neurologic involvement typically presents with meningitis or brainstem encephalitis (multiple cranial nerve palsies and confusion) in a patient with a history of rash and arthralgia. Chronic indolent disease may involve cognitive symptoms, but they are typically not acutely progressive, as they are in this patient.

Progressive multifocal leukoencephalopathy typically presents with subacute neurologic symptoms that are focal

CONT.

(unilateral weakness or numbness, aphasia, cranial nerve palsies) in an immunocompromised patient, with characteristic white matter abnormalities on MRI.

Rapidly progressive dementia, such as Creutzfeldt-Jakob disease, sometimes presents with symptoms similar to this patient's but usually is not accompanied by hyponatremia or focal seizures.

KEY POINT

- The presence of new-onset status epilepticus and progressive confusion in a previously healthy patient strongly suggests a diagnosis of autoimmune limbic encephalitis.

Bibliography

Shin YW, Lee ST, Shin JW, Moon J, Lim JA, Byun JI, et al. VGKC-complex/LGI1-antibody encephalitis: clinical manifestations and response to immunotherapy. J Neuroimmunol. 2013;265:75-81. [PMID: 24176648] doi:10.1016/j.jneuroim.2013.10.005

Item 40   Answer: C

Educational Objective: Evaluate cognitive and functional decline in a patient with depression.

This patient should undergo neuropsychological testing. She has treatment-refractory depression but also cognitive impairment and some functional deficits. Given the progression of the cognitive symptoms, additional diagnostic studies should be pursued to evaluate for cognitive impairment independent of that associated with depression. More than half of patients with late-life major depression exhibit clinically significant cognitive impairment, most frequently affecting processing speed, executive function, and visuospatial ability. Notably, late-life depression may be a prodromal feature of Alzheimer disease. A history should be obtained from the patient and someone well acquainted with the patient who can provide information on current daily functioning relative to premorbid functioning. A tool for identifying and assessing the severity of depression is the Patient Health Questionnaire (PHQ)-9. A score of 5 to 9 indicates mild depression, 10 to 14 moderate depression, 15 to 19 moderately severe depression, and 20 or higher severe depression. In a patient with possible depression-related cognitive and functional decline, a trial of antidepressant therapy is an appropriate first step. Psychotherapy (cognitive-behavioral therapy, psychodynamic therapy, and interpersonal therapy) and psychopharmacology, alone or in combination, are mainstays of treatment and can prove synergistic. Patients who do not respond to full-dose antidepressant monotherapy for 6 weeks may respond to a different antidepressant drug, either from the same or a different class, or the addition of a second antidepressant drug. If the patient does not respond to an adequate trial of therapy, other diagnoses should be considered. Because this patient has not responded to two different antidepressants, the addition of mirtazapine is unlikely to be helpful.

Neuropsychological testing can be useful in identifying a pattern or degree of cognitive impairment that is not typical of depression-related cognitive impairment. When results of neuropsychological testing are more consistent with Alzheimer disease than depression, additional diagnostic studies, such as 18F-fluorodeoxyglucose PET, could be pursued, as could a trial of cognitive enhancers (such as acetylcholinesterase inhibitors).

Although some Alzheimer disease–specific biomarkers can be detected by cerebrospinal fluid (CSF) analysis, abnormal Aβ42 peptide levels are often seen in an older population (30%-50%) in the absence of cognitive impairment. These CSF studies are most helpful in younger patients to discriminate normal from abnormal findings.

A normal head CT scan and normal MRI of the brain do not rule out an underlying neurodegenerative process, particularly if a disease is in its mild stages, and are thus inappropriate in a patient with probable depression as the cause of her symptoms.

KEY POINT

- In a patient with treatment-refractory depression who also has cognitive and functional decline, neuropsychological testing can be useful in identifying a pattern or degree of cognitive impairment that is not typical of depression-related cognitive impairment.

Bibliography

Hashem AH, Gomaa MA, Sadek MN, Khalaf OO. Late versus early onset depression in elderly patients: Vascular risk and cognitive impairment. Curr Aging Sci. 2017. [PMID: 28382870] doi:10.2174/1874609810666170404105634

Item 41   Answer: D

Educational Objective: Evaluate medically intractable epilepsy.

This patient is having ongoing focal seizures with altered awareness (formerly known as complex partial seizures) because of temporal lobe epilepsy despite taking two antiepileptic drugs and should be referred to an epilepsy center for monitoring by video electroencephalography (EEG). Because his epilepsy is medically intractable, he may be a candidate for epilepsy surgery. Video EEG is the first step in determining candidacy for surgery by confirming that the seizures seen on video EEG match the location of abnormal findings on MRI. Temporal lobectomy leads to seizure freedom in 60% to 70% of patients with temporal lobe epilepsy not helped by medication and is the best option for treating this patient.

Although levetiracetam and topiramate are reasonable options for treating this seizure type, and topiramate has the added benefit of migraine prophylaxis, the chance of seizure freedom from an additional drug is only approximately 5% to 10%. Additionally, this patient's migraines are already well controlled, so a prophylactic agent is not required.

Use of a vagus nerve stimulator is a palliative measure, is unlikely to result in freedom from seizures, and should be offered only if resection is not an option.

KEY POINT

- Video electroencephalography is first step in determining candidacy for epilepsy surgery in patients with medically intractable epilepsy.

Bibliography

Nair DR. Management of drug-resistant epilepsy. Continuum (Minneap Minn). 2016;22:157-72. [PMID: 26844735] doi:10.1212/CON.0000000000000297

Item 42   Answer: C

Educational Objective: Treat an unruptured intracranial aneurysm.

This patient should be referred for surgical intervention. She has an intracranial aneurysm in the posterior circulation (posterior communicating artery) that is unruptured but now has several features consistent with a high risk of subarachnoid hemorrhage (SAH): size equal to or greater than 7 millimeters, rapid growth, and a cranial nerve deficit, which in this patient is compression of the oculomotor nerve (cranial nerve III) on the right. Although neurosurgical intervention (with clipping or coiling, depending on local expertise) has a potential risk of adverse events, the risk of SAH without surgery is greater. A diagnostic angiogram is likely to be required for operative planning and can be obtained in conjunction with a planned coiling procedure.

The patient's blood pressure is already within the appropriate target of less than 140/80 mm Hg. Given the high risk of rupture, further control of blood pressure (with an agent such as lisinopril) at this point is unwarranted and unlikely to be effective.

Carotid artery dissection is typically recognized by the presence of unilateral pain of the head, neck, or face; partial Horner syndrome (ptosis, miosis); and cerebral or retinal ischemia. Less than one third of patients will have all three components. The patient has no headache or other features on examination that are consistent with an internal carotid artery dissection. The examination is instead consistent with oculomotor nerve (cranial nerve III) palsy. If internal carotid artery dissection were suspected, a magnetic resonance angiogram (MRA) of the neck would be an appropriate next step. It is not indicated in this patient.

A repeat MRA of the brain in 6 months also is inappropriate. This patient has now met several criteria for aneurysm surgery. Additional screening to document further changes in the size of the aneurysm will change nothing, and delaying surgery runs the risk of rupture.

KEY POINT

- Surgical treatment with clipping or endovascular coiling can be considered in patients with symptomatic aneurysms or aneurysms of 7 millimeters or greater in the posterior circulation (posterior communicating and basilar arteries).

Bibliography

Thompson BG, Brown RD Jr, Amin-Hanjani S, Broderick JP, Cockroft KM, Connolly ES Jr, et al; American Heart Association Stroke Council, Council on Cardiovascular and Stroke Nursing, and Council on Epidemiology and Prevention. Guidelines for the Management of Patients With Unruptured Intracranial Aneurysms: A Guideline for Healthcare Professionals From the American Heart Association/American Stroke Association. Stroke. 2015;46:2368-400. [PMID: 26089327] doi:10.1161/STR.0000000000000070

Item 43   Answer: D

Educational Objective: Treat psychosis in Parkinson disease.

The dopamine agonist pramipexole should be discontinued in this patient with Parkinson disease psychosis. Dopamine agonists, such as pramipexole, can be used as adjuvant therapy to limit the total dose of levodopa. Dopamine agonists are associated with higher risk of specific adverse effects, including impulse control disorder, punding, sleep attacks, ankle edema, and confusion, that may limit their use, especially in older patients. Impulse control disorder is the increased tendency for compulsive behaviors, such as excessive gambling, shopping, or hypersexuality. Punding is a complex prolonged, purposeless, and stereotyped behavior (such as collecting, sorting, cataloguing, or assembling and disassembling common objects). Sleep attacks involve falling asleep without warning. Medication-induced psychosis, especially visual hallucinations, triggered by dopaminergic medications also is a potential complication of Parkinson disease. All patients with Parkinson disease and psychosis should be evaluated for systemic triggers (such as infection and metabolic disturbance) and major depression. Reducing the dose of levodopa also can be considered after removal of the dopamine agonist, but this step may not be possible because of worsening of motor symptoms (as may occur in this patient given the recurrence of rigidity and slowness before each dose of medication). The decision to treat psychosis with medication adjustments or discontinuation should be based on the presence of distress to patient and caregivers, lack of insight in the patient, and progressive frequency of psychosis.

Pimavanserin, a nondopaminergic atypical antipsychotic agent and selective serotonin 5-hydroxytryptamine receptor 2A inverse agonist, is the only FDA-approved medication for Parkinson psychosis. Quetiapine and clozapine also can be considered in this setting, but most other atypical antipsychotic agents (including aripiprazole, risperidone, and olanzapine) and all typical (first-generation) antipsychotic agents should be avoided. Atypical antipsychotic agents should be used only after discontinuation of any non-levodopa Parkinson medication and resolution of systemic triggers.

KEY POINT

- Dopamine agonists are associated with higher risk of specific adverse effects, including psychosis, impulse control disorder, punding, sleep attacks, ankle edema, and confusion, that may limit their use, especially in older patients with Parkinson disease.

Bibliography

Samudra N, Patel N, Womack KB, Khemani P, Chitnis S. Psychosis in Parkinson disease: A review of etiology, phenomenology, and management. Drugs Aging. 2016;33:855-63. [PMID: 27830568]

Item 44   Answer: A

Educational Objective: Diagnose a subarachnoid hemorrhage.

The patient should undergo lumbar puncture. He has had a new thunderclap headache (severe headache that reaches maximum intensity within 1 minute) that has lasted 12 hours. Although a head CT scan without contrast was normal, an aneurysmal subarachnoid hemorrhage (SAH) is not always evident on CT scans and still needs to be excluded as a diagnosis. Several features of the patient's headache suggest aneurysmal SAH, including the sudden onset, nuchal rigidity, and pupillary dilation of the left eye. The latter finding can be seen with a posterior communicating artery aneurysm as it exerts pressure on the outer portion of the oculomotor nerve (cranial nerve III). Only examination of the cerebrospinal fluid (CSF) can effectively determine if this patient has such a hemorrhage. This test has a higher yield 12 hours or longer after headache onset when erythrocyte breakdown products will produce a yellow color (xanthochromia). Before then, the presence of erythrocytes can make it difficult to distinguish a traumatic lumbar puncture from an SAH. Examination of the CSF also allows for the evaluation of other potential causes, such as meningitis, although meningitis is unlikely in this patient, given the absence of fever and sudden onset of symptoms.

Magnetic resonance angiography is helpful in evaluating a carotid artery dissection, but the patient's examination findings are not consistent with this diagnosis. Clinically, carotid artery dissection is recognized by the presence of unilateral pain of the head, neck, or face; partial Horner syndrome (ptosis, miosis); and cerebral or retinal ischemia. However, less than one third of patients will have all three components. This patient has a global headache and an enlarged pupil consistent a compressive process involving the oculomotor nerve (cranial nerve III) and not Horner syndrome.

MRI is neither sensitive nor specific enough to definitively diagnose SAH. Furthermore, MRI is time consuming and not always available.

Given the patient's abnormal neurologic findings, performing no further testing to find the cause of his symptoms is inappropriate.

KEY POINT

- In a patient with a thunderclap headache and normal findings on a CT scan of the head, lumbar puncture should be performed next.

Bibliography

Thompson BG, Brown RD Jr, Amin-Hanjani S, Broderick JP, Cockroft KM, Connolly ES Jr, et al; American Heart Association Stroke Council, Council on Cardiovascular and Stroke Nursing, and Council on Epidemiology and Prevention. Guidelines for the management of patients with unruptured intracranial aneurysms: a guideline for healthcare professionals from the American Heart Association/American Stroke Association. Stroke. 2015;46:2368-400. [PMID: 26089327] doi:10.1161/STR.0000000000000070

Item 45   Answer: D

Educational Objective: Diagnose primary central nervous system lymphoma with vitreous fluid sampling.

This patient should undergo vitreous fluid sampling. He most likely has primary central nervous system lymphoma (PCNSL). PCNSL is a non-Hodgkin lymphoma that can affect any part of the central nervous system but commonly presents as a focal supratentorial lesion. Although PCNSL is commonly seen in patients with HIV infection, PCNSL is increasing in incidence among older, immunocompetent patients. An association with Epstein-Barr virus has been noted. Pathologic analysis, usually of a brain biopsy specimen, is required to make a diagnosis of PCNSL. Diffuse large B-cell lymphoma is typical. Cerebrospinal fluid (CSF) cytology can be diagnostic in 10% of patients, although repeated samples often are necessary. Ocular involvement in the vitreous or retina may be seen in 10% to 20% of patients and can be detected with a slit-lamp examination and confirmed by vitreous fluid sampling. In this patient, vitreous fluid collection with cytologic analysis may obviate the need for more invasive and potentially risky testing, such as brain biopsy. Despite being chemo- and radiosensitive, PCNSL typically recurs and has a generally poor prognosis.

Because the lesion is in the brainstem, brain biopsy can result in significant neurologic injury and is considered a high-risk procedure. Brain biopsy should be considered only if other tests have been unrevealing, including cytologic analysis of vitreous fluid.

When PCNSL is suspected, glucocorticoids should be avoided until the diagnosis is confirmed because they are lymphocytotoxic and can result in false-negative histopathologic or cytopathologic results. Although this patient has hydrocephalus, herniation and brain edema are not present, and thus glucocorticoid therapy may be delayed while the diagnostic evaluation is completed.

Lumbar puncture is contraindicated in a patient with mass effect and hydrocephalus because it may precipitate herniation. If mass effect with hydrocephalus were not present, CSF sampling would be a reasonable step because lymphomatous cells may often be present in the CSF and would establish the diagnosis of PCNSL.

KEY POINT

- Slit-lamp examination and vitreous fluid collection with cytologic analysis should be considered in patients with biopsy-inaccessible lesions who have suspected primary central nervous system lymphoma.

Bibliography

Hoang-Xuan K, Bessell E, Bromberg J, Hottinger AF, Preusser M, et al; European Association for Neuro-Oncology Task Force on Primary CNS Lymphoma. Diagnosis and treatment of primary CNS lymphoma in immunocompetent patients: guidelines from the European Association for Neuro-Oncology. Lancet Oncol. 2015 Jul;16(7):e322-32. doi: 10.1016/S1470-2045(15)00076-5. [PMID: 26149884]

Item 46   Answer: D

Educational Objective: Manage periodic limb movements of sleep.

This patient most likely has periodic limb movements of sleep, a disorder characterized by periodic leg kicks, often with a stereotyped triple-flexion phenomenology that repeats periodically during sleep. This condition can occur in otherwise healthy persons or be associated with sleep disorders, such as restless legs syndrome, sleep apnea, narcolepsy, and others. If another sleep disorder is present, treatment targeting the associated disorder also improves the periodic limb movements. If no associated sleep disorder is present (as is suggested in this patient by history and polysomnographic findings), treatment is only necessary if limb movements cause sleep fragmentation (brief arousals that occur during a sleep period). In the absence of such issues, no further testing or treatment is recommended.

Clonazepam often is used to treat rapid eye movement (REM) sleep behavior disorder, a condition associated with loss of the muscle paralysis normally experienced during the REM dream phase of sleep and typically characterized by dream enactment behavior with complex movements and vocalizations.

Electroencephalography (EEG) is indicated if nocturnal epilepsy is suspected. Nocturnal epilepsy is a major entity in the differential diagnosis of sleep-related movement disorders. However, this patient's stereotyped periodic movements are classic for periodic limb movements of sleep, and EEG is unnecessary.

Restless legs syndrome (RLS) is a common movement disorder characterized by discomforting sensations in the legs at rest or when falling asleep, an urge to move the legs, and immediate relief after moving the legs or walking. Patients with RLS should be screened for iron deficiency and receive iron supplements in the presence of deficiency or even low-normal serum ferritin levels. This patient does not have symptoms of RLS, such as sensory abnormalities or the urge to move.

KEY POINT

- The disorder periodic limb movements of sleep is characterized by periodic leg kicks that often exhibit a stereotyped triple-flexion phenomenology repeating periodically during sleep; if no associated sleep disorder is present, reassurance is the best management.

Bibliography

Aurora RN, Kristo DA, Bista SR, Rowley JA, Zak RS, Casey KR, et al; American Academy of Sleep Medicine. The treatment of restless legs syndrome and periodic limb movement disorder in adults–an update for 2012: practice parameters with an evidence-based systematic review and meta-analyses: an American Academy of Sleep Medicine Clinical Practice Guideline. Sleep. 2012;35:1039-62. [PMID: 22851801] doi:10.5665/sleep.1988

Item 47   Answer: A

Educational Objective: Diagnose epidural hematoma.

The patient has an epidural hematoma. This head injury most commonly results from a fracture of the temporal bone and subsequent laceration of the ipsilateral middle meningeal artery. Only 20% to 30% of these hematomas occur in other locations, and most follow trauma; spontaneous hemorrhages are rare. An epidural hematoma develops between the inner table of the skull and the dura mater. Lateral extension is prevented by dual attachments at the skull sutures; expansion occurs inwardly towards the brain parenchyma. Appearance on a head CT scan is biconvex or "lenticular." After a lucid interval, neurologic deterioration is rapid. Peak expansion of the hematoma occurs 6 to 8 hours after initial formation. Severe headache, nausea with vomiting, and eventual impairment in consciousness progress quickly. Ipsilateral compression of the occulomotor nerve (cranial nerve III) indicates potential uncal herniation. Subsequent ipsilateral midbrain compression results in contralateral upper motor neuron findings. Emergent surgical evacuation is required for those with anisocoria, a Glasgow Coma Scale (GCS) score of less than 9, or a hematoma volume greater than 30 mL.

Lobar hemorrhages are collections of blood within the brain parenchyma. Common causes are hypertension, anticoagulation, cerebral amyloid angiopathy, and aneurysmal or arteriovenous malformation rupture. Hemorrhage into areas of ischemic infarction or into tumors of primary central nervous system or metastatic origin also may be seen. Mass effect (from the hemorrhage) and the surrounding area of edema lead to a variety of neurologic presentations, some of which may require surgical evacuation.

Subarachnoid hemorrhage can result from trauma or, more commonly, rupture of an intracranial cerebral artery aneurysm. This hemorrhage is not confined by anatomic landmarks and typically spreads throughout the subarachnoid space.

Subdural hematomas are collections of blood between the brain and the dura mater. Most involve rupture of veins bridging the subarachnoid space. Because of cerebral atrophy and stretching of these veins, older patients are particularly vulnerable. Subdural hematomas can occur spontaneously or as a result of cranial trauma, and presentations range from acute to chronic. Those with acute subdural hematoma are at high mortality risk and require urgent surgical evacuation. GCS scores of less than 9, pupillary asymmetry, and hematomas greater than 10 mm in thickness are indications for emergent surgery.

KEY POINT

- Typical symptoms of epidural hematoma include severe headache, nausea with vomiting, and eventual impairment in consciousness with neurologic deterioration; emergent surgical evacuation is required when anisocoria, a Glasgow Coma Scale score of less than 9, or a hematoma volume greater than 30 mL is present.

Bibliography

Rincon S, Gupta R, Ptak T. Imaging of head trauma. Handb Clin Neurol. 2016;135:447-77. [PubMed: 27432678] doi: 10.1016/B978-0-444-53485-9.00022-2

Item 48   Answer: C

Educational Objective: Diagnose metabolic myopathy.

This patient has metabolic myopathy consistent with McArdle disease (glycogen storage disease V). This diagnosis is supported by a history of exercise intolerance associated with myalgia, "mild" weakness, and myoglobinuria and by laboratory evidence of chronic kidney disease (elevated serum creatinine level secondary to myoglobinuria). McArdle disease is caused by myophosphorylase deficiency and may be underdiagnosed because of the variability and intermittent nature of its symptoms. Patients with McArdle disease often do not have any muscle weakness or atrophy at baseline evaluation but may develop transient "mild" weakness after exertion. They can protect against severe exercise intolerance by eating a carbohydrate-rich diet before exercise; they also often describe a characteristic "second-wind" phenomenon by which a brief break taken after onset of cramping and fatigue allows for a higher level of exercise tolerance with much less difficulty.

Acute intermittent porphyria (AIP) is characterized by acute attacks of abdominal pain and vomiting and by central, peripheral, sensory, motor, autonomic, and enteric nervous system abnormalities. Patients may have episodes of reddish-brown urine (porphobilin and porphyrins) during an acute attack. AIP does not have a myopathic presentation and is not associated with intermittent exercise intolerance or "second-wind" phenomenon.

Limb-girdle muscular dystrophies are associated with baseline muscle atrophy and weakness and not with crises of exercise intolerance.

Myotonic dystrophy is unlikely in the absence of myotonia (delayed muscle relaxation), fixed muscle weakness, stiffness, and multiorgan involvement. Crises of exercise intolerance and myoglobinuria are not typical in myotonic dystrophy.

Symmetric painless proximal weakness of the arms and legs is the classic feature of polymyositis. Onset is acute or subacute, with disease progressing over weeks. A prolonged clinical course without baseline weakness and a history of exercise intolerance is not consistent with polymyositis.

KEY POINT

- McArdle disease is a metabolic myopathy associated with exercise intolerance, cramping, myalgia, mild weakness, "second-wind" phenomenon, and myoglobinuria.

Bibliography

Adler M, Shieh PB. Metabolic myopathies. Semin Neurol. 2015;35:385-97. [PMID: 26502762] doi:10.1055/s-0035-1558973

Item 49   Answer: C

Educational Objective: Diagnose dementia with Lewy bodies.

Rapid eye movement (REM) sleep behavior disorder commonly occurs in dementia with Lewy bodies (DLB) and can help distinguish DLB from Alzheimer disease and other cognitive disorders. This patient has cognitive and other symptoms suggestive of mild DLB. All the synucleinopathies (Parkinson disease, Parkinson disease dementia, and DLB) have a much higher rate of REM sleep behavioral sleep disorder than other neurologic and neurodegenerative diseases. REM sleep behavior disorder is characterized by the acting out of dreams secondary to loss of normal muscle paralysis during the dream phase of sleep. Symptoms may range from hand gestures to violent thrashing, punching, and kicking that may result in harm to self or bed partner. Patients also may have severe sensitivity to neuroleptic medications, which is more common in DLB than in other dementing illnesses.

Delusions occur in both Alzheimer disease (especially the later stages) and DLB; frank hallucinations are more typical of DLB. Therefore, the presence of delusions is unlikely to help distinguish Alzheimer disease from DLB.

Depression is a common symptom in most neurodegenerative dementia syndromes; it occurs in as many as 40% to 60% of patients with Alzheimer disease at some point of their disease. Its presence in this patient would not help establish a diagnosis.

Repeated falls can occur in DLB but also in vascular cognitive impairment, normal pressure hydrocephalus, and the later stages of Alzheimer disease. Therefore, this finding is unlikely to help in establishing a diagnosis in this patient.

KEY POINT

- Rapid eye movement sleep behavior disorder commonly occurs in dementia with Lewy bodies (DLB) and can help distinguish DLB from Alzheimer disease and other cognitive disorders.

Bibliography

Walker Z, Possin KL, Boeve BF, Aarsland D. Lewy body dementias. Lancet. 2015;386:1683-97. [PMID: 26595642] doi:10.1016/S0140-6736(15)00462-6

Item 50   Answer: B

Educational Objective: Treat acute intracerebral hemorrhage.

This patient should receive intravenous nicardipine. She has an acute intracerebral hemorrhage whose location suggests hypertension as the cause. Systolic blood pressure on emergent physical examination is greater than 180 mm Hg; this means she is at high risk for hematoma expansion. The systolic blood pressure should thus be lowered to a target of 140 mm Hg with a rapidly acting intravenous agent, such as intravenous nicardipine. A recently completed trial that compared systolic blood pressure targets of 120 mm Hg and 140 mm Hg noted increased adverse renal events in the treatment

CONT.

arm with lower blood pressure. Whatever intravenous anti-hypertensive agent is chosen, it should be possible to taper its dose quickly if systolic blood pressure becomes too low.

Hematoma evacuation is an inappropriate treatment because the patient's intracerebral hemorrhage is not near the cortical surface, and the clinical and imaging findings show no evidence of elevated intracranial pressure (ICP) or cerebral herniation. If she were to have neurologic decline, repeat head CT would be appropriate to evaluate for hematoma expansion. Candidates for surgical evacuation of an intracerebral hematoma include those with evidence of elevated ICP or a cerebellar hemorrhage greater than 3 centimeters in size.

Nitroprusside is not a first-line blood pressure treatment for patients with acute hemorrhagic stroke, given its potential for increasing ICP.

There is no evidence that platelet transfusion reverses the coagulopathy associated with antiplatelet agents or prevents hematoma expansion. Platelet transfusion also carries the risk of coronary stent thrombosis, volume overload, and transfusion-related reactions.

KEY POINT

- Patients who have intracerebral hemorrhage without elevated intracranial pressure whose systolic blood pressure is greater than 180 mm Hg should be treated with an intravenous antihypertensive agent, such as nicardipine, to a target blood pressure of 140 mm Hg.

Bibliography

Hemphill JC 3rd, Greenberg SM, Anderson CS, Becker K, Bendok BR, Cushman M, et al; American Heart Association Stroke Council. Guidelines for the management of spontaneous intracerebral hemorrhage: a guideline for healthcare professionals from the American Heart Association/American Stroke Association. Stroke. 2015;46:2032-60. [PMID: 26022637] doi:10.1161/STR.0000000000000069

Item 51   Answer: E

Educational Objective: **Prevent cluster headache.**

This patient should be treated with verapamil. His history is compatible with the diagnosis of cluster headache. Cluster headache is the most common of the trigeminal autonomic cephalalgias (TACs). The term "cluster" is derived from this disorder's characteristic short cycles of headache activity (weeks) interrupted by long periods of complete remission (month or years). Male sex and tobacco use are two potential risk factors. Alcohol is a commonly reported trigger during an active cycle. Episodes are common nocturnally and may occur seasonally. Attack duration is between 15 and 180 minutes. Pain is almost always unilateral and localized near the temple or orbit. Ipsilateral autonomic symptoms, such as tearing, ptosis, nasal congestion, and rhinorrhea, are characteristic. Attacks may occur one to eight times daily for several weeks or months. Brain MRI should be performed initially to exclude structural lesions mimicking cluster headache. Oxygen inhalation and subcutaneous sumatriptan are first-line therapies for acute cluster headache. The patient should be counseled to stop smoking. Verapamil is the preventive medication of choice.

Carbamazepine is the treatment of choice for trigeminal neuralgia, which most often occurs in patients older than 50 years, but has no effect on cluster headache or any of the TACs. Periorbital location of pain would be atypical for trigeminal neuralgia, as would an attack duration beyond seconds. Ipsilateral autonomic symptoms are also generally absent.

Fexofenadine, a second-generation antihistamine, has no established benefit in cluster headache. This patient has no history of allergic rhinitis or other conditions that would respond to an antihistamine.

Several indomethacin-responsive headache syndromes have been identified, but cluster headache is not among them. Chronic paroxysmal hemicrania is a TAC that responds to indomethacin. Episodes of this condition last only 3 to 20 minutes and can recur up to 40 times daily. The diagnosis also requires concomitant ipsilateral autonomic findings, such as tearing, nasal congestion, or rhinorrhea.

Propranolol is an effective migraine preventive therapy but has no benefit for cluster headache. Migraine may present with severe periorbital headache with nausea and photophobia and occasionally with autonomic features. Unlike cluster headache, which typically lasts 15 to 180 minutes, migraine by definition extends 4 to 72 hours without treatment.

KEY POINT

- Cluster headache, the most common of the trigeminal autonomic cephalalgias, is best prevented with verapamil.

Bibliography

Pareja J, Alvarez M. The usual treatment of trigeminal autonomic cephalalgias. Headache. 2013 Oct;53(9):1401-14. [PMID: 24090529] doi:10.1111/head.12193

Item 52   Answer: D

Educational Objective: **Diagnose familial amyloidosis.**

The most likely diagnosis is familial amyloidosis. His progressive sensory, motor, and autonomic axonal polyneuropathy; bilateral carpal tunnel syndrome; and family history of neuropathy and cardiac disease suggest familial amyloidosis. This disorder is diagnosed by detection of a transthyretin gene (*TTR*) mutation. Affected patients often have multiorgan involvement (diseases of the eye [glaucoma] and the neurologic, gastrointestinal, cardiac, and urinary systems), but there is wide phenotypic variation leading to delayed diagnosis. Therefore, a high level of clinical suspicion of amyloidosis is necessary in the presence of relentless progression of neuropathy, autonomic dysfunction, and positive family history of typical symptoms.

This patient has no evidence of upper motor neuron disease on clinical examination and exhibits prominent sensory and autonomic neuropathy, which are inconsistent with amyotrophic lateral sclerosis.

In this patient, the electromyographic (EMG) findings, positive family history, absence of upper motor neuron findings, and diffuse dysautonomia are inconsistent with a cervical myelopathy.

This patient's EMG findings are consistent with an axonal neuropathy, not a demyelinating neuropathy such as chronic inflammatory demyelinating polyradiculoneuropathy.

West Nile virus, which typically has an acute or subacute (not chronic) course, can cause a flaccid motor myelopathy that does not involve sensory and autonomic small fiber neurons.

KEY POINT

- Familial amyloidosis is characterized by predominantly sensory and motor peripheral neuropathy and/or autonomic neuropathy; it is diagnosed by detecting a mutation of the transthyretin gene.

Bibliography

Adams D, Lozeron P, Lacroix C. Amyloid neuropathies. Curr Opin Neurol. 2012;25:564-72. [PMID: 22941262] doi:10.1097/WCO.0b013e328357bdf6

Item 53   Answer: A

Educational Objective: Diagnose nonconvulsive status epilepticus.

The patient should undergo continuous (24-hour) electroencephalography (EEG). He has fluctuating mental status of unknown origin in the setting of a critical illness, sepsis, and multiorgan dysfunction. These findings raise suspicion of nonconvulsive status epilepticus (NCSE), which is intermittent electrical seizure activity without clinically evident seizure activity. A 20-minute EEG usually is inadequately sensitive to capture seizures, particularly if they are occurring intermittently. NCSE also is increasingly diagnosed in critically ill comatose or stuporous patients with acute neurologic or medical conditions who have not had a convulsive seizure. Similar to NCSE following CSE, NCSE in critically ill populations also is associated with increased morbidity and mortality and requires prompt attention and intervention. The diagnostic test of choice is continuous (24-hour) EEG monitoring. Most critically ill patients with nonconvulsive seizures have their first detectable seizure with EEG monitoring within 24 hours of initiating the recording, but an additional 12% have detectable seizures with 48 hours of continuous monitoring. Cefepime has been known to cause encephalopathy, coma, and status epilepticus in patients with or without epilepsy, especially those with acute kidney injury, and its use should raise the clinician's suspicion of NCSE.

Empiric treatment with fosphenytoin or lorazepam is generally not recommended until the diagnosis of NCSE or intermittent nonconvulsive seizures is confirmed by EEG. This approach differs from the treatment of generalized convulsive status epilepticus, which is diagnosed clinically and, optimally, treated without delay.

Providing no treatment is inadequate as the next step in management for this patient with altered mental status, a fluctuating level of consciousness, and other abnormalities on neurologic and laboratory testing. The diagnosis of NCSE first must be established (or excluded).

KEY POINT

- Nonconvulsive status epilepticus should be suspected in patients with critical illness who develop altered mental status; the diagnosis is confirmed with continuous (24-hour) electroencephalography.

Bibliography

Herman ST, Abend NS, Bleck TP, Chapman KE, Drislane FW, Emerson RG, et al; Critical Care Continuous EEG Task Force of the American Clinical Neurophysiology Society. Consensus statement on continuous EEG in critically ill adults and children, part I: indications. J Clin Neurophysiol. 2015;32:87-95. [PMID: 25626778] doi:10.1097/WNP.0000000000000166

Item 54   Answer: E

Educational Objective: Diagnose subacute combined degeneration due to vitamin B_{12} deficiency.

This patient's serum level of vitamin B_{12} should be measured. His examination findings are consistent with a myelopathy localizing to both the posterior columns and the corticospinal tracts of the spinal cord, and neuroimaging confirms the diagnosis. Common entities causing this pattern of weakness and sensory deficits are vitamin B_{12} deficiency, copper deficiency, and neurosyphilis. When these symptoms occur as a consequence of vitamin B_{12} or copper deficiency, the neurologic syndrome is termed subacute combined degeneration. This patient's previous chronic abuse of nitrous oxide has resulted in a functional B_{12} deficiency that is due to inactivation of the vitamin. In patients who abuse nitrous oxide, the B_{12} level also is often low or low-normal, with elevated methylmalonic acid and homocysteine levels. Not all patients with neurologic abnormalities will have anemia or macrocytosis.

Although low 25-hydroxyvitamin D levels have been associated with several conditions, including increased risk for autoimmune disease, this vitamin deficiency itself is not a cause of myelopathy.

Similarly, thiamine deficiency is associated with Wernicke-Korsakoff syndrome (nystagmus, ophthalmoplegia, ataxia, and confusion) but not with myelopathy. Wernicke encephalopathy most commonly occurs in persons with alcoholism but also has been reported in patients who have undergone bariatric surgery, have had a prolonged period of fasting, have had repeated episodes of vomiting, or have been on prolonged parenteral nutrition without adequate vitamin supplementation.

Vitamin A deficiency can cause blindness and hypervitaminosis and has been associated with benign idiopathic intracranial hypertension. Vitamin A deficiency is rarely seen in the United States but is the most common vitamin deficiency worldwide. When it does occur in resource-rich countries, it typically is associated with conditions causing fat malabsorption, such as pancreatic insufficiency, celiac disease, or certain forms of bariatric surgery. Alterations in vitamin A level do not result in myelopathy.

Vitamin B$_6$ deficiency is not common but may be associated with drugs that interfere with its metabolism, including isoniazid, hydralazine, carbidopa, and levodopa. The most common manifestations are stomatitis, glossitis, cheilosis, confusion, and depression. Both deficiency and toxicity of this nutrient can cause peripheral neuropathy. The upper motor neuron signs evident on physical examination of this patient, however, rule out a peripheral neuropathy.

KEY POINT

- Subacute combined degeneration is a myelopathy manifesting as dysfunction of the corticospinal tracts and dorsal columns that is caused by vitamin B$_{12}$ and copper deficiencies.

Bibliography

Briani C, Dalla Torre C, Citton V, Manara R, Pompanin S, Binotto G, et al. Cobalamin deficiency: clinical picture and radiological findings. Nutrients. 2013;5:4521-39. [PMID: 24248213] doi:10.3390/nu5114521

Item 55   Answer: A

Educational Objective: Treat impaired mobility in multiple sclerosis.

This patient should be given dalfampridine. She has multiple sclerosis (MS) and had a relapse more than 1 year ago that resulted in poor recovery of left leg function, which is likely now permanent. Maintenance of mobility in patients with MS is essential for maintaining overall quality of life, and maintenance of an active, healthy lifestyle can help stave off future disability. Physical and occupational therapy is useful to ensure gait safety and improve walking ability and endurance. Assistive aids, such as braces, canes, walkers, and electrostimulatory walk-assist devices, can be useful for many patients. Two recent phase III studies found that dalfampridine, a voltage-gated potassium channel antagonist, significantly improved timed 25-foot walking speeds in patients with multiple sclerosis and gait impairment. This medication theoretically helps boost conductance through demyelinated axonal pathways, which may be of most benefit for long axons, such as those providing motor signals to the legs. As a consequence of this method of action, however, dalfampridine has the rare adverse effect of seizures and should not be used in patients with kidney impairment, given the reduced clearance of the drug and resultant potentially higher rate of seizures.

Pseudobulbar affect, a less common symptomatic manifestation of MS, can act as a significant impediment to social interaction in patients with MS. This symptom manifests as uncontrolled fits of laughter or crying that occur without distinct or appropriate triggers. A successful trial of the combination agent dextromethorphan-quinidine has led to FDA approval of the use of this pharmacotherapy for pseudobulbar affect in MS. It is not effective for improving or maintaining ambulation.

Gabapentin's most frequent use in MS is to treat neuropathic pain, which this patient currently is not experiencing. There is no evidence that this medication benefits impaired mobility.

Memantine frequently is used in mild to severe Alzheimer disease to boost cognition but has not been shown to benefit cognitive dysfunction or to increase mobility in MS patients. In fact, one small study found transient worsening of MS symptoms in those taking memantine.

Modafinil also is inappropriate. This drug is frequently used to treat MS-related fatigue but has no impact on muscle strength or walking ability.

KEY POINT

- In patients with multiple sclerosis and impaired mobility, dalfampridine is the most appropriate medication.

Bibliography

Goodman AD, Brown TR, Edwards KR, Krupp LB, Schapiro RT, Cohen R, et al; MSF204 Investigators. A phase 3 trial of extended release oral dalfampridine in multiple sclerosis. Ann Neurol. 2010;68:494-502. [PMID: 20976768] doi:10.1002/ana.22240

Item 56   Answer: A

Educational Objective: Diagnose diabetic mononeuropathy.

This patient most likely has diabetic mononeuropathy. He has an elevated hemoglobin A$_{1c}$ value that is consistent with a diagnosis of diabetes mellitus and has no evidence of herpes zoster infection. Truncal diabetic mononeuropathy presents with acute or subacute pain and paresthesia in a dermatomal pattern in the thoracic or abdominal region. The area affected may be unilateral or cross the midline. Associated weakness of abdominal wall muscles can also be present and is detected by the presence of apparent abdominal swelling in the absence of palpable organomegaly. The differential diagnosis for this condition includes truncal radiculopathy caused by varicella zoster infection and thoracic myelopathy caused by demyelinating disease.

Paraproteinemic neuropathy can present as a symmetric distal sensory neuropathy or as sensorimotor, multifocal motor, and cranial neuropathies. The normal results of serum electrophoresis and serum free light chain measurement rules out this diagnosis.

Uremic neuropathy is similar to other neuropathies caused by metabolic disruptions and is associated with distal symmetric polyneuropathy. Asymmetric truncal neuropathy is not a typical presentation. Also, uremic neuropathy is often associated with a more severe degree of kidney injury than is present in this patient.

Vitamin B$_{12}$ deficiency can cause myeloneuropathy, distal symmetric neuropathy, and cranial neuropathy but typically does not present as truncal mononeuropathy.

KEY POINT

- Acute or subacute pain and paresthesia in a dermatomal pattern in the thoracic or abdominal region in a patient with diabetes mellitus and no evidence of herpes zoster is most likely due to diabetic mononeuropathy.

Bibliography

Pasnoor M, Dimachkie MM, Barohn RJ. Diabetic neuropathy part 2: proximal and asymmetric phenotypes. Neurol Clin. 2013;31:447-62. [PMID: 23642718] doi:10.1016/j.ncl.2013.02.003

Item 57   Answer: C

Educational Objective: Diagnose spinal cord compression.

This patient should undergo emergent MRI of the lumbosacral spine. His history and clinical findings suggest acute (or subacute) compression of the lower spinal cord–most likely a cauda equina syndrome–given the finding of saddle anesthesia and the absence of a sensory spinal level on physical examination. Given the elevated INR, the most likely diagnosis is a spinal epidural hematoma compressing the lumbosacral spine. MRI is the most appropriate test to localize the injury and determine its cause, both of which are necessary to make an immediate treatment plan. Of note, an MRI of the thoracic spine is not appropriate for this patient; although compression of the thoracic spine could cause an acute myelopathy, it would be unlikely to produce saddle anesthesia in the sacral pattern noted, and the lack of a thoracic spine sensory level on physical examination makes this localization unlikely. Given the suspected hemorrhagic cause of cord compression, noncontrast CT could be an alternative imaging modality in this patient.

Surgical decompression will likely be required to treat nerve root compression due to a probable hematoma. In this patient, management of the bleeding diathesis by correcting the INR also will be necessary. Glucocorticoids have no role in treating spinal cord compression caused by a hematoma. Several trials have shown a benefit of high-dose intravenous glucocorticoids administered within the first 8 hours of traumatic spinal cord injury and in the management of metastatic spinal cord compression.

A CT myelogram would be inappropriate for this patient. Although the myelogram may show compression of the cord, it does not always reveal the cause. Furthermore, this test is difficult to obtain on an emergency basis, given the interventional nature of the procedure, and cannot be used in patients with contrast dye allergies or impaired kidney function. CT myelography is useful when MRI is not feasible (as in patients with implantable devices).

A radiograph of the lumbosacral spine is unlikely to reveal an epidural hematoma or cord compression. This test would be most appropriate in traumatic injury of the spine to investigate for fracture.

KEY POINT

- In a patient with suspected compression of the lower spinal cord, emergent MRI of the lumbosacral spine is the most appropriate test both to localize the injury and to determine its cause.

Bibliography

Kelley BC, Arnold PM, Anderson KK. Spinal emergencies. J Neurosurg Sci. 2012;56:113-29. [PMID: 22617174]

Item 58   Answer: C

Educational Objective: Diagnose idiopathic intracranial hypertension.

This patient should have a lumbar puncture. The clinical picture is compatible with idiopathic intracranial hypertension (IIH), and lumbar puncture is required to confirm the diagnosis. Although most presentations of IIH occur in the context of obesity in women of child-bearing age, several other risk factors have been identified. Exposure to minocycline or other members of the tetracycline class of antibiotics has been linked to the development of IIH. Retinoic acid, estrogen and progesterone supplements, and glucocorticoids are other drugs implicated as causes of this disorder. Headaches, vision changes, and intracranial noises are the most common presenting symptoms. Visual blurring, diplopia, and brief episodic dimming (obscurations) also are common, and papilledema is characteristic; abducens nerve (cranial nerve VI) palsy occurs occasionally. Cerebrospinal fluid (CSF) analysis typically shows an elevated opening pressure (>250 mm H_2O) with normal CSF composition. The treatment of choice is acetazolamide.

Amitriptyline is the preventive medication of choice for chronic tension-type headache (CTTH). Although the headache described in this patient is similar to that of CTTH, the presence of vision changes and intracranial noises would be atypical, and abducens nerve palsy is incompatible with that diagnosis.

Of the indomethacin-responsive headache syndromes, only hemicrania continua is possible in a patient with daily headache. However, the bilateral location of the headache pain, the absence of cranial autonomic features, and the presence of papilledema and abducens nerve palsy are incompatible with that diagnosis.

Magnetic resonance angiography is indicated in cases of suspected intracranial or cervical arterial disease. Although occulomotor nerve (cranial nerve III) palsy is common with an aneurysm of the posterior communicating artery, isolated abducens nerve palsy from vascular lesions is unusual. Carotid or vertebral dissections may result in Horner syndrome or, less commonly, ophthalmoplegia but not papilledema.

Temporal artery biopsy would be indicated in cases of suspected giant cell arteritis, which most commonly presents after age 50 years. Despite classic involvement of the temporal artery, pain may occur in various head locations. Amaurosis and jaw claudication are common associated features. Although cranial nerve palsies occasionally are noted, papilledema is not.

KEY POINT

- In a patient with suspected idiopathic intracranial hypertension, lumbar puncture is required to confirm the diagnosis.

Bibliography

Markey KA, Mollan SP, Jensen RH, Sinclair AJ. Understanding idiopathic intracranial hypertension: mechanisms, management, and future directions. Lancet Neurol. 2016 Jan;15(1):78-91. Epub 2015 Dec 8. [PMID: 26700907] doi:10.1016/S1474-4422(15)00298-7

Item 59   Answer: E

Educational Objective: Treat asymptomatic extracranial carotid artery stenosis.

This patient with 60% to 80% stenosis of the left internal carotid artery should receive no further treatment or intervention. The patient's LDL cholesterol level indicates that his atherogenic dyslipidemia is adequately treated with pravastatin, a moderate-intensity statin. Although there is some evidence suggesting that his 10-year risk for a major cardiovascular event is high enough to warrant switching to a high-dose, high-intensity statin, there are no specific guidelines recommending such a change. Asymptomatic carotid artery stenosis was not included in the definition of atherosclerotic cardiovascular disease used in the latest dyslipidemia treatment targets. Data are insufficient among patients with asymptomatic disease to recommend a specific therapy beyond treatment with a statin; there is currently no consensus on which statin and what dose to use.

Carotid endarterectomy or stenting is not the best treatment for this patient. The patient has asymptomatic internal carotid artery stenosis of 60% to 80%; the risk of stroke with best medical therapy is very low. Carotid revascularization with either endarterectomy or stenting, on the other hand, has a higher risk of adverse effects, including stroke, and its absolute risk reduction of stroke in asymptomatic patients is small, particularly among patients with stenosis of 80% or less. According to previous studies, predictors of stroke with asymptomatic internal carotid artery stenosis include greater than 80% stenosis, asymptomatic infarcts on brain imaging, an abnormal transcranial Doppler ultrasound study, or rapid progression. Carotid revascularization should be considered in patients at low risk for perioperative cardiovascular morbidity who have greater than 80% stenosis only in the context of a clinical trial.

Magnetic resonance angiography (MRA) of the neck is inappropriate because an additional diagnostic test is unlikely to change medical management. The accuracy of MRA without contrast versus carotid ultrasound is likely similar, but neck MRA is associated with patient discomfort and a higher cost.

Because there is no clear evidence that clopidogrel is superior to aspirin for the primary prevention of stroke in the setting of asymptomatic internal carotid artery stenosis, replacing this patient's aspirin with clopidogrel is unwarranted.

KEY POINT

- Statin therapy is indicated for asymptomatic carotid stenosis of 60% to 80%.

Bibliography

Marquardt L, Geraghty OC, Mehta Z, Rothwell PM. Low risk of ipsilateral stroke in patients with asymptomatic carotid stenosis on best medical treatment: A prospective, population-based study. Stroke 2010 Jan; 41:e11-7. [PMID: 19926843]

Item 60   Answer: B

Educational Objective: Manage Guillain-Barré syndrome.

This patient with Guillain-Barré syndrome (GBS) who exhibits improvement after an initial course of plasma exchange should be discharged to rehabilitation. A diagnosis of GBS, an acute inflammatory demyelinating polyradiculoneuropathy, is supported by prodromal systemic infection, ascending weakness, radicular symptoms, cerebrospinal fluid albuminocytologic dissociation (elevated protein, normal leukocyte count), demyelinating changes (reduced conduction velocity) on a nerve conduction study, and areflexia. GBS is a monophasic disease with weakness reaching its nadir in less than 4 weeks. Given that this patient has already passed the nadir of weakness and is stable from a respiratory and autonomic standpoint, she should be transferred to a rehabilitation center. Rates of full recovery can be slow, but 80% of patients resume ambulation by 6 months.

In a patient with GBS who is already extubated and whose motor strength has improved by 50%, continued monitoring in the hospital is unnecessary and would not be cost-effective high value care. Additionally, early initiation of an active rehabilitation program would reduce the risk of secondary weakness caused by decompensation.

Repeating plasma exchange is indicated in GBS only if symptoms get worse after initial improvement or stabilization. This patient has experienced no deterioration.

Treatment with intravenous glucocorticoids is contraindicated in GBS and may worsen the clinical outcome.

Although intravenous immune globulin (IVIG) has the same efficacy as plasma exchange in shortening the time to recovery and reducing the duration of ventilation in GBS, serial treatment with IVIG after plasma exchange is not superior to either treatment alone and is not recommended. An exception would be if symptoms deteriorate after initial improvement or stabilization.

KEY POINT

- A hospitalized patient with Guillain-Barré syndrome who exhibits improvement after an initial course of plasma exchange should be discharged to rehabilitation.

Bibliography

Willison HJ, Jacobs BC, van Doorn PA. Guillain-Barré syndrome. Lancet. 2016;388:717-27. [PMID: 26948435] doi:10.1016/S0140-6736(16)00339-1

Item 61   Answer: B

Educational Objective: Avoid antiepileptic medications that can accelerate bone loss in patients with osteoporosis.

Lamotrigine is the most appropriate antiepileptic drug (AED) to treat this patient's focal seizures. Carbamazepine, phenytoin, and phenobarbital are all inducers of the cytochrome p450 system; these drugs increase breakdown of vitamin D, which results in increased parathyroid hormone levels, and thus cause bone loss and osteoporosis. Valproic acid also is associated with bone loss, although the mechanism of this effect is unclear. Lamotrigine and other AEDs that do not induce the P450 system, such as levetiracetam, have no recognized effect on bone turnover; therefore, of the choices listed, lamotrigine is the most appropriate AED to use in a patient with established osteoporosis.

All patients on chronic AED therapy with phenytoin, carbamazepine, phenobarbital or valproic acid should undergo initial bone densitometry testing after 5 years of therapy, regardless of age, sex, or menopausal status. Those especially at risk are nonambulatory and physically inactive patients with epilepsy who have a non–weight-bearing status. Screening should be repeated, depending on the results, but not more frequently than every 2 years.

Patients with AED-associated osteoporosis should be assessed for adequate intake of calcium and vitamin D, with initiation of supplementation if intake is inadequate or if low levels of 25-hydroxyvitamin D are noted. Otherwise, treatment for osteoporosis associated with AEDs is the same as for osteoporosis in general and usually involves administration of a bisphosphonate, such as alendronate.

KEY POINT

- Lamotrigine does not have the potential to cause or worsen osteoporosis in patients with epilepsy.

Bibliography

Schmidt D. Starting, choosing, changing, and discontinuing drug treatment for epilepsy patients. Neurol Clin. 2016 May;34(2) (2016): 363-81, viii. Epub 2016 Mar 5. [PMID: 27086984] doi:10.1016/j.ncl.2015.11.007

Item 62   Answer: C

Educational Objective: Treat subarachnoid hemorrhage with nimodipine.

This patient should receive nimodipine. She has an aneurysmal subarachnoid hemorrhage (SAH) and is at high risk for neurologic decline from cerebral vasospasm. The risk of vasospasm is greatest 5 to 10 days after SAH onset. Nimodipine is indicted for all nonhypotensive patients with SAH and is associated with improved neurologic outcomes and survival. Because nimodipine may not directly reduce the vasospasm, additional monitoring with repeat neurologic examinations and transcranial Doppler ultrasonography is indicated in a specialized ICU. The presence of vasospasm is suggested by worsening findings on neurologic examination and can be confirmed with CT angiography or catheter angiography, with the latter test having the additional benefit of providing endovascular therapy.

Glucocorticoids, such as dexamethasone, are not routinely indicated for any stroke subtype and are ineffective in reducing intracranial pressure in that setting. One randomized study of 95 patients with aneurysmal SAH treated with 3 days of methylprednisolone showed improved 1-year functional outcomes in patients. However, the preponderance of evidence does not support glucocorticoid treatment for SAH.

Magnesium sulfate therapy has been used to prevent vasospasm following SAH, but randomized trials have not shown improved clinical outcomes. A 2013 systematic review and meta-analysis concluded that while intravenous magnesium reduced delayed cerebral ischemia, there was no improvement in clinical neurologic outcomes.

Nitroglycerin is not an appropriate treatment for this patient. Given the risk of cerebral vasospasm, blood pressure often is allowed to remain elevated in such patients. If her blood pressure were to require treatment, nitroglycerin would be inappropriate because it can increase cerebral venous volume and intracranial pressure, which is a concern in patients with SAH.

Verapamil is a calcium channel blocker, as is nimodipine, but verapamil has not been shown to improve outcomes in patients with SAH or vasospasm.

KEY POINT

- Nimodipine is indicated for all nonhypotensive patients with subarachnoid hemorrhage and is associated with improved neurologic outcomes and survival.

Bibliography

Hemphill JC 3rd, Greenberg SM, Anderson CS, Becker K, Bendok BR, Cushman M, et al; American Heart Association Stroke Council. Guidelines for the management of spontaneous intracerebral hemorrhage: a guideline for healthcare professionals from the American Heart Association/American Stroke Association. Stroke. 2015;46:2032-60. [PMID: 26022637] doi:10.1161/STR.0000000000000069

Item 63   Answer: B

Educational Objective: Screen a patient with Parkinson disease for risk of falling backward.

This patient's risk of falling backward is best determined by the pull test, which is the most sensitive predictor of risk of backward falls in Parkinson disease. During this test of postural stability, the examiner throws the patient off base by pulling backward on the shoulders; the test is considered positive if the patient topples into the examiner's arms or takes more than two corrective steps. Backward falls are often related to loss of postural reflexes and resultant postural instability. Additional factors, including insufficient control of motor symptoms, dyskinesia, and orthostatic hypotension, also can contribute to falls in Parkinson disease. In this patient, history and gait assessment did not reveal any interference with balance caused by freezing of gait or lower body dyskinesia, and he had no symptoms or findings suggestive of orthostatic hypotension.

The head impulse (or thrust) test involves asking the patient to keep eyes focused on a distant object; the examiner then suddenly turns the head approximately 20 degrees. Patients with a normal vestibuloocular reflex remain focused on the object. An abnormal response, indicating a peripheral vestibular lesion, is movement of the eyes off the target followed by jerking of the eyes back to the target (corrective saccade). In this patient, the absence of vertigo and dizziness makes a vestibular cause less likely and testing unnecessary.

The Dix-Hallpike test is another bedside test for assessment of peripheral vestibular pathology and is most helpful in the presence of vertigo, which is absent here.

A positive Romberg test, defined as severe unsteadiness elicited by eye closure in a patient standing comfortably, indicates impairment of large sensory pathways at the spinal-cord or peripheral nerve level. The absence of abnormal findings on sensory and reflex examinations makes a sensory ataxia less likely in this patient.

Tandem gait, in which a patient walks on a straight line, may be intact in the early phase of Parkinson disease. An impaired tandem gait, however, can indicate cerebellar or sensory ataxia or other causes of imbalance but is not a sensitive or specific predictor of backward falls.

KEY POINT

- The pull test is the most sensitive predictor of the risk of backward falls in Parkinson disease.

Bibliography

Canning CG, Paul SS, Nieuwboer A. Prevention of falls in Parkinson's disease: a review of fall risk factors and the role of physical interventions. Neurodegener Dis Manag. 2014;4:203-21. [PMID: 25095816] doi:10.2217/nmt.14.22

Item 64   Answer: C

Educational Objective: Diagnose primary stabbing headache.

This patient most likely has a primary stabbing headache (also known as an "ice-pick" headache). The condition is characterized by transient localized stabs of head pain that occur spontaneously in the absence of organic disease and typically last seconds, with some lingering for 1 to 2 minutes; a less-localized dull ache or soreness lasting minutes may follow. The frequency of primary stabbing headache averages less than one per day in most patients, but headache attacks also can occur in series. Periods of activity and remission are common. Pain can occur anywhere on the head, including the eye, but the face is often spared. Primary stabbing headache is more common among those with a history of migraine. No cranial autonomic symptoms are reported. Indomethacin may be helpful during cycles of repeated occurrences but is rarely necessary.

Cluster headache is characterized by episodes of severe pain localized to the periorbital or temporal area with associated ipsilateral cranial autonomic features. Attacks of cluster headache may last 15 to 180 minutes and recur one to eight times daily over a span of weeks to months; the shorter duration distinguishes cluster headache from migraine. Many of the attacks are nocturnal, and some may be provoked by alcohol ingestion. The brief duration, parietal location, and absence of autonomic features in this case make cluster headache unlikely.

A new daily persistent headache is one with an identifiable and remembered onset. Pain becomes continuous and unremitting within 24 hours, a quality absent in this patient. The pain lacks many characteristic features, but the most common phenotype is similar to that of chronic tension-type headache. This disorder has no known treatment.

This patient's pain is occurring in an extratrigeminal location incompatible with the diagnosis of trigeminal neuralgia.

Of note, hemicrania continua is characterized by continuous head discomfort isolated and "locked" to one side. Some patients experience brief intense exacerbations of head pain that may be sharp and similar to that of primary stabbing headache. The condition, however, is known to display ipsilateral autonomic features not present in this patient, such as conjunctival injection, lacrimation, nasal congestion, rhinorrhea, forehead and facial sweating, miosis, and ptosis (and/or eyelid edema). An ipsilateral foreign body sensation in the eye is common. This headache is absolutely sensitive to indomethacin.

KEY POINT

- Primary stabbing headache is characterized by transient localized stabs of head pain that occur spontaneously in the absence of organic disease and typically last seconds; this headache is common among those with a history of migraine

Bibliography

Chua AL, Nahas S. Ice pick headache. Curr Pain Headache Rep. 2016 May;20(5):30. [PMID: 27038969] doi: 10.1007/s11916-016-0559-7

Item 65   Answer: A

Educational Objective: Treat focal seizures in an older patient with multiple comorbidities.

This patient should be treated with lamotrigine. He has a history of focal seizures with altered awareness (formerly known as complex partial seizures) and also has had a generalized tonic-clonic seizure. Only a few antiepileptic drugs (AEDs) (namely, lamotrigine, levetiracetam, topiramate, valproic acid, and zonisamide) are considered broad-spectrum agents and can be used to treat both generalized and partial epilepsy syndromes. Other narrow-spectrum AEDs (such as carbamazepine, gabapentin, oxcarbazepine, phenobarbital, phenytoin, and pregabalin) have the potential to exacerbate seizures in patients with generalized epilepsy. Lamotrigine is the most appropriate treatment because of the good evidence of its safety and effectiveness in epilepsy with focal seizures, especially in older patients, and is effective in generalized seizures. Lamotrigine is unlikely to cause cognitive dysfunction and does not affect blood counts, the liver, the kidney, or electrolytes. Although lamotrigine is associated with Stevens-Johnson syndrome, the drug can be titrated slowly to minimize risk; this patient's seizures are infrequent enough to allow for a 6- to 8-week titration. Although all the other drugs listed are likely effective in controlling seizures, lamotrigine also has a lower risk of adverse effects.

Oxcarbazepine is known to cause hyponatremia, especially in older patients taking thiazide diuretics, and thus should be avoided in this patient.

Phenytoin can lead to dizziness, ataxia, tremor, peripheral neuropathy, cerebellar atrophy, and agranulocytosis. Additionally, it has a narrow therapeutic window that is difficult to maintain, especially in older patients who are usually more sensitive to its zero-order pharmacokinetics at higher doses (constant absorption rate independent of concentration).

Kidney stones and cognitive impairment can be exacerbated by topiramate. The drug should be avoided in this patient with mild cognitive impairment and nephrolithiasis.

Valproic acid can cause tremor, cognitive dysfunction (including parkinsonism-associated dementia in older persons), and thrombocytopenia and thus is inappropriate for this patient.

KEY POINT

- Lamotrigine is the most appropriate treatment for epilepsy with focal seizure in older patients because of strong evidence of its safety and effectiveness.

Bibliography

Motika PV, Spencer DC. Treatment of epilepsy in the elderly. Curr Neurol Neurosci Rep. 2016;16:96. [PMID: 27628963] doi:10.1007/s11910-016-0696-8

Item 66   Answer: C

Educational Objective: Diagnose frontotemporal dementia.

This patient's age, gender, history, and cognitive evaluation findings all support a diagnosis of behavioral-variant frontotemporal dementia (FTD). FTD typically involves an alteration in personality and behavior that develops years before the onset of cognitive impairment; altered behaviors typically manifest as obsessive-compulsive tendencies, impulsivity, apathy, impaired judgment, emotional coldness, disinhibition, excessive spending, and excessive eating, particularly of high-calorie, nonnutritional foods. Amyotrophic lateral sclerosis, the major form of motor neuron disease, is found in 20% to 30% of patients diagnosed with behavioral-variant FTD. The presence of motor neuron disease generally portends a much more rapid progression of FTD but is exceptionally rare in other neurodegenerative disorders.

Classically, Alzheimer disease presents with the insidious development of recent memory loss. Forgetfulness of the details of recent events predominates early in the disease course. Aphasia is frequently seen early and is initially characterized by word-finding difficulties. Visuospatial dysfunction also is common and often presents as episodes of becoming lost in familiar environments or problems in assembling objects (constructional apraxia). Executive dysfunction may manifest as impairment of problem-solving abilities, judgment, and multitasking. Obsessive-compulsive tendencies, impulsivity, apathy, impaired judgment,

emotional coldness, disinhibition, and excessive eating are not typical of Alzheimer disease.

Core features of dementia with Lewy bodies are fluctuating cognition, recurrent visual hallucinations, and parkinsonism. Cognitive fluctuations include variations in both attention and level of arousal and can vary hour to hour, day to day, or week to week. These features are not present in this patient.

Cognitive impairments in Parkinson disease are subcortical, which implies that they primarily involve slow processing speed, impaired short-term memory, and attention deficits with relative sparing of cortical functions, such as language and declarative memory. Dopamine agonists are associated with higher risk of specific adverse effects, including impulse control disorder, punding (repetition of complex motor behaviors), sleep attacks, hallucinations, and confusion, but are not seen in untreated Parkinson disease.

KEY POINT

- Frontotemporal dementia typically involves an alteration in personality and behavior that develops years before the onset of cognitive impairment.

Bibliography

Bang J, Spina S, Miller BL. Frontotemporal dementia. Lancet. 2015;386:1672-82. [PMID: 26595641] doi:10.1016/S0140-6736(15)00461-4

Item 67   Answer: B

Educational Objective: Diagnose multiple system atrophy.

The combination of parkinsonism, cerebellar ataxia, dysautonomia, and early postural instability and falls in this patient is most consistent with multiple system atrophy, a Parkinson-plus syndrome. Typical autonomic deficits include orthostatic hypotension and urinary symptoms. Anosmia and acting out of dreams during sleep are suggestive of multiple system atrophy and Parkinson disease but not of progressive supranuclear palsy. A trial with levodopa may provide limited or partial benefit for this patient.

Corticobasal degeneration usually presents with markedly asymmetric parkinsonism and frequently is associated with dystonia, myoclonus, cortical sensory deficits, prominent cognitive dysfunction, and apraxia (impaired motor planning). MRI typically shows asymmetric posterior parietal and frontal cortical atrophy. The absence of these features makes this diagnosis less likely.

Many features of this patient's disorder are expected in idiopathic Parkinson disease, but the early prominent imbalance, recurrent falls, and cerebellar findings are atypical.

Given her early prominent postural instability, progressive supranuclear palsy is the main differential diagnosis in this patient. However, she does not have the characteristic impairment in vertical extraocular movements (supranuclear gaze palsy) that is typical. Additionally, the cerebellar features, asymmetric tremor, anosmia, and rapid eye movement sleep behavior disorder are more typical of multiple system atrophy than progressive supranuclear palsy.

Patients with vascular parkinsonism have sudden or step-wise onset of symptoms and exhibit disproportionate involvement of the lower extremities. The involvement of the upper body, gradual course, nonmotor symptoms, and brain MRI findings in this patient make this diagnosis unlikely.

> **KEY POINT**
>
> - The combination of parkinsonism, cerebellar ataxia, dysautonomia, and early postural instability characterizes multiple system atrophy, a Parkinson-plus syndrome.

Bibliography

Aerts MB, Esselink RA, Post B, van de Warrenburg BP, Bloem BR. Improving the diagnostic accuracy in parkinsonism: a three-pronged approach. Pract Neurol. 2012;12:77-87. [PMID: 22450452] doi:10.1136/practneurol-2011-000132

Item 68   Answer: B

Educational Objective: Manage an acute stroke treated with thrombolysis.

This patient should have CT angiography of the head. She has an acute ischemic stroke and was appropriately treated within 3 hours of symptom onset with intravenous recombinant tissue plasminogen activator (alteplase). The neurologic examination was consistent with an acute occlusion of the left intracranial internal carotid artery or middle cerebral artery. The patient's atrial fibrillation and subtherapeutic INR make a cardioembolic stroke subtype likely. Patients with an ischemic stroke and large-vessel occlusion have low recanalization rates with intravenous thrombolysis, and recently completed clinical trials have shown a clinical benefit from the addition of endovascular therapy, such as embolectomy, among carefully selected patients. The first step in patient selection requires the presence of a large vessel occlusion on vessel imaging, which is most quickly seen with CT angiography.

Because this patient already has received intravenous alteplase, all antithrombotics need to be held for at least 24 hours after a head CT shows no hemorrhage to prevent hemorrhagic conversion. In patients who do not receive thrombolysis, aspirin can reduce the risk of recurrent stroke within the first 2 weeks when administered within 48 hours of ischemic stroke onset.

Intravenous labetalol should not be administered to this patient. Her blood pressure does not meet the postthrombolytic treatment threshold (180/105 mm Hg). If clinical or radiographic evidence of hemorrhage is seen after treatment, lisinopril can be initiated.

MRI the area of infarction is not necessary for planning the next treatment steps. Furthermore, obtaining an MRI is time consuming and may lengthen the duration of time before an embolectomy can be performed. In acute ischemic stroke embolectomy trials, the greatest benefit occurred the faster treatment was initiated.

> **KEY POINT**
>
> - CT angiography of the head is the most appropriate test to determine candidacy for endovascular therapy in patients with a cardioembolic stroke who have undergone thrombolysis.

Bibliography

Powers WJ, Rabinstein AA, Ackerson T, Adeoye OM, Bambakidis NC, Becker K, et al; American Heart Association Stroke Council. 2018 Guidelines for the early management of patients with acute ischemic stroke: a guideline for healthcare professionals from the American Heart Association/ American Stroke Association. Stroke. 2018 Mar;49(3):e46-e110. [Epub 2018 Jan 24] [PMID: 29367334] doi:10.1161/STR.0000000000000158

Item 69   Answer: C

Educational Objective: Treat brain herniation.

This patient should receive intravenous dexamethasone. He has a primary brain tumor (most likely, a high-grade glioma) that has expanded and led to brainstem compression, as suggested by the focal ocular and limb examination findings. The subsequent development of fixed, dilated pupils in the presence of acute coma indicates brainstem herniation. His elevated blood pressure, irregular respirations, and bradycardia (Cushing triad) are typical of elevated intracranial pressure, which can be caused by herniation. His condition represents a neurologic emergency and requires immediate treatment with intravenous glucocorticoids. Dexamethasone is the preferred agent because of its lack of mineralocorticoid effects. Although glucocorticoids are generally avoided when lymphoma is suspected, the presence of brain herniation is an exception because death is likely if the herniation is not treated.

While considering more definitive treatment options, such as surgical decompression or resection, other temporizing, immediate measures also should be taken, including elevation of the head of the bed to 30 degrees, artificial hyperventilation, and (possibly) osmotic diuresis with mannitol or hypertonic saline. Because artificial respiratory alkalosis will lower intracranial pressure, herniation is an indication for emergent intubation, even in the absence of respiratory compromise. Although surgical resection is the definitive treatment for many gliomas, treatment of herniation takes precedence because of its associated mortality, and other temporizing measures, including glucocorticoid administration, are needed to stabilize the patient for necessary emergent CT to confirm the herniation and assess for its cause (for example, stroke, tumor, or hemorrhage).

Brain MRI is appropriate to further characterize the lesion and help in planning for biopsy or resection, but treatment for herniation should not be delayed while awaiting MRI results. In an emergency situation, CT is preferred because it is can be performed more rapidly and is more widely available.

Brain biopsy may be necessary eventually. However, administration of glucocorticoids is the most appropriate first step because they can be administered immediately and may be lifesaving.

CONT.

Antiepileptic drugs (AEDs), such as levetiracetam, may be considered if the patient develops seizures or needs perioperative prophylaxis, but their administration is not a first priority in this patient because AEDs have no effect on herniation, which is an immediate threat to life.

KEY POINT

- Brain herniation in a patient with a malignant primary brain tumor should be emergently treated with a glucocorticoid, particularly dexamethasone.

Bibliography

Stevens RD, Shoykhet M, Cadena R. Emergency neurological life support: intracranial hypertension and herniation. Neurocrit Care. 2015;23 Suppl 2:S76-82. [PMID: 26438459] doi:10.1007/s12028-015-0168-z

 Item 70   Answer: D

Educational Objective: Avoid using antibiotics that lower seizure threshold in patients with epilepsy.

Given his history of epilepsy, this patient should receive an injection of piperacillin-tazobactam as treatment of his hospital-acquired pneumonia. This drug has the lowest risk of triggering seizures of the drugs listed. Although all four choices may trigger seizures, piperacillin-tazobactam and non–fourth-generation cephalosporins have the weakest association with triggering seizures in patients with epilepsy (class IV evidence that seizure association is not well established in patients with epilepsy or past seizures).

Cefepime and carbapenems (such as imipenem) have class III evidence of triggering seizures in patients with epilepsy. In addition, cefepime has been known to cause encephalopathy, coma, and status epilepticus in patients with or without epilepsy, especially those with acute kidney injury.

There is class IV evidence that fluoroquinolones (such as levofloxacin) and fourth-generation cephalosporins lower the seizure threshold, including in patients with epilepsy.

KEY POINT

- Although evidence is limited, carbapenems, fluoroquinolones, and fourth-generation cephalosporins may lower the seizure threshold and thus should be avoided in patients with epilepsy.

Bibliography

Sutter R, Rüegg S, Tschudin-Sutter S. Seizures as adverse events of antibiotic drugs: A systematic review. Neurology. 2015;85:1332-41. [PMID: 26400582] doi:10.1212/WNL.0000000000002023

Item 71   Answer: B

Educational Objective: Diagnose migraine.

The patient's headaches meet the diagnostic criteria for migraine. The International Classification of Headache Disorders (third edition [beta version]) (ICHD-3) criteria require at least five episodes lasting 4 to 72 hours when untreated (or unsuccessfully treated) for this diagnosis. Pain should exhibit two of the following four characteristics: unilateral location, throbbing nature, moderate to severe intensity, and worsening with physical activity. Associated features must include either nausea or a combination of photophobia and phonophobia. Neurologic symptoms reflective of aura are described by 30% of patients with migraine. There must be no evidence of a secondary pathologic cause of the headache. Patients with chronic migraine may report milder attacks meeting tension-type headache criteria with at least some attacks meeting full migraine criteria. This patient described 8- to 12-hour severe attacks aggravated by activity with associated combined photophobia and phonophobia; her neurologic examination findings are normal. Neuroimaging is unnecessary in typical migraine presentations such as hers.

Medication overuse headache may result from overtreatment with acute medication in patients with underlying migraine or tension-type headache. Use of triptans, ergot alkaloids, opioids, or combination analgesics for 10 or more days per month or simple analgesics for 15 or more days per month constitutes medication overuse. Naproxen sodium used 8 days per month does not constitute medication overuse.

Over 90% of self- and clinician-diagnosed "sinus" headaches fulfill criteria for migraine. Acute rhinosinusitis may cause discomfort in the head or face, but headache is late in the disease course and typically a minor feature. Correlation of chronic or recurrent headaches with sinonasal pathology is without solid evidence. Weekly episodes of headache without nasal or sinus symptoms have no origins in the sinus cavities.

Episodic tension-type headache (TTH) is characterized by attacks of a nondisabling headache that lacks the typical features of migraine. Episodes may last from 30 minutes to 1 week. The pain of TTH typically is not severe or aggravated by routine physical activity. Photophobia or phonophobia may be present, but not both, according to ICHD-3 criteria. Mild nausea sometimes is noted with chronic TTH (≥15 days/mo) but not episodic TTH (<15 days/mo). Moderate to severe nausea and aura are not found with either TTH subtype.

KEY POINT

- The diagnosis of migraine requires at least five episodes lasting 4 to 72 hours when untreated (or unsuccessfully treated), with pain exhibiting two of the following characteristics: unilateral location, throbbing nature, moderate to severe intensity, and worsening with physical activity; associated features must include either nausea or a combination of photophobia and phonophobia.

Bibliography

MacGregor EA. Migraine. Ann Intern Med. 2017;166:ITC49-ITC64 [PMID: 28384749]

Item 72   Answer: B

Educational Objective: Treat ischemic stroke with antiplatelet agents.

This patient should be treated with aspirin. She most likely has a cardioembolic stroke related to atrial fibrillation. She is beyond the treatment window for intravenous thrombolysis and is not a candidate for intra-arterial therapy because of the location of the lesion in the posterior circulation and already demonstrated infarction. Therefore, medical therapy is indicated for preventing recurrent stroke. Only aspirin and heparinoids have been studied for their effectiveness in the acute stroke setting, and only aspirin has been shown to reduce the risk of stroke at 2 weeks. Therefore, aspirin monotherapy is a reasonable first-line antiplatelet regimen for secondary stroke prevention in the acute setting. For stable patients with small strokes, long-term warfarin therapy is typically administered 24 hours after hospitalization to reduce the risk of hemorrhagic transformation. Hemorrhagic transformation is more likely to occur in larger infarcts (those involving more than one third of hemispheric volume) and in infarcts with a cardioembolic cause. Warfarin is often withheld for 2 weeks in the setting of large strokes, strokes that have undergone hemorrhagic transformation, or uncontrolled hypertension.

The use of novel oral anticoagulants, including apixaban, has not been established as effective in the acute setting after a stroke. Apixaban may be a reasonable long-term option for stroke prevention at hospital discharge.

Clopidogrel has not been studied as monotherapy for acute ischemic stroke and is currently not recommended.

Intravenous heparin is not effective in reducing the risk of recurrent stroke within the acute hospitalization period in patients with all stroke subtypes, including ischemic strokes with a cardioembolic cause. Intravenous heparin can be considered in patients with a high short-term risk of recurrent ischemic stroke, such as those with mechanical heart valves, but the benefit of this approach must be weighed against the risk of hemorrhagic conversion.

KEY POINT

- In the absence of thrombolytic therapy for cardioembolic stroke, short-term therapy with aspirin reduces the risk of stroke at 2 weeks.

Bibliography

Kernan WN, Ovbiagele B, Black HR, Bravata DM, Chimowitz MI, Ezekowitz MD, et al; American Heart Association Stroke Council, Council on Cardiovascular and Stroke Nursing, Council on Clinical Cardiology, and Council on Peripheral Vascular Disease. Guidelines for the prevention of stroke in patients with stroke and transient ischemic attack: a guideline for healthcare professionals from the American Heart Association/ American Stroke Association. Stroke. 2014 Jul;45(7):2160-236. [PMID 24788967] doi:10.1161/STR.0000000000000024

Item 73   Answer: C

Educational Objective: Manage mild traumatic brain injury in an athlete.

The patient should undergo neuropsychological testing. She sustained a mild closed head injury with typical symptoms of a concussion. Loss of consciousness established the presence of mild traumatic brain injury (TBI). Headache, nausea, dizziness, and cognitive dysfunction are all typical symptoms of postconcussion syndrome. Guidelines recommend initial screening with a symptom checklist and a neurologic examination, including assessments of cognition and balance. Guidelines also recommend head CT in those with suspected hemorrhage. Neuropsychological testing provides an additional objective and more sensitive measure of cognitive function and should be part of a comprehensive TBI management strategy for patients with persistent symptoms.

Amantadine has been shown to be useful in the management of severe traumatic brain injuries. Data suggest that treatment with amantadine can accelerate functional recovery among patients in vegetative or minimally conscious states after a TBI and can effectively accelerate the pace of recovery of cognitively mediated behaviors compared with placebo. However, there is insufficient evidence to recommend amantadine in cases of mild TBI.

A brain MRI is not indicated in this patient, who has shown symptomatic improvement in the 2 weeks since injury and now has normal neurologic examination findings. Further neuroimaging is unnecessary.

Return to play before complete recovery may increase the risk of recurrent injury. Concussion symptoms should have resolved completely before the patient resumes exercise. A return-to-play program should then involve a stepwise increase in physical activity, with monitoring for recurrence of symptoms. Guidelines recommend that a patient be asymptomatic without medication both at rest and when subjected to physical exertion. The presence of continued cognitive symptoms in this patient makes return to play inappropriate at this time.

KEY POINT

- Besides initial screening with a symptom checklist and a neurologic examination, including assessments of cognition and balance, neuropsychological testing should be part of a comprehensive mild traumatic brain injury management strategy for patients with persistent symptoms.

Bibliography

Wasserman EB, Kerr ZY, Zuckerman SL, Covassin T. Epidemiology of sports-related concussions in National Collegiate Athletic Association athletes from 2009-2010 to 2013-2014: symptom prevalence, symptom resolution time, and return-to-play time. Am J Sports Med. 2016 Jan;44(1):226-33. [PMID: 26546304] doi: 10.1177/0363546515610537

Item 74   Answer: B

Educational Objective: Treat cognitive impairment in a patient with vascular cognitive impairment.

The most appropriate medication for this patient's cognitive impairment is the acetylcholinesterase inhibitor donepezil. Given her history of multiple strokes, pseudobulbar affect (a neurologic disorder characterized by involuntary outbursts of laughing and/or crying that are out of proportion to the emotions being experienced), prominent gait problems, and asymmetric neurologic findings, she most likely has vascular cognitive impairment. Treatment of vascular cognitive impairment should focus on identifying and treating cerebrovascular risk factors, such as smoking, diabetes mellitus, hyperlipidemia, hypertension, ischemic heart disease, atrial fibrillation, and hypercoagulable states. Although not yet FDA approved as treatment of vascular cognitive impairment, acetylcholinesterase inhibitors have shown modest benefit in clinical trials and are generally recommended for this type of dementia.

Citalopram and other selective serotonin reuptake inhibitors are appropriate to treat the pseudobulbar symptoms exhibited by this patient but are unlikely to improve her cognitive deficits.

Ginkgo biloba has not been found to be more effective for dementia than placebo in controlled trials. Because this herbal supplement also is associated with increased bleeding, it is contraindicated in patients taking anticoagulant or antiplatelet agents.

Methylphenidate has been shown to be effective in treating the severe apathy often associated with vascular cognitive impairment. This patient has no evidence of apathy. In addition, this agent can raise blood pressure and is inappropriate for this patient with hypertension.

KEY POINT

- Treatment of vascular cognitive impairment should focus on identifying and treating cerebrovascular risk factors; off-label use of acetylcholinesterase inhibitors has shown modest benefit in clinical trials and thus is generally recommended for this condition.

Bibliography
Ritter A, Pillai JA. Treatment of vascular cognitive impairment. Curr Treat Options Neurol. 2015;17:367. [PMID: 26094078] doi:10.1007/s11940-015-0367-0

Item 75   Answer: D

Educational Objective: Treat immune-mediated necrotizing myopathy.

This patient, whose progressive muscle weakness has persisted after discontinuation of simvastatin and who has biopsy evidence of necrotizing myopathy without inflammation, should be treated with a glucocorticoid, such as prednisone. He most likely has immune-mediated necrotizing myopathy. This condition can be triggered by previous exposure to statins but is distinguished from more common statin-induced toxic myopathies by progression of muscle necrosis and weakness after removal of the statin. The presence of antibodies to hydroxymethylglutaryl coenzyme A reductase is disease specific and can further support the diagnosis because these antibodies are absent in patients with nonnecrotizing statin myopathy or in those without myopathy who take statins. Treatment with a glucocorticoid or other immunosuppressive agents can reverse the myopathy. In patients who have

fully recovered from a previous episode of nonnecrotizing myopathy caused by a lipophilic statin, such as simvastatin, resumption of treatment with a hydrophilic statin, such as pravastatin, may be considered.

Although glucocorticoid-sparing immunosuppressive medications, such as azathioprine, are sometimes used as second-line therapy in other inflammatory myopathies (for example, polymyositis), evidence is limited with these agents in immune-mediated necrotizing myopathy. In addition, azathioprine has a delayed mechanism of action and is not immediately effective. Glucocorticoids are much more effective as first-line therapy.

Continued clinical monitoring is indicated in nonnecrotic statin myopathy, in which symptoms gradually improve in the absence of the causative agent. Progressive weakness and ongoing necrosis on biopsy should prompt suspicion of immune-mediated necrotizing myopathy, which requires immunosuppressive therapy.

The benefit of coenzyme Q10 as a protective agent against statin-induced myopathy remains controversial. No evidence suggests that coenzyme Q10 supplementation is effective against immune-mediated necrotizing myopathy.

KEY POINT

- Immune-mediated necrotizing myopathy is a form of statin myopathy that is associated with antibodies to hydroxymethylglutaryl coenzyme A reductase and biopsy evidence of muscle necrosis without inflammation; treatment with a glucocorticoid or other immunosuppressive agents can reverse the myopathy.

Bibliography
Mohassel P, Mammen AL. Statin-associated autoimmune myopathy and anti-HMGCR autoantibodies. Muscle Nerve. 2013;48:477-83. [PMID: 23519993] doi:10.1002/mus.23854

Item 76   Answer: B

Educational Objective: Manage intracranial hypotension.

This patient has intracranial hypotension and should undergo placement of an epidural blood patch (EBP). Spontaneous intracranial hypotension classically presents with an orthostatic headache. The interval between postural change and headache development is highly variable. When the headache duration is weeks to months, the orthostatic component may fade completely. Presentation may be thunderclap (maximum onset within 1 minute) or subacute. Intracranial hypotension is the result of cerebrospinal fluid (CSF) leakage that can arise as a result of lumbar puncture, surgery, or trauma or can occur spontaneously. Associated features include tinnitus, diplopia, neck pain, nausea, photophobia, and phonophobia. Clinical examination findings are typically normal but occasionally reveal a "falsely localizing" abducens nerve (cranial nerve VI) palsy. Female sex, middle age, and connective tissue disorders are risk factors. Brain MRI with contrast is abnormal in 80% of affected patients, with possible findings of diffuse nonnodular pachymeningeal enhancement, cerebellar tonsillar abnormalities, and subdural fluid collections.

Use of an EBP is the initial treatment of choice. Patients who do not respond to this treatment should undergo CT myelography for potential detection of the precise site of cerebrospinal fluid (CSF) leakage. Subsequent treatments may include a repeat EBP or surgical repair of the identified site.

Acetazolamide is indicated in patients with intracranial hypertension but relatively contraindicated in cases of intracranial hypotension.

A diagnosis of intracranial hypotension can be confirmed by a CSF opening pressure of less than 60 mm H_2O, but lumbar puncture would introduce another site of potential CSF leakage. In the presence of patient history and brain MRI abnormalities that are typical for intracranial hypotension, lumbar puncture is unnecessary and should be avoided.

Small subdural fluid collections are commonly seen in patients with intracranial hypotension and do not require surgical evacuation. Typical indications for surgical management include an acute subdural hematoma measuring greater than 10 mm in thickness, a Glasgow Coma Scale score less than 9, and pupillary asymmetry or fixation.

KEY POINT

- Placement of an epidural blood patch is the initial treatment of choice for patients with intracranial hypotension; CT myelography is appropriate for those who do not respond to this treatment.

Bibliography
Hoffmann J, Goadsby PJ. Update on intracranial hypertension and hypotension. Curr Opin Neurol. 2013;26(3):240-7. [PMID: 23594732] doi: 10.1097/WCO.0b013e328360eccc

Item 77   Answer: D
Educational Objective: Diagnose multiple sclerosis.

This patient should undergo MRI of the brain. She has signs and symptoms consistent with an episode of inflammatory transverse myelitis. Although idiopathic transverse myelitis can occur, the most common cause of a transverse myelitis event is multiple sclerosis (MS). MRI of the brain should be routinely performed in patients with new-onset transverse myelitis to evaluate for lesions consistent with MS, such as those located in periventricular, juxtacortical (or cortical), and infratentorial white matter. If these lesions are present, MS should be diagnosed if they fulfill the diagnostic criteria for dissemination in space and in time.

No MS-specific diagnostic biomarkers are available. Initial studies championed myelin basic protein as a potential marker of MS disease activity, but subsequent evidence found that this biomarker is not associated with MS disease activity and is not useful to confirm a diagnosis of MS.

Lumbar puncture to determine the presence of oligoclonal bands is not warranted. Although lumbar puncture sometimes is appropriate in the evaluation of MS, the presence or absence of oligoclonal bands is not part of multiple sclerosis diagnostic criteria because of poor sensitivity and specificity for the disease. Approximately 10% to 15% of patients with MS have normal cerebrospinal fluid on testing; additionally, oligoclonal bands are sometimes elevated in other inflammatory conditions. For these reasons, if MRI confirms the diagnosis of MS, CSF testing is unnecessary.

The erythrocyte sedimentation rate may be elevated in patients with inflammatory transverse myelitis. However, the test is nonspecific and would not lead to a diagnosis of the cause of this patient's myelitis, such as MS.

Detection of a subclinical lesion in a site remote from the region of clinical dysfunction supports a diagnosis of multifocal MS. Evoked potentials also may help define the anatomic site of the lesion in tracts not easily visualized by imaging (for example, optic nerves, dorsal columns). Evoked potential testing is reserved for situations in which the diagnosis of MS is equivocal. The best initial test remains a brain MRI.

KEY POINT

- Because multiple sclerosis (MS) is the most common cause of transverse myelitis, MRI of the brain should be performed in patients with new-onset transverse myelitis to evaluate for MS lesions.

Bibliography
Thompson AJ, Banwell BL, Barkhof F, Carroll WM, Coetzee T, Comi G, et al. Diagnosis of multiple sclerosis: 2017 revisions of the McDonald criteria. Lancet Neurol. 2017. [Epub ahead of print] [PMID: 29275977] doi:10.1016/S1474-4422(17)30470-2

Item 78   Answer: A
Educational Objective: Prevent venous thromboembolism after a hemorrhagic stroke.

This patient should begin receiving low-molecular-weight heparin. He has severe hemiparesis. Two poststroke CT scans obtained 48 hours apart show no evidence of active bleeding. The hemiparesis places him at high risk of deep venous thrombosis (DVT), which is the leading complication of hospitalization for stroke. DVT is found in 11% of immobile patients at 1 week after stroke and pulmonary embolism in about 1% of patients with stroke. Prophylaxis with low-molecular-weight heparin can be started 48 hours after hemorrhagic stroke in patients with no evidence of active bleeding on imaging. Before that time, DVT prophylaxis is possible with external sequential compression devices.

Administering warfarin without heparin is not adequate for immediate and short-term prevention of DVT because the anticoagulant effect of warfarin is delayed for 36 to 72 hours. Because of the immediacy of its action, heparin is preferred.

A randomized trial of thigh-high graduated compression stockings showed no benefit in preventing venous thromboembolism in patients with all types of stroke and

CONT.

substantial leg weakness. Skin breaks, ulcers, blisters, and skin necrosis were significantly more common in patients wearing stockings.

Aspirin should not be resumed in this patient who has no immediate indication for use of antiplatelet agents, such as an acute myocardial infarction or a history of vascular stents. There is no evidence that aspirin is effective prophylaxis for DVT in hospitalized patients. Aspirin can be resumed in patients with intracerebral hemorrhage caused by hypertension 2 to 4 weeks after stroke onset if the hematoma has resolved on imaging and there is an appropriate high-risk indication.

> **KEY POINT**
>
> - Prophylactic heparin can be started 48 hours after a hemorrhagic stroke to prevent development of deep venous thrombosis as long as there is no evidence of active bleeding on neuroimaging

Bibliography
Hemphill JC 3rd, Greenberg SM, Anderson CS, Becker K, Bendok BR, Cushman M, et al; American Heart Association Stroke Council. Guidelines for the management of spontaneous intracerebral hemorrhage: a guideline for healthcare professionals from the American Heart Association/American Stroke Association. Stroke. 2015;46:2032-60. [PMID: 26022637] doi:10.1161/STR.0000000000000069

Item 79 Answer: D

Educational Objective: Treat chronic cervical stenosis.

This patient should have physical therapy. Spinal cord compression can result from acute or chronic causes. Evaluation and confirmation of suspected acute spinal cord compression with appropriate neuroimaging studies should occur in an urgent manner. Immediate treatment may be necessary to prevent severe and irreversible neurologic injury. Patients with chronic spinal stenosis due to osteoarthritic degenerative spinal disease frequently have chronic myelopathic symptoms, most often involving the cervical and lumbar spines. This patient has chronic symptoms of cervical stenosis due to multilevel disc disease. Most patients with chronic cervical and lumbar stenosis respond well to conservative measures, such as physical therapy and pain control. However, those with symptoms of more moderate to severe disease who also have signs of myelopathy on examination, such as progressive leg weakness, spasticity, distal numbness, and bladder impairment, may require surgical intervention. The lack of these findings in this patient supports the use of conservative measures, such as physical therapy.

Gabapentin can be useful in patients with neuropathic pain. This patient, however, has none of the typical symptoms of neuropathic pain, such as burning, electrical, or frostbite-like sensations.

Immobilization of the neck in hard (or soft) cervical collar would be an unnecessary and excessive restriction for someone with chronic cervical stenosis, especially in light of potential adverse effects. A hard cervical collar most commonly is used for cervical spine stabilization after trauma,

surgery, and fractures or dislocations. It would be excessive in this patient whose clinical examination and imaging findings show no true cord compression or spinal instability.

Although some patients with spinal stenosis will eventually require neurosurgical intervention, outcomes for multilevel disc disease are generally poor, and this approach should be used only after conservative measures have been exhausted. The finding of signal abnormality within the cord may correlate with the severity of compressive myelopathy. Multiple levels of signal abnormality may be a more significant finding than single-level changes. The lack of clear cord compression on examination or signal-intensity changes on MRI indicates that this patient does not need emergent surgery.

> **KEY POINT**
>
> - Most patients with chronic cervical and lumbar stenosis respond well to conservative measures, such as physical therapy and pain control.

Bibliography
Rhee JM, Shamji MF, Erwin WM, Bransford RJ, Yoon ST, Smith JS, et al. Nonoperative management of cervical myelopathy: a systematic review. Spine (Phila Pa 1976). 2013;38:S55-67. [PMID: 23963006] doi:10.1097/BRS.0b013e3182a7f41d

Item 80 Answer: C

Educational Objective: Treat a patient with Alzheimer disease and sick sinus syndrome with memantine.

This patient should receive memantine. She has probable Alzheimer disease, moderate stage, given the degree of functional impairment she exhibits and her Mini-Mental State Examination score. The treatment of Alzheimer dementia is multifactorial and is symptom targeted. Both cholinesterase inhibitors (such as donepezil) and the *N*-methyl-D-aspartate receptor antagonist memantine are approved for treatment of moderate stages of Alzheimer disease. The cholinesterase inhibitors exert their effect by inhibiting the enzymes responsible for breaking down acetylcholine, thereby increasing the levels of acetylcholine in the neuronal synapse. No clinically significant difference in effectiveness has been shown between the cholinesterase inhibitors. Relative contraindications for their use include (but are not limited to) sick sinus syndrome, left bundle branch block, uncontrolled asthma, angle-closure glaucoma, and ulcer disease. Memantine is believed to reduce glutamate-mediated neurotoxicity in the central nervous system, is not associated with adverse cardiovascular effects, and thus is the most appropriate treatment for this patient.

Benzodiazepines (such as alprazolam) and antipsychotic agents (such as risperidone) should be used only in very limited circumstances in patients with Alzheimer disease who have severe psychosis and anxiety. At this point in her disease course, this patient has neither.

In patients with mild to moderate Alzheimer disease, donepezil and other acetylcholinesterase inhibitors have had modest benefits in improving cognitive performance without clear improvements in daily functioning. Because of this patient's cardiac history, donepezil is not an appropriate medication.

Selective serotonin reuptake inhibitors (such as paroxetine) can be helpful for improving mood and treating psychiatric and behavioral symptoms of dementia. This patient's symptoms are mild at this time, do not warrant use of this drug class, and should be treated with behavioral management.

KEY POINT

- Relative contraindications for the use of cholinesterase inhibitors in the treatment of dementia include sick sinus syndrome, left bundle branch block, uncontrolled asthma, angle-closure glaucoma, and ulcer disease.

Bibliography

Molano JR1, Bratt R, Shatz R. Treatment and management of dementia due to Alzheimer's disease. Curr Treat Options Neurol. 2015 Aug;17(8):363. doi: 10.1007/s11940-015-0363-4

Item 81   Answer: B

Educational Objective: Diagnose a secondary headache.

This patient should have a brain MRI. His development of a new headache after age 50 years, use of an anticoagulant, and progressive headache pattern are all red flags indicating a potential secondary headache condition. Other red flags for secondary headache include first or worst headache, abrupt-onset or thunderclap attack, episode associated with neurologic symptoms lasting more than 1 hour, alterations in consciousness, abnormal physical examination findings, and onset after exertion, sex, or Valsalva maneuvers. Brain MRI is the most appropriate diagnostic study for patients with a suspected secondary headache and should be performed before additional testing is considered.

Amitriptyline is the treatment of choice for prevention of chronic tension-type headache. Diagnosis of this condition, however, first requires exclusion of a secondary headache. Although features of the patient's clinical presentation may suggest a tension-type headache syndrome, the presence of red flags makes brain neuroimaging a priority.

Neck pain is a nonspecific feature common to many primary and secondary headache syndromes. Its presence does not necessarily indicate a primary pathologic abnormality in the cervical region. Neurologic examination findings do not suggest cervical radiculopathy or myelopathy and thus an MRI of the cervical spine is not indicated.

Head CT is indicated in the assessment of acute severe headache in an emergent setting. In these situations, intracranial hemorrhage often is suspected and is well-visualized by a noncontrast CT scan. Given its greater sensitivity and safety, brain MRI is recommended in the evaluation of subacute or chronic headache requiring imaging.

Temporal artery biopsy is helpful in the evaluation of suspected giant cell arteritis. Most patients with this disorder are older than 50 years. Erythrocyte sedimentation rate and C-reactive protein level are frequently elevated. Brain MRI and reversal of anticoagulation are both indicated before temporal artery biopsy.

KEY POINT

- Brain MRI is the most appropriate diagnostic study for patients with a suspected secondary headache and should be performed before additional testing is considered.

Bibliography

Nye BL, Ward TN. Clinic and emergency room evaluation and testing of headache. Headache. 2015 Oct;55(9):1301-8. [PMID: 26422648] doi: 10.1111/head.12648

Item 82   Answer: B

Educational Objective: Monitor for adverse effects of multiple sclerosis treatment.

This patient should now have regular ophthalmologic examinations. Fingolimod is a once-daily pill that results in sequestration of activated lymphocytes in lymph nodes. Fingolimod reduces relapse rates by approximately half over 2 years compared with placebo and also reduces the risk of disability progression and accumulation of new MRI lesions. In clinical trials of fingolimod as treatment of multiple sclerosis (MS), the medication was found to confer a 0.5% risk of macular edema. This adverse effect is reversible and typically resolves after discontinuation of the drug. If unrecognized, however, macular edema can result in permanent visual deficits. Therefore, regular macular examinations (that is, visual evaluation or measurement through optical coherence tomography) are recommended for patients taking this medication. Fingolimod also requires first-dose monitoring because of the first-dose bradycardia that occurs in most patients and should not be used in patients with heart block.

There have been rare reports of patients who take fingolimod as a disease-modifying therapy for MS developing progressive multifocal leukoencephalopathy (PML). However, no evidence suggests that serum antibodies to the JC virus are a useful tool for predicting this adverse effect of the drug. Extensive data do support serum testing to predict the risk of PML in patients with MS who take natalizumab, in whom PML is much more common. The overall risk is approximately 1 in 1000 but is significantly higher in patients who have previous exposure to immunosuppressant agents or chemotherapy and those who have elevated serum titers of antibodies against the JC virus. Stratification of risk by treatment history and JC virus antibody testing is thus an important step before initiating natalizumab.

Kidney complications have not been associated with fingolimod use, which makes serum creatine measurement every 6 months unnecessary.

Tuberculosis has not been reported as an adverse effect of fingolimod. Although the risk of opportunistic infections may be increased with use of this drug, tuberculin skin testing is not recommended specifically, and given this patient's office-based occupation, she has no specific expected exposures that would require such testing.

KEY POINT

- In patients with multiple sclerosis who take fingolimod as a disease-modifying therapy, regular ophthalmic examinations are necessary because of the increased risk of macular edema with this medication.

Bibliography

Jain N, Bhatti MT. Fingolimod-associated macular edema: incidence, detection, and management. Neurology. 2012;78:672-80. [PMID: 22371414] doi:10.1212/WNL.0b013e318248deea

Item 83   Answer: D

Educational Objective: Diagnose primary progressive aphasia.

The most likely diagnosis is language-variant frontotemporal dementia, also known as primary progressive aphasia (PPA). Frontotemporal dementia (FTD) comprises two distinct clinical syndromes. The first, behavioral-variant FTD, is associated with prominent changes in behavior, personality, or executive function. The second, PPA, is associated with prominent and early changes in language function and is further subclassified according to the pattern of language impairment: semantic (or fluent) aphasia, nonfluent (agrammatic) aphasia, and logopenic aphasia. Semantic aphasia, as demonstrated by this patient, is characterized by early prominent difficulty with language comprehension. Nonfluent aphasia is recognized by changes in language production. Logopenic aphasia describes hesitant but grammatically correct speech. Although language decline is common in many dementia syndromes, in PPA it is the symptom noted first, and language is often the only cognitive domain affected for years before the development of additional cognitive deterioration. Structural brain imaging typically reveals asymmetric involvement of the left temporal lobe (which controls language in most patients), as shown (*arrow*).

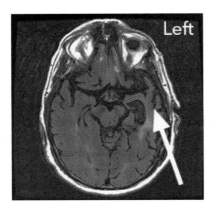

Persistent forgetfulness is the hallmark of Alzheimer disease, beginning with objects, appointments, names, and other apparently trivial items. As the disease progresses, memories are lost, and problems with word-finding ability become apparent.

The most prominent feature of behavioral-variant FTD is an alteration in personality and behavior that typically develops years before the onset of cognitive impairment. Apathy, diminished interest, loss of empathy, lack of initiative, increased emotionality, disinhibition, euphoria, impulsivity, changes in eating behaviors, and compulsiveness are the most common symptoms reported by families.

Patients with dementia with Lewy bodies may demonstrate a pattern of cognitive impairment with psychiatric features of personality change, apathy, depression, and psychosis. Abnormal dream enactment behavior during rapid-eye movement (REM) sleep in which patients fight or call out in their sleep (REM sleep behavior disorder) may precede the onset of cognitive decline or motor symptoms by years.

KEY POINT

- Primary progressive aphasia is a language-predominant neurodegenerative dementia in which language is often the only cognitive domain affected for years before the development of additional cognitive deterioration; structural brain imaging often shows asymmetric involvement of the left temporal lobe.

Bibliography

Mesulam MM, Rogalski EJ, Wieneke C, Hurley RS, Geula C, Bigio EH, et al. Primary progressive aphasia and the evolving neurology of the language network. Nat Rev Neurol. 2014;10:554-69. [PMID: 25179257] doi:10.1038/nrneurol.2014.159

Item 84   Answer: C

Educational Objective: Diagnose a medication-induced movement disorder.

This patient has tardive dyskinesia. Involuntary choreiform movements, most often involving the face and hands, can be an adverse effect of long-term exposure to dopamine-blocking agents, including neuroleptic agents and chronic antiemetic medications, such as metoclopramide. Removal of the causative medication is key to treatment, but symptoms of tardive dyskinesia can take months to resolve or may become permanent. A longer duration and higher dose of the causative medication, older age, and female sex carry a higher risk of permanent dyskinesia. The risk of tardive dyskinesia should be discussed with patients before starting chronic dopamine-blocking agents. Pharmacologic treatment of tardive dyskinesia is often unsatisfactory, but options include clonazepam, tetrabenazine, valbenazine, anticholinergic agents, and clozapine. The persistence of involuntary movements 6 months after removal of metoclopramide is most consistent with tardive dyskinesia. The initial symptoms of shuffling gait and pill-rolling tremor were likely due to neuroleptic-induced parkinsonism, a distinct movement disorder that, unlike tardive dyskinesia, is reversible with discontinuation of the causative dopamine-blocking agent.

Akathisia and dystonic reaction are both caused by exposure to dopamine-blocking agents of the neuroleptic or antiemetic class; these disorders occur acutely and do not account for the persistent symptoms described. Akathisia is a movement disorder characterized by a feeling of restlessness and an overwhelming need to be in motion manifested as pacing, rocking from foot to foot, lifting the feet as if marching in place, and crossing and uncrossing the legs; this patient does not have a need to move, and her symptoms are more limited than what is typically seen with akathisia. Acute dystonic reaction consists of sustained, frequently painful muscle contractions that can cause abnormal twisting postures, repetitive movements, and difficulty speaking. It may be limited to the head and neck, but the choreiform appearance of movements and their persistence months after removal of the offending medication make it an unlikely cause in this patient.

Withdrawal emergent syndrome is characterized by dyskinesia starting after sudden withdrawal of a dopamine-blocking agent; the disorder usually is managed by reinstitution of the causative agent (or another agent from same class) and a subsequent slow taper over few months. In this patient, the presence of dyskinesia before the offending medication was removed and its persistence for 6 months after removal is not consistent with withdrawal emergent syndrome.

KEY POINT

- Tardive dyskinesia can be caused by exposure to dopamine-blocking agents, such as neuroleptic and antiemetic agents, and may persist for more than 6 months after removal of the offending medication or become permanent.

Bibliography

Caroff SN, Campbell EC. Drug-induced extrapyramidal syndromes: implications for contemporary practice. Psychiatr Clin North Am. 2016;39:391-411. [PMID: 27514296] doi:10.1016/j.psc.2016.04.003

Item 85   Answer: C

Educational Objective: Treat a hemorrhagic stroke with an ACE inhibitor.

The patient had an intracerebral hemorrhage in the thalamus due to hypertension. Given his age and hypertension, the hemorrhage is unlikely to have had a secondary cause. During acute hospitalization for an intracerebral hemorrhage, lowering the blood pressure acutely is recommended, although achieving systolic blood pressure levels of less than 140 mm Hg is associated with increased adverse events. After the initial hospitalization, however, the risk of recurrent ischemic and hemorrhagic stroke remains increased if the blood pressure is higher than 130/80 mm Hg, according to secondary prevention trials of stroke examining the effectiveness of ACE inhibitors. There is no contraindication to starting an ACE

inhibitor, such as lisinopril, which reduces the risk of ischemic and hemorrhagic stroke regardless of blood pressure levels.

Aspirin is an inappropriate treatment for this patient who has no clear indications for secondary prevention of ischemic stroke or other ischemic cardiovascular disease events. If a patient were to require an antiplatelet agent in the setting of known atherosclerotic disease (for example), aspirin can be safely started 30 days after an initial hemorrhagic stroke if the original event was due to hypertension and the blood pressure is well controlled.

The patient does not require fluoxetine because currently there is no evidence of clinical depression. Low-dose fluoxetine was shown to be better than placebo at improving motor function after stroke, but only when the drug was administered during the acute hospitalization. In the chronic setting, fluoxetine has not been shown to improve stroke recovery, and several reports suggest a potential increase in the risk of hemorrhage with selective serotonin reuptake inhibitors.

Rosuvastatin is not appropriate as treatment for this patient, whose serum LDL cholesterol level is not elevated, who has no evidence of atherosclerotic disease or diabetes mellitus, and whose 10-year atherosclerotic risk is less than 7.5%.

KEY POINT

- After the acute phase of stroke, patients with hypertension should be treated with antihypertensive therapy to reduce the risk of recurrent stroke.

Bibliography

Hemphill JC 3rd, Greenberg SM, Anderson CS, Becker K, Bendok BR, Cushman M, et al; American Heart Association Stroke Council. Guidelines for the management of spontaneous intracerebral hemorrhage: a guideline for healthcare professionals from the American Heart Association/American Stroke Association. Stroke. 2015;46:2032-60. [PMID: 26022637] doi:10.1161/STR.0000000000000069

Item 86   Answer: C

Educational Objective: Treat Bell palsy.

Oral prednisone should be given to this patient with Bell palsy within 72 hours of symptom onset to expedite the speed and rate of full recovery. Clinical history and examination findings in this patient are classic for Bell palsy, and thus no initial imaging or laboratory testing is indicated. Unilateral facial weakness involving both upper and lower parts of the face is characteristic of peripheral facial nerve (cranial nerve VII) involvement and distinguishes this condition from a central nervous system process (such as stroke), which typically spares the upper facial muscles because of bilateral innervation. Associated features of classic Bell palsy include alteration in taste (due to involvement of the chorda tympani) and hyperacusis (intolerance of loud noise due to involvement of stapedius muscle); other common features are ipsilateral sensory paresthesia and pain without objective sensory loss. Because this patient does not have subjective or objective hearing loss or any other involvement beyond a unilateral facial nerve, initial brain imaging is not indicated.

Neither brain MRI nor intracranial magnetic resonance angiography is indicated in this patient. Sudden painless paralysis of a unilateral facial nerve is unlikely to be caused by aneurysmal compression or bleeding. These imaging tests might be appropriate if the patient had a thunderclap headache (maximum onset of pain within minutes of symptom onset), a slow progressive course of facial weakness, or progressive myoclonic hemifacial spasms.

The effectiveness of oral antiviral therapy, such as valacyclovir, in the treatment of Bell palsy is controversial. Currently, no available evidence suggests that adding antiviral therapy improves prognosis.

KEY POINT

- Oral prednisone administered within 72 hours of symptom onset expedites the speed and rate of full recovery in patients with Bell palsy.

Bibliography

Glass GE, Tzafetta K. Bell's palsy: a summary of current evidence and referral algorithm. Fam Pract. 2014;31:631-42. [PMID: 25208543] doi:10.1093/fampra/cmu058

Item 87   Answer: B

Educational Objective: Treat trigeminal neuralgia.

The patient should receive carbamazepine. She has paroxysmal facial pain typical of trigeminal neuralgia. Episodes of this disorder consist of sharp or shock-like pain and have a duration of less than 1 second to 120 seconds, with variable frequency. The maxillary and mandibular branches of the trigeminal nerve (cranial nerve V) are affected in 95% of affected patients. Attacks may be spontaneous or triggered by innocuous stimuli. Autonomic features are rare. Incidence increases with advanced age. Multiple sclerosis (MS) is present in 5% of patients with trigeminal neuralgia and is a common cause in patients younger than 50 years. Demyelinating plaques in the pontine entry of the trigeminal root may be seen. Carbamazepine is the treatment of choice; management with this agent requires serum monitoring for hyponatremia and agranulocytosis.

Acetazolamide is indicated for idiopathic intracranial hypertension (IIH). Headaches associated with this condition are phenotypically similar to tension-type headache or migraine and not to the pain of neuralgia. This patient lacks both significant risk factors for and the papilledema typical of IIH. Her afferent pupillary defect is secondary to MS.

Indomethacin is the preferred treatment for chronic paroxysmal hemicrania (CPH). As with the other trigeminal autonomic cephalalgias, CPH pain mainly involves the ophthalmic branch of the trigeminal nerve, resulting in pain localized to the orbital, supraorbital, or temporal regions. Episodes of CPH last 2 to 30 minutes and recur as many as 40 times per day. Ipsilateral cranial autonomic features are present. Attacks may be precipitated by cervical spine rotation

or compression, but facial stimulation is not provocative. Response to indomethacin is absolute.

Lamotrigine is the treatment of choice for short-lasting unilateral neuralgiform headache attacks with conjunctival injection and tearing (SUNCT), although this type of headache is largely refractory to medical management. Similarly to trigeminal neuralgia, episodes last 1 to 600 seconds and may recur more than 100 times daily. Unlike trigeminal neuralgia, attacks of SUNCT involve the ophthalmic branch of the trigeminal nerve and include the ipsilateral autonomic features of conjunctival injection and tearing.

KEY POINT

- Carbamazepine is the treatment of choice for trigeminal neuralgia; management with this agent requires serum monitoring for hyponatremia and agranulocytosis.

Bibliography

Maarbjerg S, Gozalov A, Olesen J, Bendtsen L. Trigeminal neuralgia–a prospective systematic study of clinical characteristics in 158 patients. Headache. 2014 Nov-Dec;54(10):1574-82. [PMID: 25231219.] doi: 10.1111/head.12441

Item 88   Answer: D

Educational Objective: Treat glucocorticoid-refractory idiopathic transverse myelitis.

This patient is exhibiting signs and symptoms consistent with idiopathic transverse myelitis (TM). Idiopathic TM is a monophasic inflammatory and demyelinating myelopathy affecting a portion of the spinal cord. Affected patients frequently experience a subacute onset of weakness, sensory changes, and bowel or bladder dysfunction, which is sometimes preceded by back pain or a thoracic banding sensation. Diagnostic criteria for idiopathic TM require the presence of clinical features of the syndrome, evidence of inflammation (either leukocytosis in the cerebrospinal fluid or contrast enhancement on MRI), and exclusion of other potential causes. First-line treatment for this disorder is administration of high-dose intravenous glucocorticoids. A 5-day course of high-dose methylprednisolone, however, had no beneficial effect on this patient's symptoms. The most appropriate next step is plasma exchange therapy, which has been shown to improve outcomes in patients with idiopathic transverse myelitis that is refractory to glucocorticoids.

The symptoms experienced by this patient are unlikely to be the result of tuberculosis. Tuberculosis can cause central nervous system infection and inflammation, but when it does, it most often involves the meninges, which are not affected in this patient, and spinal fluid analysis frequently shows a low glucose level and a mononuclear pleocytosis. The acute onset of symptoms also is highly unusual for tuberculosis.

Although this patient will benefit from inpatient rehabilitation, it should be delayed until all of the other treatment options have been exhausted. Transfer to rehabilitation

CONT.

without initiation of plasma exchange would not provide the patient with the best chance for recovery.

Intravenous immune globulin therapy has not been shown to provide benefit in glucocorticoid-refractory transverse myelitis and thus would be inappropriate treatment for this patient.

KEY POINT

- In a patient with signs and symptoms of idiopathic transverse myelitis in whom first-line treatment with a high-dose intravenous glucocorticoid has been ineffective, plasma exchange therapy is the most appropriate next step in treatment.

Bibliography

Scott TF, Frohman EM, De Seze J, Gronseth GS, Weinshenker BG; Therapeutics and Technology Assessment Subcommittee of American Academy of Neurology. Evidence-based guideline: clinical evaluation and treatment of transverse myelitis: report of the therapeutics and technology assessment subcommittee of the American Academy of Neurology. Neurology. 2011;77:2128-34. [PMID: 22156988] doi:10.1212/WNL.0b013e31823dc535

Item 89   Answer: D

Educational Objective: Evaluate for vitamin D deficiency in patients with multiple sclerosis.

This patient's serum 25-hydroxyvitamin D level should be measured to determine if she has vitamin D deficiency. The response to disease-modifying therapy is monitored with clinical evaluation and often with periodic MRI studies. Although she is clinically stable, the MRI shows possible new disease activity. Accumulating evidence suggests that disease activity in multiple sclerosis (MS) is highly correlated with serum vitamin D levels, with less frequent relapses and MRI lesion development in patients with high vitamin D levels. Furthermore, administration of vitamin D supplementation has now been shown to provide additional control of disease activity, with a recent trial finding less MRI activity in patients taking interferon plus vitamin D versus interferon alone. This patient is not taking any vitamin D supplementation, which may make her more prone to exacerbations. Supplementation would be indicated if she demonstrates deficiency on serologic testing.

The addition of dalfampridine to this patient's regimen would have no benefit at this time. Although this medication has shown efficacy in improving ambulatory function in some patients with MS, it has no immunologic, disease-modifying effect. Because this patient has no ambulation difficulty and is experiencing an inflammatory disease breakthrough, addition of dalfampridine would be an inappropriate choice.

Glatiramer acetate is a copolymer of four amino acids that, among other mechanisms of action, may bind major histocompatibility complex molecules and induce a shift in the immune response away from autoimmunity. Glatiramer acetate also has been shown to reduce the relapse rate by approximately one third compared with placebo and appears equivalent to the beta interferons in head-to-head studies. However, clinical trial evidence has shown that combining glatiramer acetate with an interferon beta provides no added benefit to what either drug achieves alone.

Lumbar puncture to obtain cerebrospinal fluid for JC virus testing is not appropriate. Reactivation of the JC virus in the brain can result in progressive multifocal leukoencephalopathy (PML), an adverse effect of some immunosuppressive medications and chemotherapy. PML, however, is not a known adverse effect of the interferon beta preparations, and the changes on this patient's MRI are not indicative of PML. Thus, performance of this invasive test is not indicated.

KEY POINT

- Adjuvant therapy with vitamin D supplementation in patients with relapsing-remitting multiple sclerosis provides additional disease activity control.

Bibliography

Soilu-Hänninen M, Aivo J, Lindström BM, Elovaara I, Sumelahti ML, Färkkilä M, et al. A randomised, double blind, placebo controlled trial with vitamin D3 as an add on treatment to interferon β-1b in patients with multiple sclerosis. J Neurol Neurosurg Psychiatry. 2012;83:565-71. [PMID: 22362918] doi:10.1136/jnnp-2011-301876

Item 90   Answer: A

Educational Objective: Identify Alzheimer disease as the cause of mild cognitive impairment.

Cerebrospinal fluid (CSF) analysis is likely to provide the most specific information about whether Alzheimer disease is the cause of this patient's mild cognitive impairment (MCI). This test can measure levels of soluble Aβ42 peptide and soluble tau protein, which can help identify a specific pattern consistent with a diagnosis of Alzheimer disease, namely, decreased Aβ42 and increased tau and p-tau levels. In a patient with MCI, these levels have a greater than 80% sensitivity and specificity in identifying Alzheimer disease as the cause of cognitive symptoms. With the emphasis of clinical trials targeting the earliest stages of Alzheimer disease, the use of CSF biomarkers can assist in the diagnosis and prognosis of the underlying cause of MCI and in identifying patients who could qualify for clinical trials.

Electroencephalography (EEG) detects electrical activity in the brain and is most useful in the diagnosis of epilepsy, although it also can help diagnose sleep disorders, encephalopathy, coma, and brain death. Because EEG provides only nonspecific information about brain function, it is not helpful in detecting the presence of Alzheimer disease.

Fluorodeoxyglucose (FDG) PET provides information on the metabolic function of the brain and can help identify patterns of neuronal impairment. However, these findings are not exclusive to Alzheimer disease. Any information FDG PET provides about brain function is similarly nonspecific.

MRI can provide information on hippocampal atrophy and the presence of enlarged ventricles and cerebrovascular disease. However, these features are seen in both Alzheimer disease and other unrelated syndromes. Likewise, the information MRI provides about brain structure and size is not specific to Alzheimer disease.

Serum apolipoprotein-E (*ApoE*) allele testing provides no useful information for diagnosing cognitive disorders. *ApoE* is a gene that can indicate a patient's risk for Alzheimer dementia but adds little to the prediction of progression of symptoms from MCI.

KEY POINT

- In a patient with mild cognitive impairment, decreased Aβ42 peptide and increased tau protein and p-tau levels in the cerebrospinal spinal fluid have a greater than 80% sensitivity and specificity in identifying Alzheimer disease as the cause.

Bibliography

Blennow K, Zetterberg H. Cerebrospinal fluid biomarkers for Alzheimer's disease. J Alzheimers Dis. 2009;18:413-7. [PMID: 19661632] doi:10.3233/JAD-2009-1177

Item 91   Answer: D

Educational Objective: Treat blood pressure after thrombolysis.

This patient requires no further treatment of his blood pressure at this time. He has had an acute ischemic stroke and was treated appropriately with recombinant tissue plasminogen activator (alteplase). His posttreatment blood pressure is less than 180/105 mm Hg, which is less than the guideline threshold for initiating antihypertensive therapy. Given the presence of internal carotid artery stenosis, expansion of the infarct is possible if the blood pressure is significantly lowered. Blood pressure lowering may be appropriate in patients with symptomatic intracerebral hemorrhage after thrombolysis, but this diagnosis is unlikely in this patient whose physical examination findings after thrombolysis are stable.

Amlodipine is inappropriate as treatment because this patient's blood pressure does not need to be lowered acutely after thrombolysis. Home antihypertensive agents thus should be held for most patients with acute ischemic stroke for at least 48 hours unless evidence of end-organ damage exists.

Clopidogrel is an antithrombotic agent and thus is contraindicated in this patient who has just received thrombolytic therapy. In patients with a transient ischemic attack or minor stroke, aspirin in combination with clopidogrel for 21 days may reduce the risk of recurrent stroke, although confirmatory trials are required.

Intravenous nitroprusside also is inappropriate treatment in this patient who does not require acute lowering of blood pressure. Additionally, nitroprusside is not the medication of first choice in patients with acute stroke because of its potential to increase intracranial pressure.

KEY POINT

- After thrombolytic therapy for acute stroke, antihypertensive treatment is not necessary if blood pressure is less than 180/105 mm Hg and there are no symptoms of intracerebral hemorrhage.

Bibliography

Powers WJ, Rabinstein AA, Ackerson T, Adeoye OM, Bambakidis NC, Becker K, et al; American Heart Association Stroke Council. 2018 Guidelines for the early management of patients with acute ischemic stroke: a guideline for healthcare professionals from the American Heart Association/American Stroke Association. Stroke. 2018 Mar;49(3):e46-e110. [Epub 2018 Jan 24] [PMID: 29367334] doi:10.1161/STR.0000000000000158

Item 92   Answer: D

Educational Objective: Diagnose secondary progressive multiple sclerosis, with progression and activity.

This patient's clinical course at this time can best be described as secondary progressive multiple sclerosis (MS), with progression and activity. His initial relapsing event of optic neuritis initially would have been diagnosed as relapsing-remitting MS. However, over the past 3 years, the patient has had a slow progressive decline in multiple neurologic symptoms without any clear exacerbations, which is the hallmark of progression in MS. Given the initial relapsing course followed by at least 2 years of disability progression without relapses, the patient's disease would now be considered secondary progressive. Recent revisions to clinical course descriptions in MS have been made to acknowledge that the clinical course in MS is not static and should be redefined constantly. Furthermore, these revised course descriptions have acknowledged the fact that relapses can occur in patients who otherwise have progressive MS and that MRI changes should be seen as a sign of relapsing activity in MS. In summary, clinical relapses or MRI evidence of new or enlarging lesions define "activity," whereas the gradual accumulation of neurologic deficits independent of relapses defines "progression." In light of this patient's recent gradual decline in neurologic function (progression) and MRI changes (activity), his disease status is best described as secondary progressive with progression and activity. If, at a later time, the patient exhibits a pattern of no new neurologic deficits, experiences no relapses, and has no new lesions on MRI, his disease status can then be described as secondary progressive without progression or activity.

The patient's initial symptoms involved an acute demyelinating event (optic neuritis), with signs of disability progression coming later. He is not among the 15% of patients with MS who never experience a relapse but instead have progressive disability accumulation from the time of disease onset; these patients have primary progressive MS. Therefore, it would be inaccurate to describe the current status of this patient's MS as primary progressive.

Although this patient's initial clinical course was relapsing, the progressive decline with absence of improvement in the past 3 years indicates a transition to progressive MS. The clinical course of his MS thus cannot be described as relapsing remitting, with activity.

KEY POINT

- The three core phenotypes of multiple sclerosis can be modified by the presence of activity (clinical relapse or new/enlarging MRI lesion); primary and secondary progressive multiple sclerosis can be further modified as "progressive" if there is ongoing accumulation of neurologic deficits independent of clinical relapses.

Bibliography

Lublin FD, Reingold SC, Cohen JA, Cutter GR, Sørensen PS, Thompson AJ, et al. Defining the clinical course of multiple sclerosis: the 2013 revisions. Neurology. 2014;83:278-86. [PMID: 24871874] doi:10.1212/WNL. 0000000000000560

Item 93   Answer: B

Educational Objective: Treat generalized epilepsy in a patient with psychiatric disease.

This patient should receive lamotrigine instead of valproic acid to control his seizures. No single antiepileptic drug (AED) is recommended for the initial treatment of epilepsy. Approximately 50% of patients with this disorder will respond to the first AED administered. Choosing an AED for an individual patient depends on several factors, including his or her epilepsy syndrome, age, sex, and comorbid medical conditions and the drug's adverse-effect profile and cost. Lamotrigine is commonly prescribed in women with childbearing potential and is also a good option for older patients or those who have depression or other mood disorders. This patient has generalized epilepsy that is not controlled with valproic acid. Lamotrigine is the most appropriate medication to use instead, not only because of its effectiveness as treatment for generalized tonic-clonic seizures, but also because of its mood-stabilizing effects. Lamotrigine is FDA approved for maintenance treatment of bipolar I disorder, and clinical trials have demonstrated its efficacy in the treatment of depersonalization/derealization disorder.

Ethosuximide is used only to treat absence seizures, not other types of generalized seizures. Therefore, the medication is inappropriate for this patient with tonic-clonic seizures.

Although often used as a first-line treatment of generalized epilepsy, levetiracetam can worsen depression and should be avoided in this patient who has depression with psychotic features.

Topiramate also is not appropriate for this patient because it can cause or worsen psychosis.

KEY POINT

- In a patient with generalized epilepsy and psychiatric disease, lamotrigine is an appropriate medication to use not only because of its effectiveness as treatment for generalized tonic-clonic seizures, but also because of its mood-stabilizing effects.

Bibliography

Thigpen J, Miller SE, Pond BB. Behavioral side effects of antiepileptic drugs. US Pharm. 2013;38(11):HS15-HS20.

Item 94   Answer: D

Educational Objective: Diagnose myoclonus.

This patient's clinical history and clinical examination findings are most consistent with myoclonus. Myoclonus consists of rapid, nonsuppressible, shock-like, jerky movements that can result from metabolic, endocrine, toxic, infectious, epileptic, autoimmune, and other causes. Posthypoxic myoclonus (Lance-Adams syndrome) occurs in patients with a history of hypoxic brain injury (suggested in this patient by his previous cardiopulmonary arrest) and is characterized by prominent action-induced myoclonus that impairs ambulation because of a combination of positive (rapid jerky movements) and negative (lapses in muscle tone) myoclonus. Other examples of negative myoclonus include hiccups and asterixis.

Ataxia is associated with wide-based gait, incoordination, and dysmetria. However, rapid shock-like movements and brief lapses of muscle tone are not features of ataxia. Ataxia is a hallmark of cerebellar damage and can be seen in posthypoxic settings.

Chorea consists of random, nonrepetitive, flowing, dance-like movements, unlike the abnormal movements exhibited by this patient. Choreiform movements are not rapid or shock-like.

Dystonia involves sustained muscle contractions leading to stereotyped and directional twisting and posturing movements that are absent in this patient.

An orthostatic tremor is a high-frequency, rhythmic tremor that emerges in the legs only during standing and resolves with sitting or ambulation. This does not describe the patient's movements, which are nonrhythmic and jerky.

KEY POINT

- Posthypoxic myoclonus, which occurs in patients with a history of hypoxic brain injury, is characterized by prominent action-induced myoclonus that impairs ambulation because of a combination of positive (rapid jerky movements) and negative (lapses in muscle tone) myoclonus.

Bibliography

Mills K, Mari Z. An update and review of the treatment of myoclonus. Curr Neurol Neurosci Rep. 2015;15:512. [PMID: 25398378] doi:10.1007/s11910-014-0512-2

Item 95   Answer: D

Educational Objective: Evaluate a patient who has minor cognitive difficulties and daytime sleepiness with polysomnography.

This patient should have polysomnography. He has minor symptoms of cognitive impairment, such as memory lapses and calculation difficulties at work. To exclude a slowly progressive dementia and identify any potentially reversible causes of his symptoms, the patient's examination should consist of a neurologic examination, including a cognitive screening evaluation, and evaluation for depression, sleep disorders, alcohol abuse, and family history of dementia. The patient does not use alcohol and has no family history of dementia. His score on the Montreal Cognitive Assessment is borderline abnormal, which would be unlikely if Alzheimer disease or another progressive dementia were the cause of his symptoms, and several depression scales provide no evidence of depression. Because depression and a primary neurodegenerative disorder are unlikely in this patient, additional diagnostic testing is necessary. His hypertension, obesity, and self-reported daytime sleepiness are consistent with a diagnosis of obstructive sleep apnea (OSA). Other neuropsychiatric symptoms of OSA include mood alterations, difficulty concentrating, and problems completing tasks at school or the workplace. Objective testing is required for the diagnosis of OSA.

The traditional gold standard of in-laboratory, technician-attended polysomnography is being replaced by portable technology designed for use by the unaccompanied patient and is referred to as out-of-center sleep testing (OCST). This portable testing is typically limited to measurement of oronasal airflow, chest wall excursion, body position, and pulse oximetry, whereas in-laboratory polysomnography also measures brain waves (electroencephalography), muscle activity (electromyography), and heart rhythm (electrocardiography) and occurs in the presence of a technician in case of technical difficulties. OCST performs comparably to polysomnography in patients without comorbid cardiopulmonary disease who have a high pretest probability of moderate to severe OSA.

Given the patient's normal findings on neurologic examination and relatively minor neurologic symptoms, cerebrospinal fluid analysis, fluorodeoxyglucose PET scanning, and mild structural brain imaging with MRI are likely to be of low yield.

KEY POINT

- Polysomnography should be performed in a patient with minor symptoms of cognitive impairment and self-reported daytime sleepiness who scores normally on cognitive and depression assessments.

Bibliography

Gagnon K, Baril AA, Gagnon JF, Fortin M, Décary A, Lafond C, et al. Cognitive impairment in obstructive sleep apnea. Pathol Biol (Paris). 2014;62:233-40. [PMID: 25070768] doi:10.1016/j.patbio.2014.05.015

Item 96   Answer: A

Educational Objective: Treat cognitive dysfunction in multiple sclerosis.

This patient should be referred for cognitive rehabilitation therapy. Cognitive dysfunction occurs in at least 50% of patients with multiple sclerosis (MS). The most common deficits involve short-term memory, processing speed, and executive function. Cognitive disability has a significant effect on the employability of patients with MS and can reduce their overall quality of life. To this point, however, no pharmaceutical agent has been shown to improve these symptoms in patients with MS. In contrast, cognitive rehabilitation approaches, such as the development of accommodative strategies and training with challenging cognitive tasks, have shown this benefit and should be pursued in this patient.

Depression also is a common symptom in patients with MS, and the suicide rate is elevated in these patients compared with patients who have depression for other reasons. The depression that occurs in MS is likely multifactorial, involving the emotional response to dealing with a chronic disease, the consequences of demyelinating lesions and inflammatory cytokines, and the adverse effects of treatments (such as the interferon beta formulations). Clinicians should be vigilant for signs of depression and have a low threshold for initiating antidepressants and offering referrals to psychiatry. This patient has not had any severe worsening of depression. Therefore, increasing the dosage of the selective serotonin reuptake inhibitor fluoxetine is unlikely to improve any cognitive deficits.

In trials of their effectiveness in improving cognitive deficits in MS, donepezil, memantine, and methylphenidate have shown no benefit. Donepezil has shown modest benefits in cognitive performance in patients with mild to moderate Alzheimer disease, and memantine has shown a similar benefit in patients with moderate to severe Alzheimer disease. Methylphenidate is a central nervous system stimulant used in the treatment of attention deficit hyperactivity disorder and narcolepsy.

KEY POINT

- Cognitive rehabilitation approaches, such as the development of accommodative strategies and training with challenging cognitive tasks, have been shown to improve symptoms of cognitive deficits in patients with multiple sclerosis.

Bibliography

Benedict RH, Zivadinov R. Risk factors for and management of cognitive dysfunction in multiple sclerosis. Nat Rev Neurol. 2011;7:332-42. [PMID: 21556031] doi:10.1038/nrneurol.2011.61

Answers and Critiques

Index

Note: Page numbers followed by f and t denote figures and tables, respectively. Test questions are indicated by Q.